Preface

The inter-comparison of specific skills as represented by performance on neuro-psychological tests is at the heart of the neuropsychological assessment process. However, there is a tendency to regard the interpretation of single tests as a process that is independent of performance on other tests, with integration of test information representing a summary of these individual test performances. As neuropsychology has become increasingly sophisticated, it has been recognized that many factors influence the performance on any given test. The meaning of the same score may vary considerably from one person to another, depending on his or her performance on other neuropsychological tests. Thus, a low score on the Halstead Category Test may indeed reflect frontal lobe damage, but only if we first rule out the influence of visual–spatial problems, emotionality, attentional issues, motivation, fatigue, and comprehension of the instructions. Simplistic interpretations that assume a common interpretation based on a specific score will invariably lead to errors in interpretation and conclusions.

The purpose of this book is to provide each test that is described with a compendium of the possible interpretations that can be used with a variety of common tests that are often included in a neuropsychological test battery. The first chapter discusses some of the pitfalls and cautions when comparing the tests, while the second chapter examines administrative and scoring issues that may be unclear or unavailable for a given test. This is not an attempt to reproduce the test manuals, but rather to highlight those areas in which there are scoring or administrative issues with which the reader may not be familiar.

The remainder of the book focuses on the analysis of the interpretive issues for each of the tests, with the tests divided into such sections as Intelligence, Sensory–Motor, Spatial, Language, Achievement, Executive Functions, and Memory and Attention. Each chapter is designed to present day-to-day interpretive issues for each test in a succinct format. This, in turn, may generate questions for the examiner to address while interpreting the test results. It is hoped that this will lead to quick analysis of each test, as well as raise questions when appropriate, indicating the need for additional tests to be included in the battery.

We have selected those tests that we found through the literature and interviews with clinicians that we concluded were likely to be most useful to the practitioner. We have, of course, not included all available neuropsychological tests, but we believe these are a representative sample of the tests in use. As a result, the interpretive strategies we cite can be used with other tests that focus on similar skills and abilities.

Contents

Chapter 1
INTRODUCTION: COMPARING NEUROPSYCHOLOGICAL TESTS   1

Normative Populations   1
Cutoffs   3
Optimization   3
Discriminant Analysis   4
Cutoffs from Normal Distributions   4
Age and Education Corrections   5
Culture and Ethnic Diversity Issues   6
Pattern Analysis   7
Observations   9
Premorbid Baseline   9
Summary   10

Chapter 2
ADMINISTRATION AND SCORING   11

Halstead–Reitan Neuropsychological Battery (HRNB)   11
Wechsler Adult Intelligence Scale (WAIS)   14
Wechsler Memory Scale—Form III   14
California Verbal Learning Test (CVLT)   17
Peabody Picture Vocabulary Test-Revised (PPVT-R)   17
Test of Line Orientation   18
Bender-Visual Motor Gestalt Test (Bender)   19
Peabody Individual Achievement Test-Revised (PIAT-R)   20
Standard Progressive Matrices (SPM)   21
Rey Auditory Verbal Learning Test (RAVLT)   21
Clock Drawing Test (CDT)   22
Benton Visual Retention Test (BVRT)   23
Wisconsin Card Sorting Test (WCST)   25

Purdue Pegboard 26
Rey Complex Figure Test (CFT) 27
Stroop Color and Word Test 29
Boston Naming Test (BNT) 30
Controlled Oral Word Association Test (COWAT) 31
Visual Form Discrimination Test (VFDT) 31
Hooper Visual Organization Test (HVOT) 32
Luria–Nebraska Neuropsychological Battery II (LNNB) 32
Test of Variables of Attention (TOVA) 47
Intermediate Visual and Auditory Continuous Performance Test (IVA)   48
CONCLUSIONS 49
REFERENCES 50

Chapter 3
INTERPRETATION 51

Section I: General Intelligence 52
   Wechsler Adult Intelligence Scale-III (WAIS-III) 52
   Charles J. Golden
   Peabody Picture Vocabulary Test-Revised (PPVT-R) 58
   Jason King
Section II: Visual–Spatial Tests 60
   Block Design Subtest (WAIS-III) 60
   Samantha Devaraju-Backhaus
   Bender-Visual Motor Gestalt Test (Bender) 65
   Jennifer Selden
   Raven's Matrices 69
   Liane Dornheim
   Test of Line Orientation 74
   Liane Dornheim
   Tactual Performance Test (TPT) 78
   Charles J. Golden
   Clock Drawing Test (CDT) 82
   Mary L. Mahrou
   Benton Visual Retention Test (BVRT) 85
   Elaine Karbonik
   Matrices (WAIS-III) 89
   Charles J. Golden
   Visual Form Discrimination Test (VFDT) 94
   Barbara Garcia
   Hooper Visual Organization Test (HVOT) 97
   Ruby Natale

Section III: Verbal Tests 99
  Reitan Aphasia Examination 99
  Charles J. Golden
  Information (WAIS-III) 103
  Charles J. Golden
  Comprehension (WAIS-III) 105
  Samantha Devaraju-Backhaus
  Boston Naming Test (BNT) 108
  Steven M. Essig
  Similarities (WAIS-III) 112
  Charles J. Golden
  Speech–Sounds Perception Test (SSPT) 114
  Jennifer Selden
  Expressive Speech Scale (C6, LNNB) 115
  Judith Migoya
  Receptive Speech (C5, LNNB) 118
  Doyle Patton
Section IV: Nonverbal Tests 121
  Picture Arrangement (WAIS-III) 121
  Derrick Blanton
  Digit Symbol (WAIS-III) 124
  Charles J. Golden
  Picture Completion Subtest (WAIS-III) 126
  Charles J. Golden
  Seashore Rhythm Test 128
  Mary L. Mahrou
Section V: Motor and Sensory Tests 130
  Finger Tapping Test (FTT) 130
  Patricia Espe-Pfeifer
  Purdue Pegboard Test 133
  Sonal K. Pancholi
  Grip Strength Test 137
  Patricia Espe-Pfeifer
  Motor Functions Scale (LNNB) 141
  Tanya Pospisil and Patricia Espe-Pfeifer
  Sensory–Perceptual Examination (HRNB) 144
  Charles J. Golden
Section VI: Achievement Tests 146
  Peabody Individual Achievement Test (PIAT-R) 146
  James D.D. Bradley
  Wide Range Achievement Test (WRAT) 151
  Charles J. Golden

Reading Scale (C8, LNNB) 154
Sarah Zimmerman
Writing Scale (C7, LNNB) 156
Sarah Zimmerman
Arithmetic Scale (C9, LNNB) 158
Judith Migoya
Section VII: Executive Skills 160
Controlled Oral Word Association Test (COWAT) 160
Doyle Patton
Wisconsin Card Sorting Test (WCST) 163
Rhiannon Thomas
Halstead Category Test 167
Rhiannon Thomas
Trail Making Test (TMT) 171
Rhiannon Thomas
Stroop Color and Word Test 174
Charles J. Golden
Section VIII: Memory Tests 177
Wechsler Memory Scale-III 177
Charles J. Golden
Digit Span (WAIS-III) 183
James D.D. Bradley
Spatial Span (WMS-III) 185
Charles J. Golden
Rey–Osterrieth Complex Figure Test (CFT) 187
James D.D. Bradley
Rey Auditory Verbal Learning Test (RAVLT) 192
Ernest J. Aucone
California Verbal Learning Test (CVLT) 195
Ernest J. Aucone
WMS-III Logical Memory Subtest 200
James D.D. Bradley
WMS-III Verbal Paired Associates Subtest (VPA) 204
James D.D. Bradley
WMS-III Faces I and Faces II Subtests 208
Patricia Espe-Pfeifer
Family Pictures (WMS-III) 214
Charles J. Golden
Intermediate Memory Scale (C12, LNNB) 215
Jennifer Selden
Memory Scale (C10, LNNB) 217
Jennifer Selden

Section IX: Sustained Attentional Tests 219
  Test of Variables of Attention (TOVA) 219
  Robert Leark
  Intermediate Visual and Auditory Continuous Performance Test (IVA)   224
  Samantha Devaraju-Backhaus
  Paced Auditory Serial Addition Test (PASAT) 227
  Patricia M. Joyce
Section X: Test Batteries 229
  The Luria–Nebraska Neuropsychological Battery 229
  Charles J. Golden
  Halstead–Reitan Neuropsychological Battery (HNRB) 234
  Charles J. Golden

Appendix: Score Translations for Neuropsychological Data 239

Index 241

1

Introduction
Comparing Neuropsychological Tests

Although the comparison of neuropsychological test results is recognized as an especially valuable method of inferring the presence and type of brain injury in a client, there are many pitfalls in such comparisons that can lead to serious errors. In this chapter we discuss some of these issues, as well as those integrative procedures we recognize as being the most useful in interpreting a battery of tests. All of these issues should be kept in mind when interpreting any kind of extensive test battery.

NORMATIVE POPULATIONS

One of the most substantial pitfalls in the comparison of tests is trying to compare tests that were normed on different samples. The samples upon which different tests were normed may vary considerably in terms of important variables, the most significant of which are age, education, and culture. Differences in these variables can dramatically change how a test score is interpreted.

For example, if Test A was normed on a group of 50-year-olds with a 10th grade education, a score by a 30-year-old with 14 years of education and with a moderate brain injury may appear to be normal. However, if Test B were normed on a group with an average age of 24 and with 18 years of education the 30-year-old's score is likely to appear abnormal. This may lead to the conclusion that the client is more impaired on Test B, when, in fact, the difference is due solely to the differences in the original norm groups. The examiner must be aware of such differences for any tests he or she utilizes.

The aforementioned is a concern primarily with regard to those tests that do not provide age or education norms or corrections. However, even when those corrected norms are available, they are often either age-corrected or education-corrected, but not both. In such a case, some tests may include age populations who do not have comparable education levels, or other tests may present norms based on education but with different ages. None of this creates insurmountable problems, but one must consider such deviations before comparing the results of two tests.

Another related issue is that of the time that has elapsed since the norms were generated. For the most part, research has found that norms collected in the 1950s and 1960s are not comparable to those gathered more recently. In general, the more complex the test, the more we need to question the results, as examinees today tend to outperform previous generations on the same version of a given test. In such cases, what was borderline performance in the past may now be clearly indicative of deficits in a given area.

Cross-cultural issues are also substantial. Data collected on different cultural and ethnic groups cannot be generalized to other groups, regardless of whether the tests are verbal or nonverbal. While differences are often more apparent on verbal tests (whether translated into another language or not), there are also differences on "nonverbal" tests that may reflect differences in style, in the meaning of age and education corrections, in cultural experiences, and other factors. Although some specific problems that arise from focal brain injuries (such as severe construction dyspraxia, dysfluency, loss of receptive skills, paralysis) are indeed universal across cultures, performance on more complex standardized tests does not hold up as well without renorming and reanalysis.

Gender correction is also an important issue, although the magnitude of the influence of gender on most neuropsychological tests is much smaller than that of age, education, culture, or when the results (i.e., norms) were collected. Gender discrepancies must be attended to on those tests for which there is a documented gender influence. For example, many normative samples come from VA populations that are entirely male.

Problems arise when comparisons are made between tests that use different levels of correction for any number of factors. Thus, if we compare the age-, education-, and gender-corrected norms of the Halstead Category Test to uncorrected norms on the Rey figure, we may again get differences that are due solely to the scoring procedures rather than to real neuropsychological findings. One can see how reliance on results that are fundamentally incompatible can produce serious errors in data interpretation.

Correcting for these issues is not a simple task. In all cases, there should be an attempt to use norms that are properly adjusted for age, education, and gender when these factors influence test performance. In the absence of such norms, the possible impact of these variables must be evaluated before any clinical conclusions are reached.

CUTOFFS

A second issue has been the tendency in neuropsychology to focus on "cutoffs" rather than on the degree to which a score deviates from the norm. This has arisen from the desire to identify only those scores that represent brain injury, rather than just a deviation from the population average. Cutoffs are used to classify clients as either "brain injured" or "normal." They fail to tell us the severity of a problem and often fail to tell us the likelihood of misclassification. Although cutoffs can be useful, the ways in which they are determined may vary, making comparison of performance across tests difficult.

OPTIMIZATION

A common method for establishing cutoffs is identifying the point in a sample of normal and brain-injured clients that optimizes correct classification of these individuals. The difficulties with such a procedure lie in three major areas. First, the cutoff is dependent on the exact sample used. For example, if one test's cutoff is determined between a matched sample of above average controls and brain-injured clients, the same cutoff will not result if a sample of matched below average normals and brain injured clients is used. The efficacy of the cutoff will vary greatly depending on how appropriate it is for the client being considered. Cutoffs often are not adequately cross-validated across different populations, again leaving their efficacy in question. When we attempt to compare two tests using such cutoffs, differences in results may occur primarily from the characteristics of the sample, which determined the cutoff, rather than from the presence of real deficits.

A second problem is that cutoffs will differ in how many brain-injured individuals are misclassified as normals and how many normals are misclassified as brain-injured. Test A may reach an optimal cutoff by classifying 100% of brain-injured correctly, but only 60% of normals correctly (for an 80% hit rate), while Test B may classify 100% of normals correctly but only 60% of brain-injured (for an 80% hit rate). When used in practice, Test A is much more likely to call someone brain-injured while Test B is more likely to call someone normal. In such cases, finding a pattern of brain-injured performance on Test A and normal performance on Test B may not reflect differential performance of the client, but rather the ways in which the cutoffs were selected.

Third, cutoffs are usually based on samples of "very normal" normals who have been screened for psychiatric problems, any history of neurological problems, learning problems, etc., and on very clearly brain-injured clients with well-documented injuries. Unfortunately, such samples represent the easiest form of distribution and do not address real life clinical scenarios in which the situation is much more ambiguous (e.g., did the person with severe depression who was not paying attention while driving get hurt in the automobile accident?). While such normative studies meet rigorous, traditional research standards, their results might not translate into real life. Studies that use individuals with other illnesses (such as orthopedic illnesses or psychiatric disorders) as controls will offer more conservative but perhaps more relevant cutoff points.

DISCRIMINANT ANALYSIS

Discriminant analysis is similar to the hand optimization level technique for establishing cutoff points, except that the former determines cutoffs using a statistical procedure. This statistical procedure is heavily influenced by sample characteristics and can vary widely with changes in the sample and sample size (especially in situations where sample sizes are uneven). When multiple groups are involved (e.g., normal, depressed, and brain-injured), the weightings of each group can heavily influence outcome. Also, seemingly small changes in running discriminant computer programs can lead to substantial changes in the results. Such programs are unconcerned with the types of errors made, and subsequently lead to cutoffs that yield very skewed results. Formulas generated to make discriminations based on groups of tests may be overly influenced by chance and not easily replicable across populations. While again discriminant analysis can be a useful technique, cutoffs that arise from it must be regarded with caution.

CUTOFFS FROM NORMAL DISTRIBUTIONS

Increasing numbers of tests use cutoffs based on the normal distribution. Such studies simply identify the mean and standard deviation of normal individuals and then select a point on the normal curve that is said to indicate brain injury. This point may be as much as two standard deviations from the mean, a very rigorous criterion, but most often it is one standard deviation or slightly more. Such studies may present a single cutoff, or ideally they might offer multiple cutoffs adjusted for age, education, and gender.

These cutoffs also have disadvantages. First, cutoffs based on normals do not tell us how well the test will identify brain-injured clients (which will also be influenced by the point on the normal curve that defines the cutoff). In some cases, a one standard deviation cutoff may identify 80% of brain-injured individuals or only 60% or 30%. This depends on the distribution of the scores in brain-injured clients, which in turn is influenced by how skewed or flat both the normal and brain-injured sample curves are and by their relative positions to one another.

Such issues are important in neuropsychological data because distributions are often skewed and not even truly normal, owing to floor and ceiling effects, as well as the basic nature of the measures employed. In these situations, cutoffs that appear equal in sensitivity actually vary greatly.

Second, classification according to such cutoffs may be affected by minor changes in scores, which are ultimately overinterpreted. Thus, the difference between a "normal" T-score of 40.01 and an "abnormal" T-score of 39.99 may indeed be minuscule and not worthy of the sudden interpretive emphasis given to the lower score. Cutoffs will clearly vary if we choose one, two, or some other number of standard deviations to indicate the cutoff points for different tests. Even using the same cutoff point (e.g., one standard deviation) across tests will result in differing levels of sensitivity and specificity, thus influencing overall accuracy.

Finally, as with all cutoffs, sample characteristics may substantially influence results and lead to questionable generalizability.

AGE AND EDUCATION CORRECTIONS

The importance of considering age and education issues in adult samples is obvious. However, these issues have the potential to produce several difficulties, some of which are obvious and others that are more subtle. First, different test norms and cutoffs may address age, education, a combination of both, or none of these. This, of course, makes direct comparison of results on different tests difficult, although these scores may be regarded as equivalent by the user. When a test that corrects for age and education is compared to one that corrects only for age, then apparent differences in scores may again be illusory. In general, tests that correct for both of these factors are viewed as more conservative in diagnosing brain injury in populations with higher age and lower education, but more liberal in populations with higher education and lower age.

A second problem arises from how age and education corrections are made. Vastly different results may emerge from samples that correct for "over 45" and "under 45" versus those that correct by year using regression formulas. Similarly, bunching of education in groups of "9–11" or "16+" may cause similar problems. In samples that use bunching techniques, sample characteristics among normative groups for each education level may cause variations in norms that are unrelated to brain injury. However, regression formulas, which assume linear relationships between test performance and demographic variables, may err if the underlying relationship is, in fact, not linear. In all of these cases, the magnitude of the effect of age, education, or other demographic factors influences the importance of these issues.

In some cases, however, age and education corrections can lead to serious problems when the age or education correction corrects for brain injury itself. In many samples of older normals, we may see a decline because of unidentified neurological factors or as a result of systemic disorders (e.g., diabetes, peripheral joint disorders, etc.) that act to bias norms toward the impaired side, masking real problems. Similarly, a group of individuals with only a sixth grade education may have been unable to go any further because of a neurological disorder, while others dropped out for economic reasons. The overall effect is that the test is less sensitive to actual (although preexisting) disorders.

CULTURE AND ETHNIC DIVERSITY ISSUES

Although not extensively researched, cultural and ethnic diversity issues are extremely important in neuropsychological test interpretation. The administration of tests to ethnic minorities and to groups whose primary and original language is not the language in which the test was normed is questionable, even in the case of so-called nonverbal tests. Our own work (e.g., Demsky, Mittenberg, Quintar, Katell, & Golden, 1998) suggests that even nonverbal tests yield different results in normal populations of different ethnicities, let alone brain injured samples. Unless a test is appropriately standardized for a group, the use of the test's norms and cutoffs must be done very cautiously and with strong attention to these factors.

It is the authors' belief that simply including a group in a more general normative sample does not make the norms culture-fair or accurate. While we may represent ethnic group X in the normative sample in the same 3% ratio in which it exists in the U.S. population, the resultant norms are no more valid for that specific group. However, it would make the norms more representative of the true population if we tested everyone in the United States, but this is irrelevant to the question of neuropsychological dysfunction. Only if the norms are appropriately evaluated with a representative sample from a specific group can we state if the norms are fair or not.

The issues involved in such norms are complex. For example, when working in Hawaii, the senior author found that norms for second-generation Japanese residents were not equivalent to those for third-generation Japanese residents. Norms for Spanish speakers from Cuba may not be the same as for Spanish speakers from Mexico. Norms for a client who is truly bilingual may not be the same for someone who speaks in a new language but still thinks predominantly in his or her native language. These issues are, unfortunately, endless yet they must be considered when selecting tests and interpreting the results.

When analyzing the results of "translated tests," differences of up to two thirds of a standard deviation (10 standard score points) may be seen in "nonverbal" tests, while differences twice as large (four thirds of a standard deviation or up to 20 points) may be due solely to issues of translation and culture. If a test is translated inappropriately or in an idiosyncratic manner, the expected changes in norms, even in normals, may be larger.

PATTERN ANALYSIS

Although cutoffs give us rough ideas of the level of performance of a client, pattern analysis across tests is a much more powerful tool by which to reach clinical conclusions. Pattern analysis ignores cutoffs and instead focuses on internal variations in the client's own test results with respect to the client's own baseline of current and previous performance. This is especially helpful in more subtle cases or in those cases in which we wish to understand the true deficits that underline a brain injury. This technique ideally translates all raw scores into a standard score system with appropriate demographic corrections.

Translation of the scores into a common system is made difficult by the presence of many scoring systems utilizing demographically corrected and uncorrected scores, such as T-scores, standard scores, z-scores, raw scores, Wechsler scale scores, and percentiles. The Appendix table presents the common transformations between standard scores, T-scores, inverted T-scores (where high scores represent more pathology or poorer performance, such as some tests scored for errors), percentiles, and z-scores. Raw scores must be translated into scores so they can be compared to other scoring systems.

All of these transformations are based on the assumption that the underlying distributions are normal, which is not always the case with neuropsychological measures. Instead they may reflect very skewed performances in normals. This Appendix table also does not address those few tests whose normative samples are brain-injured clients rather than normals; such scores cannot be directly compared to scores that utilized normals for their standardization samples.

A review of the table also shows problems related to the use of percentiles. As can be seen, percentiles change rapidly in the middle of the distribution, suggesting differences that may not be clinically significant; percentiles change slowly at the extremes of the distribution, hiding differences that may be real. The latter scenario is particularly serious, as variations in the low range may have great significance. In general, few tests rely on the use of percentiles alone, and percentiles should not be used for the purpose of neuropsychological interpretation.

Some tests address the problem of skewed distributions by using forced normal distributions. In such cases (such as the Wechsler tests, or the Heaton, Grant, and Matthews (1991) norms for the Halstead–Reitan), extreme scores are forced into a distribution that varies approximately 3 standard deviations on either side of normal, creating a ceiling effect at the high end and a floor effect at the low end. This floor effect may mask significant differences between clients, which have substantial neuropsychological implications for diagnosis and treatment. In such cases, the inspection of the underlying raw scores may reveal differences that are important to the case analysis.

Client Profile

Once scores have been converted into a common scoring system (usually standard scores or T-scores), client profiles can be plotted or analyzed to look for score differences that suggest neuropsychological significance. Such analysis must consider the issue of individual variation. When looking at an overall profile, one can calculate the individual's average scores across all tests administered. In general, research on test batteries suggests that scores for normals will vary about 1 standard deviation from this average score (15 points for standard scores on either side of the average, 10 points for T-scores). Profiles in which scores show less variation are generally considered within the normal range (although this does not prove that someone is normal). Profiles with greater variations suggest an unusual degree of variation, which may indicate the presence of cognitive problems.

Variations between Scores

Below the level of overall profile differences, scores can be compared directly to one another. The degree of difference between scores that is necessary for neuropsychological significance varies depending on the underlying relationships of the tests, as well as variations in the normative samples employed. The easiest comparisons are between scores representing identical motor or sensory performance on opposite sides of the body. These scores should be very similar to one another and are usually normed on the exact same population with the same scoring methods, thus minimizing sample or scoring errors. Therefore, differences of as little as one-half of one standard deviation may be significant.

The second class of test comparisons include those tests that are moderately correlated with one another (Verbal and Performance IQ, performance on two similar drawing tests, etc.). If both sets of scores have similar normative populations, then a difference of one standard deviation between scores is usually neuropsychologically significant. If the tests use very different normative populations or different correction methods (e.g., one corrects for education, one does not) a more conservative difference of one and one half standard deviations should be used.

The third class are tests that are independently normed but represent areas that theoretically overlap, such as achievement and IQ, executive performance and IQ, or spatial reasoning and construction skills. Comparison of such tests typically requires a difference of one and one half standard deviations before neuropsychological differences can be reliably implied. In limited cases, a more liberal difference of one standard deviation can be applied, but only when there is clear research to back up such an assumption.

The final class of test comparisons include those that are generally unrelated (Block Design and Grammatical skills) and normed on different populations. These comparisons call for the most conservative criterion of two standard deviations. If scores on two dissimilar measures are more than 2 standard deviations apart, a deficit may be implicated.

OBSERVATIONS

In addition to an analysis of scores, much information can be gained from the qualitative analysis of how a client achieved a score. Although it can be argued that an extensive test battery could be organized so that many or even most qualitative variations would be reflected in the quantitative scores, the state of testing at the present time does not have a research base that allows us to demonstrate this argument. Differences between tests as discussed in the preceding, as well as simple error variance, obscure fine differences in client performance. Such problems have less effect on simple classification of performance as "impaired" but have many more implications as we attempt to make finer discriminations as to specific problems or etiologies.

Under these circumstances, qualitative observations become an important source of collateral information, which should be integrated with the actual data. It is important to recognize that neither quantitative nor qualitative data are either better or more perfect, but that both offer insights that, when combined, create a more accurate and detailed description of the client. Thus, such observations should be made routinely, along with testing the limits of procedures when they can further elucidate the reasons behind a client's behavior. All individuals who administer tests, whether doctoral psychologists or technicians, should be trained in making and reporting such observations.

PREMORBID BASELINE

While level of performance measures compare a client's results to population norms and pattern analysis looks at current intra-individual variations, there has always been a desire to compare the client to the client's own premorbid level of functioning. This has traditionally been attempted in two ways: using formulas to estimate premorbid levels and using current performance on "hold" tests to estimate premorbid levels.

The use of formulas has generally focused on the prediction of Full Scale IQ as a measure of "g," to which all other test scores can be compared. These systems have many problems, as they tend to lump clients into heterogeneous groups that are not adequately descriptive of the individual. Most of the success of such formulas lies in classifying those in the middle of the normal distribution as being in the middle, but this adds little beyond simply assuming that everyone is normal. When these scores are used, errors of up to 15 standard score points from baseline must be assumed, with scores needing to deviate an additional 15 points before one can reach conclusion that a score has changed.

The second method involves estimation from "hold" tests, typically a test of reading recognition (such as the WRAT-III or PIAT-III) or vocabulary (such as the PPVT-R or Vocabulary from the WAIS-III). These tests offer adequate correlations with "g" and are easy to administer. In the absence of aphasia or severe visual problems, they offer reasonable estimates of the premorbid level, especially when combined with historical information on a person's actual accomplishments. However, even in the best of circumstances these scores are accurate only within 5–7 standard score points at the 68% confidence level and 10–12 points at the 95% confidence level. This range of error must be considered in any comparisons.

A final caution stems from the issue of the appropriateness of these baselines. Although they may provide some useful information about premorbid general IQ, they do not predict performance on tests of motor performance, drawing, attention, and other important areas. Thus, care should be taken before generalizing estimated baselines to the aforementioned tests, as the accuracy rate may drop and deviations as great as 20–30 standard score points may appear. There is a paucity of research on the relation of these areas to premorbid scores, and one must be cautious before making any generalizations, taking into account the other issues discussed in this chapter.

SUMMARY

Although there are many issues to consider when interpreting a comprehensive test battery, such an approach remains by far the most accurate and useful method of neuropsychological evaluation. When quantitative and qualitative information are properly integrated, and when one gives consideration to the various issues described above, valid and useful descriptions of client deficits may be identified. Once again, this description and comparison of specific skills is at the heart of neuropsychological assessment.

Administration and Scoring

Most of the tests presented in this book are well known and are described in depth in published test manuals, so little comment on their administration or scoring is required here. We have, however, given more detail on those tests where there is less consensus or for which we have adopted alternate scoring techniques to aid in interpretation. Please refer to the original sources for details on these individual tests as that information should be mastered before any test is employed.

HALSTEAD–REITAN NEUROPSYCHOLOGICAL BATTERY (HRNB)

We have included many of the HRNB subtests in this book. These are best described by Reitan and Wolfson (1993) in terms of administration and scoring. The tests are briefly described here for those unfamiliar with the HRNB. We have included the following HRNB measures: Tactual Performance Test, Category Test, Speech–Sounds Perception Test, Seashore Rhythm Test, Finger Oscillation/ Finger Tapping Test, Sensory–Perceptual Examination, Aphasia Examination, and the Grip Strength Test. In addition to Reitan's standard scoring of these tests, we also refer to the Heaton, Grant, and Matthews (1991) norms, which are a comprehensive set of norms for conversion of raw scores to T-scores, thus improving the ability to compare to other tests. These T-scores are corrected for age, education, and gender. We have generally adopted the Reitan and Wolfson administration procedures.

Tactual Performance Test (TPT)

The TPT consists of a standard form board in which a client can place 10 shapes into similarly shaped cutouts. The board is placed at a 45-degree angle on a stand. The client must place the forms into the proper cutouts while blindfolded, and is thus required to rely on touch rather than sight. The task is repeated three times. The first trial is performed with the dominant hand only, the second with the nondominant hand, and the third with both hands. After the three trials are completed, the board is hidden and the client is asked to draw on a piece of paper what the forms were (Memory Score) and where they were located (Location Score).

The original Halstead (1947) procedure allowed 15 minutes for each trial, but we use 10-minute trials for each hand. We use a time per block measure in addition to the overall times reported for the dominant hand, nondominant hand, both hands, and total time. Each of these times must be divided by the number of blocks completed on each trial to yield the time per block.

Category Test

The Category Test consists of seven subtests. Each consists of a series of slides or cards that suggest a number from 1 to 4. In the easiest subtest, the items are simply the Roman numerals from 1 to 4 (I, II, III, IV), while in the second easiest subtest the number is determined by counting the number of objects on the slide. In the most complex subtests, the spatial location or orientation of an odd item or a specific item signals the correct number. It is the responsibility of the client to guess the strategy necessary to solve the items in each of the seven subtests. The client is allowed only one guess per item. In the original version, the response to a right answer is the sound of a bell, while a wrong answer generates a buzzer sound. In later versions, the examiner may say "right" or "wrong." Using this feedback, the client must alter his or her analysis until he or she can consistently determine the correct answer. The score is the number of errors accumulated on all seven subtests.

Speech–Sounds Perception Test

This test consists of 60 multiple-choice items. The client hears from a tape a nonsense word such as "theets" and must match it against one of four choices (all of which have the internal "ee" sound). Scoring is simply done by totaling the number of failures to find the correct match.

Seashore Rhythm Test

This test consists of 30 pairs of tonal patterns. The client must listen to each pair and then write down whether they are the "same" or "different." The test requires the client to keep track of where he or she is in the sequence of pairs; success therefore demands sustained concentration. Traditional scoring is counting the number correct, although some clinicians report the number of errors.

Finger Oscillation/Finger Tapping Test

This test consists of a simple finger tapping device attached to a counter. The client moves a lever up and down with his or her index finger as quickly as possible in 10 seconds. The counter records the number of taps. Five trials are given for the dominant hand and five for the nondominant hand. Additional trials are given if some of the scores vary more than five taps from the other same-hand trials. Two scores are produced, which are the averages of the five trials for each hand.

Sensory–Perceptual Examination

This consists of a series of sensory tests adapted from traditional neurological examinations. The client is given 20 trials on each hand of Finger Agnosia (identifying which finger is touched based on touch alone) and Finger Tip Number Writing (identifying the numbers written on each finger tip). The exam also includes double simultaneous stimulation in which the client is touched in two places at the same time. This evaluates one's ability to feel only one, rather than both, of the touches. Extinction for double visual and auditory stimulation is also examined. For each of these procedures, the score is simply the number of errors on the right and left side of the body. A final procedure asks the client to recognize simple shapes (circle, square, triangle, and cross) by touch (stereognosis). Each hand is scored for errors and for total time to do the individual tasks.

Aphasia Examination

The aphasia examination consists of a series of short commands and tasks designed to screen for basic language deficits. The tasks include: (1) naming simple objects and shapes; (2) reading simple words; (3) spelling; (4) following simple commands; (5) following complex commands; (6) simple word fluency (pronouncing words and sentences correctly); (7) construction skills (drawing a cross and a key); (8) following instructions involving the identification of right and left; (9) demonstrating the use of an object; and (10) arithmetic.

Grip Strength

This task uses a dynamometer to measure grip strength in each hand. Each hand is measured twice with the average used as the client's score (i.e., two scores are calculated).

WECHSLER ADULT INTELLIGENCE SCALE (WAIS)

These tests follow exactly the WAIS-R or WAIS-III manuals (Wechsler, 1986, 1997). Scores reported are age-adjusted scaled scores which allow for a more accurate comparison of intra-individual differences, especially in the elderly. The interpretations hold relatively well for both the WAIS-R and WAIS-III, but we encourage use of the WAIS-III, which offers more current norms and the added subtests (Matrices and Letter–Numbering Sequencing).

WECHSLER MEMORY SCALE—FORM III

This book discusses the use of the new version of the Wechsler Memory Scale (Form III) (Wechsler, 1997). We have focused on the following subtests: Logical Memory I and II, Faces I and II, Family Pictures I and II, Paired Associates I and II; and the measures of working memory, Letter–Number Sequencing, and Spatial Span. All test scores are reported as scaled scores. It should be emphasized that on this test (as well as on other memory tests), the client should be encouraged strongly to guess even when he or she is not sure, for there is no penalty for guessing. In general, "I don't know" answers will lower scores and affect the validity of the interpretations.

This version of the WMS-III offers several new subtests not seen on previous versions. The new Logical Memory offers an additional trial to examine learning over trials on a new story. Another new task, Faces, is a forced choice procedure in which a client must try to recognize 24 faces presented out of 48 possibilities. Family Pictures requires the client to remember and describe four "everyday" scenes involving an extended family. Visual Span involves reproducing a visual pattern of taps on a series of spatially random blocks. Number–Letter Sequencing involves remembering a mixed list of numbers and letters (of increasing length) that must be repeated in an altered order with the letters (in alphabetical order) followed by the numbers (in numerical order).

Logical Memory (LM) I and II of the WMS-III have undergone several noticeable alterations in format and scoring procedures. The first story administered (Story A) is almost identical to Story A of the WMS-R with the alteration of only one phrase ("city hall station" changed to "police station"), most likely done to make the story more current with modern linguistic expressions. However, Story B is new and bears no resemblance to Story B of the WMS-R.

The administrative procedure of Story B has also been altered. On the WMS-R, both stories were administered at an initial time to obtain an assessment of recall ability (LM I), and were then readministered 30 minutes later to assess delayed recall memory (LM II). On the WMS-III, the examinee is administered both stories, and then asked to recall each. Directly following the recall portion of

LM I, Story B is then administered a second time. The addition of this procedure allows for the calculation of a learning slope to assess improved performance across repeated exposures to verbally presented conceptual material. LM II of the WMS-III follows the same format as seen in the previous edition, aside from the addition of a recognition phase. The recognition trial is useful, for it provides information regarding delayed memory for verbally presented material when an examinee prompted, and it also provides an assessment of delayed verbal memory in a manner that is far less incumbent upon the ability to produce complex speech.

Along with these alterations in administrative procedures, there have been some notable changes in scoring procedures as well. In scoring the recall and delayed trials of Stories A and B, the examiner must quantify two elements of the examinee's verbalizations: the reproduction of exact elements of the story and the expression of thematic elements. The scoring of exact reproductive elements has been altered from previous editions by making the scoring criterion clearer and more flexible. Scoring for the retention of thematic elements (both immediate and delayed) is new to this subtest. Although this score is not incorporated into any of the WMS-III index scores, it does have age-corrected scale scores. These provide another means for the examiner to assess memory for verbally presented material so that performance is not heavily reliant on the subject's ability to produce lengthy verbalizations. Also, the employment of both scoring techniques provides a means for the examiner to assess the memory process at different levels of complexity and specificity.

Several changes transpired in the format and design of the Verbal Paired Associates (VPA) subtest. In the third edition, VPA I has a set number of trials (four) to be administered, rather than a variable number of three to six trials depending on performance. Another noteworthy change is the level of difficulty of items administered. In both editions of the WMS, eight word-pairs are administered with each trial. In the revised edition, these eight pairs consisted of four easily associated word-pairs (e.g., baby–cries) and four difficult associations consisting of word-pairs not normally associated (e.g., cabbage–pen). In the third edition, all eight word-pairs are new and consist of only the more difficult variety. Weschler (1997) reports that this alteration was made on the basis of research showing that performance on difficult associations has been found to be more highly correlated with other measures of verbal memory and is more sensitive to cerebral dysfunction.

The reliability data surrounding this subtest has improved quite drastically from the prior version. The split-half reliability of this subtest has risen from an average r of .60 to an r of .92 for VPA I, and from an average r of .40 to .86 for VPA II. This improved split-half reliability demonstrates the greater internal consistency of this subtest. This drastic level of improvement is most likely accounted for by the fact that there are no longer two different types of items in each trial. Instead, all items are of the more difficult type and are therefore much more likely to be assessing the same construct. Test–retest reliability of this subtest demonstrates a large improvement over the prior version. Reliability estimates rose from a range of .52–.68 (WMS-R) to a range of .81–.82 (WMS-III) depending upon the age group. VPA II demonstrated similar findings, as test–retest reliability rose from a range of .52–.68 (WMS-R) to a range of .81–.82 (WMS-III) depending upon age.

The addition of new administrative and scoring elements has brought about new index and composite scores. The total recall score of Logical Memory I goes into the computation of the Immediate Memory Index. As this index is made up of performance on two visually mediated and two verbally mediated recall subtests, index scores can also be seen for each modality individually (Auditory Immediate & Visual Immediate). The combination of scores across Logical Memory and Verbal Paired Associates is employed to create a number of indices, as both of these subtests are measures of memory for verbally presented material. The recall scores from the initial phases of both subtests comprise the Auditory Immediate Memory Index. The total delayed recall of both make up the Auditory Delayed Index, and the scores across the delayed recognition portion of each are used to compute the Auditory Recognition Delayed Index. The WMS-III has also added several composite scores that examine various aspects of auditory processing and are all computed by combining various aspects of performance on the Logical Memory and Verbal Paired Associates subtests.

For the administration of Faces I and Faces II, the following test material is required: WMS-III Stimulus Booklet 1 (Faces I), Stimulus Booklet 2 (Faces II), and a record form. The client should be seated across from the examiner. For each part of the subtest, the appropriate stimulus booklet should be placed in front of the client so that he or she has an adequate view of the test stimuli. Individuals who have visual deficits, such as age-related macular degeneration (a loss of central vision in both eyes caused by pathological changes in the macula lutea and characterized by spots of pigmentation or other abnormalities), should be instructed to adjust their heads so that they have an appropriate view of the stimuli.

At the start of Faces I, the examiner tells the client, "I am going to show you some pictures of faces, one at a time. Look at each face carefully and remember what it looks like." The client is then presented a series of 24 faces, for 2 seconds each, while being verbally prompted to remember each face (i.e., the examiner says, "Remember this one"). The client is then provided the following instructions: "Now I am going to show you some more pictures of faces, one at a time. I want you to look at the face on each page carefully. Say *Yes* if the face is one that I asked you to remember or *No* if it is not." The examiner is allowed to repeat or rephrase the instructions if the client does not understand the task. Forty-eight pictures of faces are then presented to the client and he or she is required to identify each face as being either one they were asked to remember or a new face (i.e., not previously presented). The examiner records the client's response in the record form by circling one of two choices, Y (yes) or N (no). Each correct response is worth one point and incorrect responses earn zero points. After the 48 items are administered, the examiner instructs the client to try and remember the first group of faces (i.e., the initial 24 faces that were presented) because he or she will be asked to identify them during a later portion of the WMS-III test. After the 48 items are administered, a recognition total score (ranging from 0 to 48 points) is calculated.

The Faces II subtest should be administered 25–35 minutes after the Faces I subtest has been completed. The subtest begins with the following instructions: "Now I'm going to show you some more pictures of faces. I want you to look at each face carefully. Say *Yes* if the face is one that I asked you to remember earlier or *No* if it is not." These instructions can be repeated and/or rephrased if the client does not understand the task. The client is then shown a series of 48 faces and required to indicate whether or not the picture was one that he or she was asked to remember during the Faces I subtest. The examiner records the client's responses on the record form in the same manner that was described for Faces I. A recognition total score is calculated by adding together the number of correct responses (1 point is earned for each correct response, 0 points earned for incorrect responses), with the range in scores being a minimum of zero points to a maximum of 48 points.

CALIFORNIA VERBAL LEARNING TEST (CVLT)

The CVLT consists of a related-unclustered word list (List A) presented over five learning trials. Immediately following these five learning trials, a second distracter word list (List B) is presented. Following free recall of List B, trials of short-delay free recall, short-delay cued recall, long-delay free recall, and long-delay cued recall of List A are presented. The long-delay free recall and long-delay cued recall trials are administered after a 20-minute delay interval in which nonverbal testing occurs. Finally, a single trial of long-delay recognition for List A words is presented. Each list (i.e., Lists A and B) consists of 16 words representing four semantic categories with four words per category. The words are read to the client so that a given word is never followed by another word from the same semantic category.

Scoring of the CVLT can be done either by hand or by using the CVLT® Administration and Scoring System. However, because the scoring is cumbersome to compute manually, it is recommended that CVLT scoring software be used for such purposes.

PEABODY PICTURE VOCABULARY TEST-REVISED (PPVT-R)

The PPVT-R is a simple test, requiring 10–20 minutes for administration. It is commonly used as a quick screening test for general mental ability and cognitive impairments. The PPVT-R assesses the ability to integrate right hemisphere visual stimuli with left hemisphere word knowledge. Thus, the PPVT-R assesses a complex and multifaceted skill that may be related to overall neurological integrity or to more specific types of damage (Kaufman, 1990).

Like the original edition, the PPVT-R (Dunn & Dunn, 1981) is an individually administered, norm-referenced test of receptive vocabulary. Available in two alternate forms, designated L and M, the test is comprised of five practice items and 175 test items arranged in order of increasing difficulty. Each item consists of four black-and-white, clear, bold-lined illustrations that have been updated from the earlier version for more appropriate racial, ethnic, and gender balance.

The PPVT-R is quite simple to administer, with each item having a multiple-choice format. After the examiner names a stimulus word (object, action, or concept), the client selects the one out of the four picture choices that best illustrates the meaning of the word. Clients have the option of either pointing to the selected picture of orally naming the number of the picture that they wish to select. If neither of these response styles is possible, such as when testing an extremely handicapped individual, it is permissible for the examiner to point to each of the responses asking the question, "Is this the one?" The client may then respond by head nodding or a predetermined signal, such as eye blinking.

Although the test consists of 175 items, the client must answer only about 40 items matched to his or her specific level of ability. Items that are much too easy or hard are not administered. The score recoding forms provided by the publisher contain starting point guidelines for chronological age when subjects are thought to be of average ability.

Several cautions are in order when using the PPVT-R with adults. The PPVT-R was standardized nationally on a sample of 5028 individuals—4200 children and adolescents, and 828 adults between the ages of 19 and 40 years. Although the sample of children and adolescents was matched to 1970 U.S. Census data, the adult standardization sample falls well short of this level. Dunn & Dunn (1981) report that the adult sample was closely matched to Census data only for occupation. In addition, only Form L was used for the development of the adult norms. Further, the norms for adults stop at age 40. When assessing individuals over the age of 40, the norms for the highest age group (35-0 to 40-11) may be used with the understanding that the standard score is an estimate. In spite of these limitations, the PPVT-R demonstrates good repeated measures of reliability, alternate forms reliability, and split-half reliability.

TEST OF LINE ORIENTATION

The test developed by Benton, Hannay, and Varney (1975) consists of five practice items and 30 test items. For each item, the client is presented with a semicircle divided into 11 numbered radii with two solutions of a pair of angled lines to be matched to the display. Two parallel forms of the test exist, presenting the same items in different order. Norms are available for adults from age 16 to 74, and for children from age 7 to 14. Score corrections for age and gender are provided (Benton, Hamsher, Varney, & Spreen, 1983; Eslinger & Benton, 1983; Mittenberg, Seidenberg, O'Leary, & DiGiulio, 1989). Scoring is simply based on the number of correct matches.

The client is presented with each item and asked which of the numbered radii in the semicircle matches the same angle as the item. The examiner records the answer. This is a simple and objective test with high scoring reliability because of its simplicity.

BENDER-VISUAL MOTOR GESTALT TEST (BENDER)

The Bender, a very well known test, includes a total of nine cards, each with a geometric figure or design on one side and blank (apart from numbers or letters with which the clinician orders the cards) on the other side. In addition, the client has access to several sheets of plain white paper and a no. 2 pencil with an eraser.

Administration of the test begins with card A. Some clinicians choose to use this merely as a sample, while others include it in the scoring. The clinician instructs the client to copy the figure onto paper just as he sees it on the card before him. Consequently, the card should be placed squarely before the client, and attempts to rotate the card or paper should be discouraged, so that any deviations in rotation of the copied figure are due to the client's perception, not to the orientation of the test apparatus. Instructions to copy the figure exactly are the only ones given, without any mention as to spacing the figures on the paper or to using more than one piece of paper, etc. Through this paucity of guidance, the clinician receives clues about the client's decision-making, spatial tendencies, temporal performance, and the like.

Cards are presented to the client one after the other, and each remains in the client's field of vision until he finishes copying his version of the figure. Some clinicians note the time it takes the client to begin drawing after being presented with each card, and complete each drawing. The former represents the rate at which the client makes decisions and plans the steps necessary to replicate the figure; the latter gives some indication as to how exactly and with how much ease or difficulty the client makes his attempts at copying the figures. Other clinicians introduce memory trials into the test, asking clients to recall a figure immediately after the card has been removed or after some period of delay.

Following suit, scoring methods for the Bender are many and varied, but Hain's (1963, 1964) scoring method stands out for neuropsychological purposes, for it offers norms for brain-damaged versus normal individuals. Fifteen different categories of errors exist, and a single violation of a given error type satisfies the requirement for having committed it. In other words, one need commit the error type only a total of once on all nine cards to be penalized, and multiple instances of the same error type do not raise the score. Error types are assigned their scores based on the level to which they suggest organicity. A single instance of perseveration, rotation or reversal, and/or concretism earns 4 points; added angles, separation of lines, overlap, and distortion receive 3 points each; embellishments and partial rotations get 2 points each; and omission, abbreviation of designs 1 or 2, separation, absence of erasure, closure, and point of contact on figure A get 1 point each. Scores can range from zero for a perfect presentation to a maximum of 34 for the presence of each of the 15 types of errors. Utilization of a cutoff score of 9 allows for the correct identification of 80% of clients (Lezak, 1995).

PEABODY INDIVIDUAL ACHIEVEMENT TEST-REVISED (PIAT-R)

The PIAT-R consists of the same five subtests seen in the original version with the addition of a sixth subtest (Written Expression). The test kit comes with four volumes consisting of three easels for the administration of subtest items in both visual and verbal format, as well as a test manual containing instructions on test administration and scoring, plus normative data.

The subtests are as follows in the order of administration:

1. General Information: This subtest is aimed at assessing a person's global fund of information. Items are administered orally and the client is required to give an oral response.
2. Reading Recognition: This subtest is designed to assess the fundamental skills of reading (e.g., phonemic and discrimination). The client is presented with written words and is asked to read each word aloud. Credit is given for correctly pronounced words only.
3. Reading Comprehension: The client is shown a page containing a sentence and is asked to read it silently. After the client indicates that he or she has completed reading the sentence, the next page is shown, which contains four picture choices. The client is then asked to point to the corresponding picture that best depicts the meaning of the sentence.
4. Mathematics: The client is asked to perform mathematical calculations mentally, without the use of paper or pencil. Questions are administered orally and visual cues or information is provided at the top of each stimulus page. Below this are four answer choices from which the client chooses the appropriate answer.
5. Spelling: The examiner reads a word to the client, uses it in a sentence, and then reads the word again. The client is then asked to point to the correct spelling of the word from a list of four choices on the stimulus page.

6. Written Expression: This subtest is designed to assess an individual's writing ability. It is divided into two parts. Level I is aimed at assessing basic writing skills, as the client is required to write his or her name, as well as write out letters, words, or sentences presented orally. Level II is administered to clients in the second grade or above. For this section there are two pictorial prompts. The client is then given 20 minutes to write a story about the scene in the pictorial prompt. The client's performance is quantified based upon his or her use of writing mechanics, grammar, and punctuation. The manual details the exact administration and scoring procedures.

STANDARD PROGRESSIVE MATRICES (SPM)

The Standard Progressive Matrices (also known as Raven's Matrices) consists of 60 items grouped into five sets (A to E). Each item represents a pattern problem with one part missing and six to eight possible solutions of which only one is correct. The examinee points to the pattern piece selected as correct (individual administration) or writes its number on the answer sheet (group administration). Administration takes between 40 and 60 minutes. Scores are converted into percentiles. Norms are available for age range 6–65.

REY AUDITORY VERBAL LEARNING TEST (RAVLT)

A predecessor to the CVLT with many similarities, the RAVLT consists of an unrelated word list (List A) presented over five learning trials. Immediately following these five learning trials, a second distracter word list (List B) is presented. Following free recall of this distracter list, a trial of short-delay free recall of List A words is presented. Long-term retention is generally assessed after 30 minutes. After administration of this long-delay recall trial, a trial of recognition memory occurs. A third list (i.e., List C) is available should either List A or List B presentations be spoiled by interruptions, improper administration, or premature response on the client's part (Lezak, 1983). Each list (i.e., Lists A, B, and C) consists of 15 semantically unrelated words.

To give the test, the examiner introduces the test and its purpose. After the examiner is sure that the examinee understands the instructions, he or she reads the stimulus words of List A aloud at a rate of one word per second. After the list is completed, the client is asked to repeat the words with the exact order recorded. Each response is coded as either repeated (R); (RC) if the client corrects herself/himself; (RQ) if she/he questions whether she/he has repeated the word but is unsure; (EC) if the word was confabulated; or (EA) if the word was the product of phonemically or semantically related errors. In addition, intrusions from List A into the recall of List B (i.e., proactive interference) are errors that are coded (A), and intrusions from List B into the recall of List A (i.e., retroactive interference) are errors that are coded (B). List A is administered five times using a similar procedure.

Following the fifth presentation of the List A words, the examiner presents the immediate free recall trial of List B items by telling the client that he or she is to learn a new list of words. These are presented in the same manner as Trial I of List A. When recall of List B is complete, the examinee is asked to recall as many words as he or she can from the first list (i.e., List A).

Following this short-delay free recall trial of List A words, the long-term retention is tested after an additional 30 minutes. During the 30 minutes it is recommended that the individual engage in nonverbal tasks so as to minimize interference from other verbal material.

The score for each trial of the RAVLT is simply the number of words correctly recalled. A total score (e.g., the sum of trials 1–5) can also be calculated, and a learning curve can be formed based on the number of correctly recalled words for each of the five trials. In addition, the number of words learned after the first trial (highest score for a trial minus the score on trial 1), the number of words forgotten over the interference trial (trial 5 minus trial 7), the percentage of words forgotten (number of words forgotten divided by the score on trial 5), and the number and types of errors can be calculated. Rey (1964) provides norms for trials 1–5 for adults, adolescents, and children. Savage and Gouvier (1992) provide norms for 30-minute delayed recall, for errors on delayed recall, and for recognition using the story format with 134 healthy participants ranging in age from the late teens through the seventh decade.

CLOCK DRAWING TEST (CDT)

The CDT is a paper-and-pencil test. There are several methods for administering the CDT (Brodaty & Moore, 1997). In the Shulman method (Shulman et al., 1993), subjects are given a piece of paper with a predrawn circle on it and asked to add in the numbers of a clock face. They are also asked to set the hands of the clock at 10 after 11. Scoring for the CDT ranges from 1 to 6, with a score of 1 being a perfect clock, a score of 2 indicating mild visuospatial errors, a score of 3 indicating errors in denoting the specified time, a score of 4 representing moderate visuospatial disorganization, a score of 5 suggesting severe visuospatial disorganization, and a score of 6 signifying no reasonable representation of a clock.

The Sunderland method (1989) requires the subject to draw a clock with all the numbers on it with the hands reading 2:45. This method requires that the subject draw the circle as opposed to giving him or her a predrawn circle. The scores are as follows: 10 equates hands being in the correct position, 7 signifies that the placement of hands is significantly off course, 4 represents further distortion of the number sequence, and 1 indicates that either no attempt, or an uninterpretable attempt was made.

In the Wolf-Klien method (Brodaty & Moore, 1997), the subjects are only asked to draw a clock on a predrawn circle. Time setting is not assessed in this administration method. The scoring system pertains to the spacing of numbers: a score of 10 is normal, a score of 7 shows very inappropriate spacing, a score of 4 shows counterclockwise rotation, and a score of 1 shows irrelevant figures. Brodaty and Moore (1997) found the Shulman method to be the easiest to follow and most reliable.

BENTON VISUAL RETENTION TEST (BVRT)

The BVRT test consists of a stimulus book with three sets of 10 cards containing geometric designs. Each set of 10 cards is an alternate form of the test. Depending on the form administered, the client will either copy the design while looking at the card or reproduce the design from memory immediately after presentation or following a 15-second delay. The three alternate forms of the BVRT may be administered by any of four methods, as described below. Any of the alternate forms may be given using any mode of administration and in any order. Many of the cards have more than one figure, and most consist of a three-figure design that is sensitive to unilateral spatial neglect.

For all administrations, the client is provided with 10 blank sheets of paper and a pencil with an eraser. Erasures and corrections are permitted. A stopwatch or a watch with a second hand is required for administration. The designs should be presented at an angle of about 60 degrees from the table surface, and should not be placed flat on the table.

For Administration A, the client is advised that he will be shown a card containing one or more figures that he may study for 10 seconds. When the card is removed, he is to draw the figure(s) as accurately as possible. The cards are to be presented without comment by the examiner, with the exception of Design III, which is the first card to contain a minor peripheral figure in addition to two major figures. The examiner should introduce this card with a reminder to draw everything present. This may be repeated on the next card if the client omits the peripheral minor figure in the reproduction of Design III.

Administration B is identical to that of Administration A except that the client views each design for only five seconds and then immediately reproduces the design from memory. Administration C is a copying task in which the client reproduces each design while viewing it. This is often administered first to assess the quality of a client's drawings and to familiarize the client with the three-figure format.

During Administration D, the subject views each design for 10 seconds and then reproduces the design following a 15-second delay. To ensure that the subject does not begin drawing before the delay interval is over, the paper and pencil should be handed to the subject at the end of each delay interval rather than at the beginning of the test. After the subject completes each design, the drawing and the pencil are both taken away.

The number of correct designs, as well as the number of errors, are scored. The Number Correct Score is determined on an all-or-none basis. If the reproduction contains no errors, it is scored as Correct and given one point. If the reproduction contains any errors, it receives a score of 0. The Number Correct Score for any of the alternate forms of the test (10 designs) ranges from 0 to 10 points.

The Number Error Score is composed of six categories of errors: omissions, distortions, perseverations, rotations, misplacements and size errors. Within these categories are 56 specific types of error. Although the Number Error score has a wide range, the typical protocol typically contains fewer than 24 errors (Benton, 1974). The scoring system for errors is complex to learn but relatively simple to apply. Once the scoring system is learned, each form of the test can be scored in about 5 minutes.

Scoring criteria for this test allow a wide margin of error, for the test is designed to measure the client's capacity to retain a visual impression rather than his or her drawing ability. For example, the size of the total reproduction is of less concern to the examiner than is the size of each individual figures relative to one another within the design.

Errors are scored according to the following categories:

1. Omission errors consist of the omission of any single figure of a design. These errors are coded by the significance of the figure omitted, the placement (right or left) of the figure, and the addition of figures not present in the stimulus.
2. Distortions are defined as inaccurate reproductions and are coded by the significance of the distorted figure, placement (right or left), substitution (e.g., square for triangle), or the omission, addition, or misplacement of an internal detail of the figure.
3. A perseveration is a substitution or addition that is a reproduction of a figure from the previous stimulus design, or when a peripheral or major figure in a design is drawn identical to a major figure in the same design. However, a perseveration is not recorded if the major figure appears to be a perseveration of a peripheral figure in the same design, as this is scored as a distortion. In addition, when a perseveration is scored, no

    other type of substitution, addition, or rotation error is recorded for the same figure.

4. Rotations are scored based on the degree to which the figure is rotated, and they are coded according to which figure in the design is rotated.
5. Misplacements represent the distortion of spatial relationships between figures of a design. Only one misplacement error may be scored for each card.
6. Size errors reflect distortions of the size of figures relative to other figures in the same design.

WISCONSIN CARD SORTING TEST (WCST)

    The standard WCST consists of four stimulus cards and two response decks. The stimulus cards are comprised of one red triangle, two green stars, three yellow crosses, and four blue circles. The two response decks consist of 64 cards each, totaling 128 cards, containing geometric shapes that vary according to features of form (e.g., circle, square, triangle, or cross), color (e.g., red, green, blue, or yellow), and number of shapes on each card (e.g., one, two, three, or four). The 64 cards in each deck are unique and reflect all possible combinations of color, form, and number.

    The client is instructed to match each consecutive card from a total of two response decks of 64 cards each, to one of four stimulus cards. The test requires the client to determine the current sorting principle and to sort the cards according to one of the three features (e.g., color, form, or number) based solely upon the examiner's feedback of "correct" or "incorrect" when the test is administered in a manual fashion, or upon the computer's feedback tones when the test is automated. Clients are not informed as to the strategy or method for sorting, but must generate hypotheses and utilize examiner feedback to modulate response patterns.

    Upon every 10 consecutive cards correctly sorted by the client, the examiner changes the criterion or sorting principle (e.g., color, form, number). The client must shift to the new sorting strategy that is cued only by the feedback of correct or incorrect from the examiner. The test begins with color as the initial sorting principle, changing to form and then to number and returning to color. The test is terminated when the client has completed six runs of ten correct placements.

    Various scores have been reported for the WCST including measures of success, perseverative tendencies, scores concerning nonperseverative errors, and measures of conceptual ability and learning effect. The manual WCST is scored by circling all incorrect responses. The total number of errors, the total number of correct responses, and the number of categories (each criterion run of ten consecutive correct responses) completed (for which zero to six are possible) are then totaled. Perseverative responses are then identified. A perseverative response is defined as one that would have been correct under a previous criterion principle. Scoring rules for perseverated response are many and complex and should be attended to with care. Other scoring criteria include "nonperseverative errors" and "percent perseverative errors." These latter scores appear less useful than the basic perseveration score.

There are two measures of conceptual organization. One is the number of "trials to complete the first category;" the other is the "percent conceptual level responses" score. The final scores obtained are the "failure to maintain set" and the "learning to learn."

PURDUE PEGBOARD

The Purdue Pegboard consists of a board with two parallel rows of holes into which cylindrical metal pins (pegs) are placed by the examinee. Each row contains 25 holes. The top of the board has four cups in which pins and other components of the instrument are placed. The pins are placed in the extreme right and extreme left cups of the board. In the center two cups, metal collars, and washers are placed. The test involves a total of four trials. Each of the first three trials is 30 seconds long. During each trial the examinee places as many pins as possible into the holes on the board. In the first trial, the client is required to use only the preferred (dominant) hand when placing pins into the holes. During the second trial, the nonpreferred (nondominant) hand is tested, and in the third trial both hands are used. The fourth trial lasts for 60 seconds. During the fourth trial the examinee is asked to build assemblies consisting of a pin, a washer, a collar, and then another washer using both hands and then placing them in the board.

Administration of the test begins with a demonstration of each of the four trials. Then the client is allowed to practice each trial until the examiner is confident that the client understands the requirements of each trial. Generally, only a single practice trial is necessary for each of the four trials. The first trial is conducted using the preferred hand, the second trial tests the nonpreferred hand, and the third trial tests both hands simultaneously. When testing the right hand, the examinee is asked to select pins from the extreme right side cup and place them, as quickly as possible, in the right side column. The examinee is told to start at the top and work downward without skipping any holes. The trial is stopped at the end of 30 seconds. The same procedure is used when testing the left hand. Before the third trial, the pins from both columns are removed. In the third trial, both hands are used simultaneously. The examinee selects pins with each hand from the same side cup and places them in the respective side's column. Again, the examinee begins at the top of each column and works downward during a 30-second period. The pins are then removed.

The fourth trial, which is the assemblies trial, also requires the use of both hands. In this trial, the examinee is asked to use both hands in a continuous alternating motion, such that the first one picks up a pin, the second one picks up a washer, the first one picks a collar and so on, in order to build the assemblies. The examinee constructs the assembly and then places it in the board, repeating the sequence as quickly as possible within a 60-second time limit.

In practical use, many administer and score only the first two trials of the test. When all four trials are administered, scores are obtained for each of the four trials. The number of pins placed in the holes during the 30-second periods is the score for each of the first two trials. The score for the third trial, during which both hands are used, is the total number of pairs of pins placed in the board. The total number of parts assembled is the score for the fourth trial. These scores are compared to the average scores of the appropriate normed population. It should be noted that practice effects have been found on this measure. The practice effect is greater in younger populations (in the 25–33-year-old age range) as compared to that in older populations.

REY COMPLEX FIGURE TEST (CFT)

The CFT requires the client to draw directly from a figure and from memory a complex figure that is not easily verbally encoded. It involves drawing and memory skills beyond those tested by simpler drawing tests, such as the Bender or BVRT. To administer the CFT, the examiner will need a reproduction of the figure and three blank sheets of paper. The first section of this test is called the Copy Phase. In this phase, the examiner sets a blank sheet of paper in front of the client and places the stimulus sheet (containing the figure) directly above it. The examiner must not allow the client to rotate either sheet during testing and should make no indication that there will be readministrations at later time intervals. The subject is then asked to copy the figure onto the blank piece of paper. There is no time limit for copying the figure. When the client finishes, the stimulus page and answer sheet are removed and put in a place where they cannot be viewed for the remainder of the testing period.

The Immediate Recall phase of the test is administered approximately 3 minutes after the Copy Phase is completed. However, administration of the copy phase as soon afterward as 30 seconds has been shown to have no significant effect on the results (Meyers & Meyers, 1995). The examiner places a blank sheet of paper in front of the client and the client is asked to draw the design as best he can from memory. Again there is no time limit and the answer sheet is to be removed upon completion. The last phase administered is the Delayed Recall phase, and administration follows the same format as the Immediate Recall phase. The client is asked to reproduce the figure from memory. This delayed readministration typically occurs 30 minutes after the initial administration. However, findings indicate that varying the time interval between the Immediate Recall and Delayed Recall phases (15, 30, or 40 minutes) has no significant effect on the score. However, omission of the Immediate Recall phase has been found to have a significant impact on performance of the Delayed Recall phase (Meyers et al., 1995), likely because an additional consolidation trial was omitted.

If the examiner wishes to gain insight into the strategy used by the client for purposes of qualitative analysis, additional administrative procedures have been recommended. One easy way to do this is to have the client use different colored pencils or pens after completion of each section of the drawing. When using this procedure, the examiner must record the order in which each colored pencil was given to the client. This will yield a record of the order in which the client reproduced the drawing, giving the examiner additional insight into the order in which the client recalled and reproduced various sections of the figure. Other methods for recording order of response have also been recommended.

Several scoring procedures have been developed for use with the Rey-Osterrieth Complex Figure Test (Denman, 1984; Hamby, Wilkins, & Barry, 1993; Kaplan, 1993; Lezak, 1995). The 18-point scoring system developed by Rey & Osterrieth (as cited in Lezak, 1995) is discussed in detail in this section, as this is the scoring method of primary use in the field of research and clinical practice. The Rey-Osterrieth scoring method includes 18 individual scoring criteria. Each considers the presence of a figural element. For each of these 18 elements, a verbal description and visual representation of the key element are offered (Taylor, 1959; Lezak, 1995). Each of these key elements is to be considered separately and is given a score of 2, 1, .5, or 0. The first thing for the clinician to consider upon examining each element is whether the element in question is "correct." For an element to be considered correct, it must be reproduced in its entirety, easily recognizable without distortions, and complete. If it meets these criteria, as well as being placed in the proper position in relation to the elements of the figure, then the client will earn a score of two points. If it meets the criteria for a correct response but is poorly placed, it earns only one point. If the key element is distorted or incomplete, yet can still be recognized by the examiner as an attempted reproduction of that element, then the client may still qualify for partial credit. If the distorted or incomplete element is recognizable and properly placed, the examiner is to give a score of 1. If the element is poorly or improperly placed, a score of .5 is given.

The examiner evaluates each of the 18 key elements in this manner. As the client may earn from 0 to 2 points on each of the scored elements, the total score may range from 0 to 36 for each phase of the test. A list of the key scoring elements for the Rey-Osterrieth and Taylor Complex Figures are provided by both Taylor (1969) and Lezak (1995). Once raw scores for the Copy and Recall phases of the examination have been calculated, percentile scores can be obtained from normative data. Sources of normative data are available in Lezak (1995), Osterrieth (1944), Taylor (1969), and Spreen and Strauss (1991).

Based on findings that the standard 18-point scoring procedure was unable to discriminate hemispheric involvement in patients with temporal lobe epilepsy, Loring, Lee, and Meador (1988) developed an 11-point scoring system intended for this purpose. This scoring system follows scoring procedures similar to those previously discussed.

STROOP COLOR AND WORD TEST

The test consists of three pages. The first page is a list of color names (e.g., RED, GREEN, and BLUE) repeated in a random order and printed in black ink. The second page consists of a nonmeaningful pattern (XXXX) printed in the same ink colors as the color names on the first page. The third page consists of the color names on page 1 printed in colored ink in such a manner that the color of the ink and the word does not match. Thus this page includes the word RED printed in green or blue ink, the word BLUE printed in green or red ink, and the word GREEN printed in blue or red ink. In all cases, the pattern of items is random, except that a given word or color cannot follow itself. Each page typically consists of 100 items. There are various versions of the tests available that may depart from these specifics, but all have the same common format.

Administration of the test may be done in two ways that provide equivalent information. The preferred method measures how many items a client can read out loud from each page in 45 seconds. The client is instructed on the first page to "read as many words as quickly as possible until you are stopped." On the second page, the client is similarly instructed to "name as many colors as quickly as possible." On the third page, the client is told the page "consists of the words on the first page printed in the colors on the second page, but the word and the color do not match. On each of these items, you are to ignore the word and name only the color of the ink that the word is printed in. For example, the first item is the word RED printed in blue. Your answer would be blue for the color of the ink. Remember, name as many colors as you can as quickly as possible until I tell you to stop."

On each page, the examiner says "Go" and begins timing. At 45 seconds, the client is told to stop and the number of items completed in the 45 seconds is recorded. If the client makes any errors during the test, he or she is stopped and told to reread the item. There is no need to count errors as there is a penalty for the additional time to identify the item correctly. (Some users of the test do, however, record the number of times the client is corrected.)

The alternate administration involves the same general instructions, but in this case the client is urged to identify all 100 items and the time to complete 100 items is recorded rather than the number of items completed. The drawback of this approach is that it takes much longer, especially for a slow reading or impaired client who in some cases may take 10 minutes or more to finish the last page.

Results derived from either method may be converted to time per item measures which are essentially equivalent for the different methods. Golden (1978) presents T-scores for the number of items completed in 45 seconds. Three basic scores are generated by the test: Word (the number of items completed on page 1 in 45 seconds), Color (the number of colors identified in 45 seconds on page 2), and Color–Word (the number of colors identified in 45 seconds on page 3).

A number of researchers have suggested the use of calculated Interference scores that measure the overall interference of word naming on the color naming process. There is some controversy regarding the best methods of calculating the interference score. According to Golden (1978), two methods are most frequently used. The first of these is simply to subtract the Color score from the Color–Word score, with the difference representing the loss due to interference. The weakness in this method is that it dos not take the strength of word naming into account. As word naming skills increase, it is expected that it will interfere more with color naming. As a result, individuals who are very strong on word naming are often misrepresented as showing abnormal interference when that is not the case.

The second method uses a formula to derive an expected Color–Word score from the Color and Word scores. This expected score is subtracted from the actual score. Scores that are negative reflect less than expected performance (suggesting higher levels of interference) and scores that are positive suggest better than expected performance (and less interference). The formula for estimating the expected Color–Word score is: (Color * Word)/(Color + Word). The second method is generally preferred and is used in the explanations below because it is easier to interpret and understand. Norms for the test may be found in Golden (1978).

BOSTON NAMING TEST (BNT)

The Boston Naming Test (BNT), developed by Kaplan et al. (1983), is, as its name implies, a measure designed to test a client's ability to name objects following visual presentation of representations of the objects. The stimuli consist of 60 line drawings of objects, the names of which range from simple, high-frequency words (e.g., "tree") to rare words (e.g., "abacus"). Cards containing the drawings are presented to the client one at a time. An item is passed if the client names the pictured object within 20 seconds. For adults, the first card presented is number 30 (harmonica). If any of the succeeding eight items are missed, the test continues backward from item 29 until eight consecutive items are answered correctly. Once this criterion has been met, the test proceeds in a forward direction until the subject commits six consecutive errors.

The BNT allows for the administration of two types of cues to clients. First, in those instances in which it is clear that the client has misperceived the item pictured on the card, he is informed that the picture represents something other than what was stated. For example, if, when the client is presented with the picture of a harmonica he states that it is a picture of a building, he is given the semantic "stimulus cue" and informed that it is a picture of a musical instrument. If, after receiving the semantic cue, the client correctly identifies the item within 20 seconds, he is given credit for a correct response and it is noted that the semantic cue was provided. The second type of cue is given whenever a client is unable to correctly identify the depicted item within 20 seconds. This "phonemic cue" consists of telling the client the phoneme with which the name of the object begins. For example, if the client cannot name the mushroom, he is told that it begins with the sound "mu." The client's response is then recorded as either correct with a phonemic cue or as incorrect, and no credit is given. Norms for the test are provided in the test manual.

CONTROLLED ORAL WORD ASSOCIATION TEST (COWAT)

The purpose of the Controlled Oral Word Association Test (COWAT) is to evaluate the spontaneous production of words beginning with a given letter or belonging to a given category within a limited amount of time. In brief, the test is administered by instructing the individual to produce as many words in 1 minute as he or she can think of that begin with the given letter of the alphabet excluding proper nouns and the same word with a different suffix. The most commonly used letters are FAS, although CFL and PRW are commonly used as alternatives. Another alternative that is usually given in addition to letters, but that can be substituted for them, is the use of conceptual categories for which words must be generated. For example, the subject can be instructed to name as many fruits and vegetables or animals within a minute. However, the category alternative is considered to be somewhat different than the letter version because it allows the subject to draw on a conceptual category that may permit a form of fluency that is enhanced by cues inherent to the conceptual category. The basic idea here is that the conceptual category may better activate verbal associations and therefore allow for greater access to appropriate responses.

VISUAL FORM DISCRIMINATION TEST (VFDT)

The VFDT is a 16-item multiple choice test of visual recognition for one-dimensional designs (Lezak, 1995). Each item consists of one card with a target figure, presented to the patient at a 45 degree angle, and a multiple-choice card containing four figures, lying flat on the table below the target. On the target item, a peripheral design appears to the right of the two major figures on eight items and to the left of the major figures on the other eight items. Each multiple-choice item contains the correct design and three incorrect designs containing either a displacement or rotation of the peripheral figure, a rotation of one of the major figures, or a distortion of the other major figure (Benton, Ivan, Hamsher, Varney, & Spreen, 1994).

According to Benton et al. (1994), the administration procedures are as follows: Beginning with the first of two initial demonstration items, the examiner points to the target design and says: "See this design? Find it among these four designs" (pointing to the multiple-choice card). Then the examiner asks: "Which one is it? Show me." The patient can signify a correct response by either pointing to or calling out the number of the design on the multiple choice card that is identical to the target design. If the patient fails either demonstration item, the examiner is to show him or her the correct design, point out the errors on the other choices, and then proceed with the test. If both demonstration items are passed, the examiner continues on to the rest of the test without further instruction. There is no time limit for the administration of the test but if no response is offered after 30 seconds, the examiner says: "Which one do you think is the same; what is your best guess?" Scoring is based on a 3-point system as follows: 2 points for fully correct responses, 1 point for peripheral errors, and 0 points for major rotations and distortions (Lezak, 1995).

HOOPER VISUAL ORGANIZATION TEST (HVOT)

The Hooper Visual Organization Test (HVOT) was developed to identify patients in mental hospitals with organic brain conditions (Hooper, 1958). The test consists of 30 pictures of readily recognizable objects on $4'' \times 4''$ cards. Each object has been cut up into two or more parts and rearranged. The examinee is instructed to name what the object would be if it were put together in one piece. The examinee can either name the object verbally (if given individually) or write the name of the object in spaces provided in the test booklet (if given in a group format). All 30 of the items are administered. However, Wetzel and Murphy (1991) found that discontinuing the test after five consecutive failures does not significantly change the scoring of this test. Scoring ranges from 0 to 30. The time required for administration is approximately 10–15 minutes.

LURIA–NEBRASKA NEUROPSYCHOLOGICAL BATTERY II (LNNB)

The Luria–Nebraska Neuropsychological Battery is a method that integrates the qualitative information generated by the techniques of A. R. Luria with traditional American psychometric procedures. This hybrid approach takes elements from both significant traditions. The test has been found to have both a strong psychometric base as well as to provide the clinician with the opportunity to make numerous and valuable qualitative observations and discriminations of highly specific problems in clients that cannot be easily made with traditional psychometric instruments. The test battery itself provides a brief but comprehensive evaluation in less than 3 hours, which makes it practical to use in situations in which time is limited and with impaired clients whose ability to be tested over long time periods is limited.

The LNNB provides a framework for Luria's evaluative style by adding an objective scoring system and standard administration procedures. This structuring provides a foundation of items that can be given to all clients, scored in an objective and reliable manner, and evaluated for systematic effectiveness across different populations. At the same time, Luria's qualitative and flexible administration is retained around this framework, yielding an instrument that can be studied psychometrically while at the same time used in a purely clinical and impressionistic manner.

To reach these dual goals, it was necessary to carefully modify the administration of the test. First, instructions for items were made flexible so that the clinician could be assured that the client understood the instructions. In the case of many "standardized" instructions, clients make errors because they do not understand the task requirements. The LNNB allows paraphrasing and repeating instructions, answering client questions, and offering examples to ensure that the client understands what is required. Simultaneously, the process of client information is garnered in this communicative process. For example, if the client learns only from examples, or rapidly forgets instructions and needs frequent repetition, information directly relevant to the client's condition and learning style is gained. Attention to this communicative process throughout the test can assist in making an accurate diagnosis and description of the client.

Second, "testing of the limit" procedures are encouraged throughout the evaluation. While such procedures are built into the items themselves, the test organization allows the clinician to add these procedures without affecting the validity of the standard scores. An important aspect of this flexibility is the emphasis on scoring and the client's underlying mechanism of performance. Any item on any test, regardless of the simplicity, can be missed for a variety of reasons. A full understanding of the client's condition can be achieved only with comprehension of the client's failure.

Further, qualitative observations are encouraged throughout the test. These observations not only focus on the question of "why" an item was missed, but also on behavior between items throughout the test. The need and nature of such redirection, while not scored in any item, becomes a significant part of the evaluation. In traditional tests, client errors are often misinterpreted in terms of item content rather than the attentional process. Through clinician involvement in the testing process, the LNNB separates the content issues of the items from such conditions as arousal, attention, concentration, emotionality, frustration, motivation, and fatigue.

Finally, the emphasis of the LNNB is on obtaining optimal client performance. Many traditional tests encourage suboptimal performance in brain-injured clients through minimal feedback, excessive testing times, misunderstood instructions, and other similar features. Such procedures maximize differences between the brain-injured clients and normals, increasing "hit rates" but decreasing individual differences among brain injured clients. Many of these tests may end up maximizing the manifestations of client impairment.

The LNNB, Form II, consists of 279 items organized into 12 basic scales (Golden, Purisch, & Hammeke, 1985). Because many of the items have more than one subpart, the actual number of procedures in the test is approximately 1000. The LNNB scales are nontraditional because the same procedure or question is not asked repeatedly at different levels of difficulty. The purpose of the LNNB is not to stratify individuals as "average" or "superior" but rather to address basic functions, which underlie all complex behavior. Each scale is organized to test different aspects of behavior within each area evaluated. While the items differ from one another in a variety of ways, they all have a common theme such as "memory functions" or "language functions." The 12 scales include: Motor, Rhythm, Tactile, Visual, Receptive Language, Expressive Language, Writing, Reading, Arithmetic, Memory, Intelligence, and Intermediate Memory.

Item Scoring

All items on the LNNB are scored as either a 0 (indicating normal performance), 1 (borderline performance), or 2 (impaired performance). For items that are scorable only as right or wrong, a 0 represents right and a 2 represents wrong. For those items (such as motor speed items) that involve counting of responses, the raw score is translated into a 0, 1, or 2 score using norms given on the test form. The use of this common scoring procedure allows for statistical and clinical inter-item comparisons.

Scale Scoring

Each scale is scored by adding up the 0, 1, 2 scores from each of the items. A total raw score is generated that is converted into a T-score using the table in the test form. The T-scores have a mean of 50 and a standard deviation of 10. High scores reflect poorer performance. These scores are classified as normal or impaired by reference to a cutoff score called the critical level (CL), which is individually determined by the client's age and education using a table in the test form. Scores above the cutoff are considered impaired performance. The average cutoff is 60, but may vary from 50 to more than 70 depending on the age and education of the client.

Qualitative Scoring

In addition to the item and scale scoring, the LNNB includes 60 qualitative scoring categories, which can be scored at any time during the test, including in between items. It is not within the scope of this chapter to review all of these indices, but a sample can be discussed to show their usefulness.

In general, qualitative indices represent recording of observations by the tester during the course of the examination. These reports generally fall into the categories of (1) problems related to inadequate client comprehension of procedures; (2) observations that explain why the client is missing an item; (3) unusual behaviors between items that impact the testing; and (4) problems that manifest during an item performance but are not related to the objective scoring of the test.

Problematic client comprehension generally involves confusion, insufficient vocabulary, attention deficits, arousal problems, fatigue, and motivation. Observations during the item that clarify errors differ depending on the scale but will include paralysis, motor slowness, motor awkwardness, hearing difficulties, attentional problems, tactile sensation loss, visual difficulties, visual agnosia, inability to comprehend speech, naming problems, slowness in comprehension, inability to attend to the left side of stimuli, dysarthria, slowness of speech, word substitutions in speech, sound substitutions in speech, syllable substitution in words, inability to progress from one sound to another, perseveration, concreteness, dyslexia, failure to recognize letters, failure to recognize sounds, failure to recognize number, visual–motor problems, memory problems, fatigue, and so on.

Unusual behaviors may include distractibility, inability to recall instructions, inappropriate emotional reactions, excessive fatigue, hyperactivity, lack of cooperation, poor arousal, seizures, and other related problems. The final category can include any problems seen when the person responds correctly but still shows a problem. For example, an individual may correctly describe an object but fail to name it correctly, thus demonstrating dysnomia. An individual may be literate, but only in a dysfluent manner, suggesting expressive speech problems such as dysarthria.

The LNNB may be administered as an entire test or scales or items may be removed to be used to measure specific skills. When used as a full test battery, the test generates T-score profiles that can be used to estimate the type, degree, location, and extent of brain injury. When only selected parts are used, they can be employed to augment a more comprehensive test battery to gain a more detailed or specific analysis about skills in a specific area or to act as a screening device for possible problems in a specific area. Used in this latter manner, the test offers a very flexible format and can be added to other tests with a minimum of additional time yet allow for more detailed skill evaluation in motor and nonmotor visual areas and language areas.

Some additional data are supplied for each of the scales individually included in this book for administration separately from the rest of the battery. More detailed information may be found in the test manual (Golden, Purisch, & Hammeke, 1985).

Motor Scale (Scale C1)

The administration of the C1 Motor Scale entails that the client be given detailed instructions for each of the 51 items. The verbal instructions may be altered to communicate to the client what is desired. With the exception of the items that require the client to perform motor movements in response to verbal instructions, the motor behaviors can generally be modeled. The motor movements involve the client's arms and hands and for clarity, the fingers are numbered 1 through 5, beginning with the thumb. The finger tip is described as the region between the tip of the finger and the last joint. The palm and the back of the hand are also clarified.

Items 1 through 4 are primarily measures of motor speed. For these items the client is allowed to practice the items until they are done smoothly at least twice in a row. These items are timed and once the client can perform the item accurately, his or her performance will be scored on how fast the item is correctly done. According to the number of completed sequences, a score of 0, 1, or 2 will be given quantitatively in addition to the appropriate qualitative scores.

For items 5 through 8, the client is blindfolded for the first time in the battery. The examiner will put the client's hand in a certain position and after returning his or her hand into a relaxed posture, the client is asked to repeat the position. For example, the client's hand is turned palm up by the examiner and the palmer surface of the right thumb is pressed against the fingertip of the second finger for 2 seconds. After the manipulation is complete the hand is returned to a relaxed position and the client must imitate the original position. If item 5 is done correctly a score of 0 is earned; an incorrect response yields a score of 2. Motor Awkwardness (MA) as well as other qualitative scores can be assigned.

Items 9 through 18 allow the examiner to evaluate the ability of the client to mimic gross motor activities. Specific, static movements (such as raising the hand to the height of the head) are demonstrated by the examiner, who tells the client to copy him or her and do exactly the same movement. These items are presented with the examiner sitting across from the client. As a result, some clients will mirror-image the examiner's hand position (e.g., raise the left arm when the examiner's right arm is raised). Because the intent of these items is to determine primarily motor response ability and only secondarily visual–spatial skills, the clients who make this error have a second opportunity.

Items 19 and 20 involve movements similar to the preceding items: however, the focus is on the ability to perform motor movements according to verbal directions rather than motor imitation. Items 21 through 23 represent evaluations of bilateral motor skills. These are trained and administered as in the unilateral motor speed items (items 1–4).

Item 24 is the first of the drawing items. The presence or absence of motor perseveration is the focus. The Patient Response Booklet is placed in front of the client and he or she is asked to draw the given figure as quickly as he or she can. Erasures are not permitted on any of the drawing or writing items.

Items 25 through 27 evaluate the ability of the client to perform imaginary motor acts without props. In each case, both motor skills and ability to perform in the absence of normal objects are of interest. If the client is asked to "Show me how you would hammer a nail into a wall," then the response would need to include all the motor actions necessarily as if the props were physically there. Anything missing would receive a score of 2, indicating an incorrect response.

Items 28 through 35 involve oral–motor skills. The items in this section can be demonstrated to the client along with the verbal instructions, except for items 34 and 35. Instructions including "Puff out your checks" will be given and a score of 0 will indicate the correct response while an incorrect response will be scored as a 2.

Items 36 through 47 represent the remaining drawing items. There are six drawing tasks, each of which receives two scores, one for quality and one for speed. It is important in the instructions to emphasize that the drawing is to be done "as quickly as possible without lifting your pencil from the paper." If the pencil is lifted before completion of the figures, the item may be readministered with timing starting over. The scoring criteria are based on the presence of listed violations such as an incomplete circle or a significant overlap in the lines.

The last four items of the scale (items 48–51) involve the verbal control of simple motor behaviors. In each of these cases, what the examiner does is at odds with what the client does or expects. For example, the item may require the client to knock hard when the examiner knocks gently, while others require a motor response to a purely verbal stimulus.

Intermediate Memory (Scale C12)

Although all of the C12 items are based on other items on the LNNB, no forewarning is given at the administration of the original items in their respective scales. Therefore, the client is not likely to rehearse the material in preparation for C12. As a result of this lack of preparation as well as the recall nature of many of the C12 items, clients will, on occasion, respond with material from previous items other than those that were intended. In these instances, the contaminated response is not scored as a perseveration unless the same incorrect response is offered several times.

When a client is unable to answer a C12 recall item correctly, the examiner can present the question to the client in a recognition format. Here, the examiner would list an incorrect answer and ask the client if it is the correct answer; the examiner would then follow with the true correct response and ask if it is correct. In this manner, a clinician gains qualitative information and tests the client's limits.

In cases in which one wishes to administer this subtest independent of the remainder of the LNNB, it is necessary to give just those items on which the test is based: items 1–4, 40, 42, 44, 56, 76–79, 82, 84, 87–91, 223, 234, and 235. Scale C12 should be administered 30 minutes after the completion of item 235. The 30 minutes should be filled with other testing procedures.

Expressive Speech (Scale C6)

The Expressive Speech Scale consists of 42 items that progress in level of complexity. Items 133 through 142 of this scale are very simple. They ask that the client repeat sounds or words as stated by the examiner. The following section, beginning with item 143, is very similar to the previous one in that it asks that the client repeat sounds or words, this time by reading them rather than hearing them. The purpose of this section is to determine whether a client's speech deficits (if any) are due to receptive or expressive problems, depending on what section of the scale created difficulties for the client. Items 154 through 156 require the client to repeat increasingly more complex sentences.

On items 157 and 158, the client is asked to name objects and body parts, respectively, as seen in varied stimulus cards. Item 159 requires the client to name an object from a description rather than from a visual presentation of the object. The following section (items 160–163) examines the client's automatic speech by asking him or her to count from 1 through 20 and to say the days of the week, first forwards and then backwards.

The next six items assess the client's ability to generate spontaneous speech after looking at a picture (items 164 and 165), hearing a story (items 166 and 167), and being given a topic of discussion (items 168 and 169). The last items (items 170–174) analyze higher forms of speech and complex systems of grammatical expression and, as such, can be dubbed "intellectual–expressive" items. These items require that the client fill in missing words in a sentence and make up a sentence using either a set of three words or words that are mixed up.

This scale is not designed to examine vocabulary or reading skills, and, as such, administration and scoring instructions attempt to minimize the impact of such factors on the individual's performance. Consequently, the examiner is allowed to repeat directions or stimulus items if the client appears not to have understood or heard correctly. Furthermore, the client is given the same considerations when his or her error appears to be nonarticulatory in nature. In other words, if the client's response is fluent and pronounced correctly, but does not match that required by the item, it is helpful to repeat the given stimulus and/or even ask the client to watch the examiner's lips as the words are being said so as to assist in inputting the information. It is also useful to record the client's answer verbatim so that, in case an incorrect response is given, the quality of the error can be later analyzed.

Memory Scale (C10)

For items 223 through 225, the examiner reads aloud a list of seven words. During presentation of these words, the examiner should deliver each one at the rate of one word per second. No special emphasis or intonation should be given to any of the words, as this might make the word more readily remembered. The client then repeats as many words as he can from the list, and the clinician informs him of how many of the seven words were repeated correctly. Next, the client makes a prediction about how many words he will recall correctly on the following trial. This sequence of list presentation, client recall, feedback, and client prediction continues until the client remembers all seven words for two consecutive trials or until five trials are completed.

If the client suffers from a disability that precludes him from speaking the words back during the five trials, he can respond by writing the list on paper. In either format, mispronunciation or misspelling of the word is acceptable as long as the word remains recognizable. The first seven words the client repeats are those that count toward his score, so if two intrusions occur with the first seven words, the client is told he responded correctly with five words. When a client gives seven words, pauses for more than 5 seconds, or cannot conjure up another word, the next trial commences.

Item 226 requires the client to indicate whether the image on a second card is the same as that presented on the original stimulus card before interference. The client need only respond "yes" or "no," and any means of doing so (e.g., nodding) will suffice. For item 227 the client must redraw from memory an image from a stimulus card; drawing skills should not influence the score here, so long as the figure and its details are recognizable. During the rhythm item (228) the client may use his hands, voice, feet, or other device to replicate the stimulus rhythm. For item 229 the client must use one hand (which one is not specified) to repeat the sequence of finger positions correctly.

The remaining six items target verbal memory. Although all six ask for oral responses, written answers are acceptable when speech is not possible. As with the seven-word word list from items 223–225, once the specified number of stimuli words to be recalled is attained, no additional words count toward the client's score; only the specified number of words is counted, even if intrusions are present among them.

Immediate spontaneous corrections, on the other hand, are allowed on all items on this scale. When spontaneous correction does take place, the initial response should be noted for the purpose of qualitative analysis. Guessing, too, is permitted and even encouraged on memory scale items. In instances in which the client is reluctant to guess, the clinician may "test the client's limits" by altering the recall task to a recognition one so that the client can choose the correct answer from a series of distracters.

Reading (C8)

The Reading Scale is a short, simple test consisting of three basic tasks that progress in level of complexity. First, the client is asked to generate sounds from letters that the examiner reads out loud. Second, he or she is asked to name simple letters, read simple sounds, and read simple words and letter combinations that have meaning. Last, the client must read entire sentences as well as paragraphs.

Because the focus of the test is on the internal conversion process rather than the quality of the motor output, clients should not be penalized quantitatively for articulation disorders. They should be penalized only for actual reading disorders. If a client's reading is difficult to understand because of an articulation disorder, he or she should be instructed to repeat the response.

In the event that a client has a peripheral visual problem, he or she can usually be aided by adjusting his or her distance from the stimuli, enlarging the cards, or using a magnifying device. Central visual impairments can be more problematic. In most cases, however, the client self-adjusts and provides adequate scanning of the items. Nevertheless, in some cases, the client will read only half of the stimuli and subsequently miss items. Such neglect of the left side should be noted qualitatively, and missed areas should be pointed out to the client. He or she should be allowed to try again without being quantitatively penalized. The timer should be restarted and missed items should be attempted once more.

Regional or cultural variations in pronunciation, accents, and so on are acceptable and should not be scored as errors. Any reasonable pronunciation of the syllables or words is acceptable. If a client sounds out a word, he or she should be instructed to repeat what he or she thinks the word is. The client must give a common English pronunciation of a word rather than an interpretation. However, if the client's first language is not English, this needs to be taken into consideration.

Each item of the subtest has provided instructions that should be read verbatim to the client. In addition, each item has a time limit of 10 seconds, with the exception of the last item which has a 30-second time limit. The client should be cautioned against impulsive reading and encouraged to read the items carefully. If he or she is unsure of an answer, he or she should be encouraged to guess. All items are scored both quantitatively and qualitatively.

For all but the last subtest item, quantitative scoring is based on the correct pronunciations, letters, and/or words provided in the Administration and Scoring Booklet or the Manual. Any deviations from what is considered acceptable would result in error. When qualitatively scoring the subtest items, there are more elements to consider. For example, if the client produces sounds that have nothing to do with the letters, a score of Grapheme Recognition (GR) should be given. If the client gives a letter substitute that sounds like the correct letter, an Auditory Discrimination (AU) should be scored. If the client attempts to visualize the sequences by writing the letters with his or her hands in the air or on a table, Gestural and Visual Cueing (GV) should be given. Verbal Cueing (VC) should be scored if the client attempts to repeat the letters to himself or herself aloud. Perseveration (PE) can be scored if the client gives the number of letters or continually repeats the letters or words aloud. Elaboration (EB) may be given if the client attempts to make a word out of letters, such as "cro" to "Cro-Magnon" or "ply" to "plywood." These categories pertain to all subtest items.

More specifically, in item 190, Additional Responses (AD) can be scored if the client adds extra letters beyond what is presented. Unilateral Neglect (UN) should be noted if the client ignores letters on 1 side of the card. If the client is unable to recognize the symbols as letters, Letter–Number Recognition (LN) should be given. These categories should be applied, when appropriate, to all subsequent items.

Additionally, for qualitative scoring of item 194, Perseveration (PE) should be given if the client is unable to read the letters individually and insists on reading the as a single word. Also, Gestural and Visual Cueing (GV) should be scored if the client attempts to cover up the letters to read them more effectively. Such behavior should not be allowed to continue.

Item 198 is intentionally difficult so that the context of the material does not facilitate prediction of later words in the sentence. For example, "The orange trees blossom in winter" may be said by the client as "The orange trees blossom in summer." In this case, the error scored would be Context Confabulation (CC). If the client omits articles in his or her sentence response(s), he or she may receive a score of Dropping of Articles (DA).

For the last item, the time required to read the paragraph in item 199 needs to be recorded. If the client has not finished reading the paragraph within 30 seconds, the time recorded should be 31 seconds. Quantitative scoring is based on completion time.

Writing (C7)

The Writing Scale is a straight forward test consisting of items that progress in level of complexity. First, the client is asked to copy simple letters and combinations of letters and words, and write his or her first and last names. Second, he or she is instructed to write dictated sounds, words, and phrases. Last, the client must write a few sentences on a given topic. Following administration, the client obtains a total raw score for both the spelling and motor writing responses.

For all subtest items, spelling is always scored. Any mistake in the client's spelling ability is recorded as an error. Motor writing is scored only when a written response is requested. At times, it may be difficult to determine whether the client has made spelling or motor writing errors when lettering appears clear and even and shows no obvious motor problems. In cases of spelling mistakes and writing illegibility, the client should be instructed to spell aloud the word that he or she intended to write. When, for example, the client has written certain letters or words illegibly and he or she cannot spell aloud, the client should be instructed to point to provided letters in order written. The examiner can also read the letters or words as they appear and ask the client if that is what was intended. By following these procedures, one should be able to determine spelling and motor writing errors or the presence of both. This subtest can be rescored following administration to obtain scores for spelling and motor writing performance.

Each item of the subtest has provided instructions, which should be read to the client verbatim. All subtest items are scored quantitatively and qualitatively. Specifically, item 175 has a time limit of 10 seconds per word and is quantitatively scored in terms of number of incorrect letters. Qualitatively speaking, item 175 can be given a score of Gestural and Visual Cueing (GV) if the client attempts to write the word in the air. If the client attempts to spell the word aloud, Verbal Cueing (VC) should be noted. If the client anticipates the question by responding before the examiner has given and task, Anticipation (AN) may be scored. Irrelevant Associations (IR) should be noted if the client responds with extraneous, impertinent information. If the client repeats the question to himself or herself, Repetition (RT) should be scored. Failure to Comprehend Instructions (FC) should be noted if the client tries to spell the word rather than give the number of letters. If the client starts to give the number of letters but then starts to spell the words, Confusion (C) should be given.

For item 176, quantitative scoring is based on number of incorrect responses. There is a time limit of 10 seconds per trial. Qualitative errors that may be scored in addition to the categories previously mentioned are Auditory Discrimination (AU) and Circumlocution (CR). (AU) is given if the client substitutes a letter for a letter-sound that is similar. (CR) is recorded if the client starts to describe the letter proper. In addition, if the client decides to write the response rather than say it, the motor writing categories discussed in the following item may be applied. Inability to say a letter should be scored as a disorder of articulation with the specific problem determining the category.

For items 177 and 178, the time limits are 20 and 30 seconds, respectively. Quantitative scoring is based on misspellings, illegibility, or on incomplete responses. If the client's writing is uneven, shows tremors, or if letters are not recognizable, an error should be scored. With regard to qualitative scoring, if errors are due to not completing all the letters within the time limit, Time Delay (TD) should be scored. Such difficulty is usually a result of motor impairment.

Motor Awkwardness (MK) should be noted if the client, while maintaining writing speed, makes writing errors by either substituting letters for one another, adding unnecessary lines or curves, or closing letters incorrectly, rendering them unrecognizable. If tremors are apparent, Tremors (TR) should be noted. Micrographia (MC) should be scored if the client's writing is exceptionally small. Macrographia (MA) should be scored if the client writes over a half inch in height. If the client's writing is not fluid and smooth, Stiff Motor Movement (SM) can be scored. Such writing can be identified by the client's slow and labored process and by his or her difficulty in producing the letters. Paralysis (PS) and Peripheral Impairment: Motor (M) can be diagnosed when appropriate. Care should be taken with clients who have peripheral impairments such as arthritis, other problems related to the aged, or problems resulting from traumatic accidents. Elaboration (EB) may be scored when the client not only writes the letter he or she is supposed to, but also incorporates it into a word. An example would be writing "glad" instead of just writing "g." If the client writes the same letter repeatedly, Preservation (PE) should be scored.

Item 179 has a time limit of 30 seconds and is quantitatively scored in the same fashion as the previous item. However, if the client initially forgot a word or could only spell aloud, no credit is given for this item even though it may be given for the same items in the optional, separate spelling and motor writing subtests. Qualitative scoring is the same as for previous items. However, with this item and subsequent items involving words, if the client spells a word in a way that is wrong but is phonetically reasonable, no further errors should be scored other than the ones already described. Grapheme Recognition (GR) should be scored if the client spells the word in a meaningless manner (e.g., spelling the word "Antarctic" as "krft" or other spelling that could not possibly represent the word.)

The time limits for items 180 and 181 are 15 and 10 seconds, respectively. There is no time limit for item 182. These items are all quantitatively and qualitatively scored the same as previous items. Items 183 and 184 also have no time limit and are similarly scored. One should note, however, that the qualitative score of Grapheme Recognition (GR) should not be given in item 183 if the silent letter is dropped.

For item 185, again with no time limit, the spelling and writing of each word in each group or phrase should each be quantitatively scored. Qualitative scoring does not differ from previous items. An additional category to consider is Sequence Error, which is scored when the client writes the correct words but in the wrong sequence.

The examiner should allow 60 seconds for item 186. Qualitative scoring, again, does not differ from previous items. With regard to quantitative scoring, grammar, spelling, and content are rated for the entire expression, including anything written after the time limit.

For the grammar rating, if the expression is missing any punctuation, is expressed in phrases rather than sentences, begins with lowercase rather than capital letters, or contains any other grammatical letters, the grammar should be scored as 1. The spelling rating should also be scored 1 if there are any misspellings, not including acceptable abbreviations. If the content is illogical, incoherent, or irrelevant to the topic, the content rating should be recorded as 1. The total raw score is obtained by totaling the three ratings of grammar, spelling, and content.

The last item, item 187, is scored quantitatively only. The examiner should count the number of words written, in 60 seconds, for item 186. The symbol ampersand (&) is included as a word.

Arithmetic (C9)

Items in this scale increase in level of complexity. The initial part of this scale (items 201–209) involves simply writing down both Arabic and Roman numerals from dictation. Several multidigit items have been employed for the purpose of looking for possible spatial deficits. Items 210 and 211 require that the client compare numbers. In the next section, beginning with item 212, the client is asked to do simple arithmetic problems that most individuals can usually do from memory. On items 215 throughout 217, the client's task consists of performing more complex addition and subtraction problems that cannot be done from memory. On items 218 through 220, the client is asked to perform difficult mathematical manipulations, such as filling in a missing number or sign. Finally, the last section (items 221–222) involves the presentation of serial 7s and 13s.

Because many individuals tend to have difficulty with mathematical items, and thus react to these items with fear and anxiety, it is important that the examiner be alert to the presence of such reactions and behave in a manner that is comforting and gentle while persistent. Instructions must be read as written on the test booklet while presenting the client with the response booklet and/or stimulus card as required. Some items allow the examiner to paraphrase the instruction and/or provide examples. The examiner must record all oral responses given by the client and, if an incorrect response is given, even investigate the client's reasoning process to determine the qualitative nature of the client's deficits. Furthermore, the client must not be allowed to erase incorrect answers, as these often provide important qualitative cues. Instead, the client may rewrite his or her new response next to the incorrect answer.

All items are scored both quantitatively and qualitatively. Each number, group of numbers, computation, or manipulation within an individual item is scored separately, and the total number of errors is added for a quantitative score for that specific item. In general, qualitative scoring is similar for all items of this scale, although some qualitative scores apply only to specific items.

Time limits vary across the scale. Items 201 through 219, for example, have a 10-second time limit for each operation within the item or for the entire item, as specified. Time limits for items 220, 221, and 222 are 20 seconds, 30 seconds, and 45 seconds, respectively. Time limits are based on the client starting his or her response within the specified time limit, except for those items involving only the motor writing of number, which should be completed within the required time limit. Responses to those items involving both motor writing and calculation must be started within the time limit; however, when necessary, the client may be allowed extra time to finish producing his or her response. Additional time may also be allowed when testing limits.

For items 201 through 209, instructions and visual stimuli may be repeated and presented in a variety of ways, except for those items for which oral or visual presentation is specified. The answers to items requiring oral presentation must be given orally. However, the client is not penalized for expressive difficulties as long as the answer given is correct and begun within the time limit. Similarly, clients must respond in writing to items asking for a written response, although errors are scored only for numerical and not for motor writing mistakes. If the written response is not recognizable, the examiner may ask the client to verbally clarify the response. The examiner is also allowed to provide examples for items that involve reading multidigit numbers (such as 158) as a single, whole number as long as the example does not include actual test items. Similarly, the examiner may provide examples if a client indicates unfamiliarity with roman numerals. If after being presented with an example the client remains unable to comprehend the instructions or otherwise solve the problem correctly, the client's answer is scored as an error. In general, on this section, any mistake in reading or writing a number, other than misarticulation and motor errors, is scored as an error.

For items 210 through 220, the mode of presentation and responses may be varied as necessary. The use of paper and pencil to do calculations is allowed only in some items (items 212–215). However, for items 216 through 220, the client is instructed to perform the problems from memory, without the use of paper, fingers, or any other gestural or visual cue. For items 216, 217, and 220, to test the client's limits and separate attention/concentration from calculation difficulties, the client may be allowed to perform on paper those problems that he or she could not figure out from memory alone. However, those answers would still be scored as errors.

The last two items (items 221 and 222), which involve the subtraction of serial 7s and 13s, differ from that used in the standard mental status exam in that clients are not allowed to proceed to the next subtraction until the previous one has been correctly achieved. In other words, if a client cannot subtract 7 from 100 correctly, the examiner must say "No, that is not correct. Try again. What is 100 minus 7?" The client must attempt this subtraction until a correct answer is given or the time limit is reached. Again, the client's limits can be tested by allowing additional time to complete the item and/or permitting completion of item using pencil and paper. Nevertheless, credit is given only when the correct answer is given on the first try. Scoring is based on the first six subtractions, where any answer that is not correct on the first try or that is not given within the 30-second time limit is scored as an error.

Receptive Language (C5)

Scale C5 of the LNNB is a simple test that is used to screen for deficits in the functional system of receptive speech. Consistent with conventional views about the specific brain anatomy thought to be correlated with receptive speech, C5 is generally used as a means by which to detect damage to the left hemisphere and the left temporal lobe in particular, given the subject is right-handed and his or her brain functions are lateralized in a typical manner. However, many items on C5 tap abilities that extend beyond the left temporal lobe to include the widespread anatomical sites involved in various levels of receptive speech. Materials for the C5 scale consist of items 100 through 132 on the LNNB, which are printed in the Administration and Scoring Booklet, and corresponding answer spaces for items 101, 103, 105, and 123 in the Patient Response Booklet. Verbal instructions that the examiner reads to the examinee are printed in bold lettering. Supplementary instructions and administration cues for the examiner are printed in normal lettering.

Perhaps the first and foremost task to be completed before assessing a client with scale C5 is to ascertain whether the peripheral auditory system is adequately intact. If it is not intact, assessment of receptive speech is precluded. If intact, assessment can commence. During administration of scale C5, the examiner stands behind the examinee to reduce the possible influence of visual cues. Instructions may be said while looking at the examinee to ensure proper comprehension of task demands. In fact, instructions can be presented in practically any manner deemed necessary to make sure that the examinee understands. However, because the scale is designed to assess receptive speech (i.e., as opposed to undifferentiated communication), it is imperative that stimulus items be presented in a way that minimizes the possibility of reception and interpretation by alternate means. An additional administrative issue to bear in mind is that it is essential that the examinee is paying adequate attention as each stimulus item is administered. Again, because the goal is to detect deficiencies in receptive speech, stimulus items cannot be repeated. To do so would increase the possibility of masking receptive speech deficits. Therefore, it is crucial to eliminate, as best as possible, fluctuations in attention that might otherwise erroneously be interpreted as receptive speech difficulties.

C5 items evaluate the ability to understand receptive speech, from simple phonemic discrimination to the understanding of complex sentences with inverted English grammar. The examinee is instructed to respond in a number of different ways including verbally, graphically, and via hand signals. Examinees generally are not penalized quantitatively for responses given in a form other than that requested, as long as adequate receptive speech is indicated. Rather, such deviations are recorded qualitatively and are used to enhance interpretations of failures on other portions of the LNNB. Individual items can be analyzed to determine at what level in the receptive speech functional system the breakdown occurs. Typically, errors at a lower level (e.g., phonemic discrimination) represented by items at the beginning of the scale will result in errors at higher levels represented by later items (e.g., word comprehension, following complex directions, etc.). However, this is a rule of thumb and is not always the case. Failure at higher levels may have no implications for lower level skills.

TESTS OF VARIABLES OF ATTENTION (TOVA)

Test of Variables of Attention (TOVA) (Greenberg, 1985) is a continuous performance test using non-language-based stimuli. The tests measure a cognitive element of attention (Corman & Greenberg, 1996). There are two stimulus versions available for the test, visual (the TOVA) and auditory (TOVA-A). The subject is presented a target and then presses a microswitch button one time when the target is recognized as quickly as possible. Both tests utilize the same two-condition test format over a duration of 21.6 minutes. Each also has the same 2-second interstimulus (ISI) condition throughout the test (thus, every 2 seconds a stimulus appears, the target or a nontarget). The two conditions are (1) target infrequent and (2) target frequent. The target infrequent is defined by a 3.5:1 nontarget to target ratio. Quarters one and two are the target infrequent conditions. The target frequent condition is defined by a 3.5:1 target to nontarget ratio. Quarters three and four are the target frequent conditions. The testing scenario represents a test–retest trial over each condition. This analysis is important to understanding the test interpretation strategies and will be expanded upon for each variable.

The test stimuli are not language dependent. The visual test stimuli are a box within a box. The target is defined as the inner box at the top, the nontarget defined as the inner box at the bottom. When the subject sees the target, the subject presses the button on the microswitch. For the TOVA-A, the nontarget is defined by a middle C tone, the target is defined by a G above middle C tone.

Each subject receives a practice test prior to the standardized test. The practice test is a 3-minute target infrequent condition trial. Standardized instructions are provided in the manuals (Greenberg, 1996; Leark, 1996). The practice test was administered in the norm development phase of the test, given to all subjects in the norm base. During the practice test, the examiner is encouraged to use prompts as needed to encourage the best performance. The practice test is automatically scored by the software scoring system, with results given instantaneously. If the practice test is poorly done, or if the examiner believes that a further practice trial is warranted to ensure that both the instructions are understood and the subject understands the task of the test, the practice test should be redone. It is essential for the subject to understand that the microswitch button is to be pressed when the target appears on the screen, and it must be pressed as quickly as possible after the target is recognized.

The basic scales for the TOVA are Omission, Commission, Response Time, and Response Time Variability. Omission is defined by an omission (i.e., failure to identify the target) response by the subject. The Omission score is determined by the percentage of target responses correctly identified. Commission is defined by the subject pressing the button for a nontarget (i.e., an error of commission). The Commission score is determined by the percentage of nontargets correctly identified. Response Time (RT) is defined as the average (i.e., mean) of the response time for correct responses. Response Time Variability (RTV) is defined as the variance around the mean for the response time for correct responses. The Response Time and variance are recorded in milliseconds. These raw scores are transformed to standardized scores as derived from the standardization norm sample. These calculations are computed by age and by gender.

Each test (TOVA and TOVA-A) has independent norms. The TOVA has norms developed for years 4 through adulthood. For years 4 through 19, norms are stratified by year and by gender. Over age 19, norms are stratified by decade (i.e., 20–29, etc.) and by gender. Subjects aged 4 and 5 receive an shortened format of the test (11.3 minutes). The younger aged format consists of one trial for each of the target infrequent and target frequent conditions. The practice test is also given to the younger aged subjects. The TOVA-A is developed for years 6 through 19 with norms stratified by year and gender. The TOVA-A is currently in the process of norm development for individuals over 19 years of age.

INTERMEDIATE VISUAL AND AUDITORY
CONTINUOUS PERFORMANCE TEST (IVA)

The Intermediate Visual and Auditory (IVA) Continuous Performance Test (CPT) assesses difficulties in attention and impulsivity. This computerized test measures reaction times and error rates while different conditions are presented. It was developed to aid in the diagnosis of Attention Deficit Hyperactivity Disorder (ADHD). It requires one to sustain attention to a series of stimuli that tend to be boring, as well as inhibit one's response after a certain paradigm has been established. It assesses areas of performance including speed, stamina, vigilance, prudence, consistency, and off-task behaviors.

This 13-minute test requires the examinee to click a mouse only when he or she sees or hears the target "1," but not when he or she sees or hears the foil "2."

Because this is a relatively simple task, it can be quite boring and requires sustained attention. The test measures errors of commission (impulsivity) and errors of omission (inattention). It incorporates four CPTs into one by combining impulsivity and inattention in both the auditory and visual modalities.

In the beginning and the end of the test, the "Warm-up" and "Cool-down," a brief sensory–motor subtest assessing simple reaction times is presented. The main part of the IVA consists of 5 sets of 100 trials each, with each set consisting of 2 blocks of 20 trials each totaling 500 trials. Each trials lasts 1.5 seconds. The visual targets and foils are presented for 167 milliseconds (ms), while the auditory stimuli are presented for 500 ms.

In the main section of the tests, 42 out of the first 50 trials are "1"s (84%) intermixed with eight "2"s. The examinee is required to inhibit his or her response when the "2" appears or is verbalized, but is expected to respond when the series of "1"s are presented. There are 50 trials in the first block. The second block, consisting of 50 trials, assesses errors of omission by presenting fewer "1"s than "2"s. Now the ratio of "1"s is 16%.

The stimuli are presented in a pseudo-random fashion of mixed visual and auditory stimuli, making it a demanding task. It requires cognitive flexibility and the examinee cannot predict how the stimuli will be presented. The keyboard is controlled by the examiner and must be placed to one side. The examinee should sit in front of the monitor and the mouse should also be placed in front of the monitor, so the subject can comfortably use it. Administration and scoring should be followed exactly according to the IVA manual.

Test-taking behavior is one of the first things that should be evaluated. Double-clicking of the mouse signifies hyperactive behavior. Test comprehension and motivation to do well should be established at the beginning to ensure a valid test.

All scores are reported as standard scores with a mean of 100 and a standard deviation of 100. The label of Mildly (<90), Moderately (<80), Severely (<70), and Extremely Impaired (<60) can be applied to any of the global scales, response control scales, attention scales, or sensory/motor scale. The labels of Average (≥90), Above Average (≥110), Superior (≥120), or Exceptional Ability (≥130) can also be given. Quotient scale scores can be given percentile ranks. The table for quotient scores, standard deviation, and percentile ranks are presented in the IVA manual.

CONCLUSIONS

The preceding summaries provide only general information on administration and scoring and are not intended to be complete. Please refer to the appropriate test manuals and the general reference articles listed before administering any of these tests.

REFERENCES

Benton, A. L. (1974) *Revised Visual Retention Test manual* (4th ed.). New York: The Psychological Corporation.

Benton, A. L., Hamsher, K., deS., Varney, N. R., & Spreen, O. (1983). *Contributions to neuropsychological assessment*. New York: Oxford University Press.

Benton, A. L., Sivan, A. B., Hamsher, K., Varney, N. R., & Spreen, O. (1994). *Contributions to neuropsychological assessment: A clinical manual* (2nd ed.). New York: Oxford University Press.

Corman, C. L., & Greenberg, L. M. (1996). *Medication Guidelines for use with the Test of Variables of Attention*. Unpublished manuscript. Los Alamitos, CA: Universal Attention Disorders.

Denman, S. (1984). *Denman Neuropsychology Memory Scale*. Charleston, SC: S. B. Denman.

D'Elia, L. F., Boone, K. B., & Mitrushina, A. M. (1995). *Handbook of normative data for neuropsychological assessment*. New York: Oxford University Press.

Dunn, L. M., & Dunn, L. M. (1981). *Peabody Picture Vocabulary Test-Revised: Manual for Forms L and M*. Circle Pines, MN: American Guidance Service.

Golden, C. J. (1978). *Stroop Color and Word Test*. Chicago, IL: Stoelting.

Golden, C. J., Purisch, A. D., & Hammeke, T. A. (1985). *Luria–Nebraska Neuropsychological Battery: Forms I and II Manual*. Los Angeles: Western Psychological Services.

Greenberg, L. (1996). *Test of Variables of Attention: Clinical Guide*. Los Alamitos, CA: Universal Attention Disorders.

Halstead, W. C. (1974). *Brain and intelligence: A quantitative study of the frontal lobes*. Chicago: University of Chicago Press.

Heaton, R. K., Grant, I., & Matthews, C. G. (1991). *Comprehensive norms for an expanded Halstead–Reitan battery: Demographic corrections, research findings, and clinical applications*. Odessa, FL: Psychological Assessment Resources.

Hooper, H. E. (1993). *The Hooper Visual Organization Test-Manual*. Beverly Hills, CA: Western Psychological Services.

Kaplan, E. F., Goodglass, H., & Weintraub, S. (1983). *The Boston Naming Test* (2nd ed.). Philadelphia, PA: Lea & Febiger.

Kaplan, E. (1993). Neuropsychological Assessment. In T. Boll & B. K. Bryant (Eds.). *Clinical neuropsychology and brain function: Research, measurement, and practice*. Washington, D.C.: American Psychological Association.

Kaufman, A. S. (1990). *Assessing adult and adolescent intelligence*. Boston: Allyn & Bacon.

Kolb, B., & Wishaw, I. O. (1996). *Fundamentals of human neuropsychology*. New York: W. H. Freeman & Company.

Lezak, M. D. (1995). *Neuropsychological assessment* (2nd ed.). New York: Oxford University Press.

Osterrieth, P. A. (1994). Le test du copie d'une figure complexe. *Archives de Psychologie, 28*, 206–356.

Reitan, R. M., & Wolfson, D. (1993). *The Halstead–Reitan neuropsychological test battery: Theory and clinical interpretation* (2nd ed.). Arizona: Neuropsychology Press.

Spreen, O., & Strauss, E. (1991). *A compendium of neuropsychological tests: Administration, norms, and commentary*. New York: Oxford University Press.

Spreen, O., & Strauss, E. (1998). *A compendium of neuropsychological tests: Administration, norms, and commentary* (2nd ed.). New York: Oxford University Press.

Weschler, D. (1997). *Wechsler Memory Scale—Third Edition*. San Antonio, TX: The Psychological Corporation.

Wilkinson, G. S. (1993). *Wide range achievement test (WRAT3): Administration manual*. Wilmington, Delaware: Wide Range.

3

Interpretation

As can be seen from the Introduction, interpretation of neuropsychological tests is a complex process that requires extensive knowledge, on one hand, of how the brain functions, and, on the other, how neuropsychological tests work and interact with one another. This section aims to bring out the major interpretive issues with each test presented in terms of patterns to look for within and between tests. This is a difficult task, as the possible patterns of neuropsychological test results are nearly infinite and dependent on the tests selected and the unique performance of the individual client.

The following sections of the book are best used by reading thoroughly the section on each test you have administered or are interested in. If you are looking at actual data, the appropriate paragraphs can then be selected that apply to your data. In addition to the possible interpretations, the paragraphs may suggest the usefulness of specific patterns with other tests. If these have not been given, it is often useful to look at the sections for those tests as well and consider including them in the test battery. In general, the wider the range of tests that can be administered, the more precise the conclusions that can be reached.

Although an attempt has been made to cover the major combinations with each test, for the sake of brevity and comprehensibility of the sections not all possible combinations between pairs of tests have been included. Thus, additional information will be gained by covering the section on each test that has been given.

The results of an analysis as suggested here will ultimately rest on identifying consistent patterns in the data that can be related to our knowledge of how the brain functions. In many cases, however, the presence of premorbid deficits (or even multiple injuries) will result in several overlapping patterns of findings that may affect one another so that results are not "textbook." In such cases, it is essential that the individual discrepancies be identified and explained in any detailed analysis of a client's data. Such discrepancies, if seemingly unexplainable, may reflect errors in assumptions (such as premorbid status), logic, integration, or may suggest that some of the data are invalid due to an error in administration or scoring, the use of inappropriate norms, or the lack of full effort on the part of the client (whether deliberate or the result of an outside factor such as medication).

Assessment itself is the art of explaining and reconciling these discrepancies as they are at the heart of the very individual differences we seek to identify and understand. The effort involved in doing this is much greater than for a simple "cookbook" approach to interpretation, but is rewarded by increased accuracy and better patient care. The interpretations suggested here should be viewed as only a beginning in the effort to fully comprehend the strengths and weaknesses of the client. These must in turn be combined with a knowledge of how the brain works and a full understanding of brain–behavior relationships before any definitive diagnostic conclusion can be reached.

Section I: General Intelligence

WECHSLER ADULT INTELLIGENCE SCALE-III (WAIS-III)

The Wechsler Intelligence Tests are without question the most widespread measures of intelligence in use today. As such, they assume great importance in any comprehensive test battery. Interpretation can be conducted on two levels: the summary scores and the individual subtest scale scores. This section focuses on the interpretation of the index scores, while later sections focus on individual subtests under their appropriate topic.

Interpretation

1. The Full Scale IQ (FSIQ) ideally is interpreted as an excellent measure of the individual's average general level of functioning. It is expected that other cognitive skills will group around this score, with two thirds falling within one standard deviation and 95% within two standard deviations of these scores. However, individual abilities may vary widely from this average.

2. Interpretation of the FSIQ should be cautious when there is a difference of more than 15 points between the Verbal and Performance IQs. In such cases, scores on verbal tests should be compared to the Verbal IQ (VIQ) and nonverbal tests to the Performance IQ (PIQ), rather than to the FSIQ.

3. FSIQ does not imply or rule out brain injury under any conditions. Brain injury may occur, regardless of IQ. Even when the FSIQ is at expected levels, an injury may still have occurred. Similarly, scores

below expected levels may reflect errors in expectations rather than brain injury.

4. Traditionally, PIQ–VIQ differences greater than 15 points are seen as clinically significant. However, the frequency of such differences increases greatly with IQ. At IQ levels below 80, the likelihood of a 15-point difference in controls is only about 7%; at IQ levels above 120, such differences occur almost one quarter of the time. As a result, a difference of 20 points is more acceptable for higher IQs (occurring about 10% of the time in normals).

5. A significant difference between VIQ and PIQ in which PIQ is higher than VIQ is rarely associated with a recent brain injury. It may be related to poor education or observed in an individual whose native language is not English. It may also be linked to childhood injuries (usually before age 6) that impaired the development of language functions. Exceptions are injuries that cause serious damage to the language areas of the dominant hemisphere (most often a stroke, open head injury, or head trauma with substantial bleeding in this area).

6. A significant difference between VIQ and PIQ in which Verbal IQ is higher is more commonly seen after head injuries to the nondominant hemisphere or subcortical areas of the brain. However, this pattern of scores may also occur after dominant head injuries because of motor impairment that slows performance on Digit Symbol and Block Design. Such deficits will also occur with peripheral motor deficits, which can be seen with non-neurological disorders (such as arthritis) or neurological disorders (such as multiple sclerosis). In these cases, the deficits cannot be reliably interpreted as indicating a cognitive problem.

7. PIQ may be lower in clients with poor vision whether or not there is a neurological component.

8. Comparisons of Perceptual Organization (PO) and Verbal Comprehension (VC) indices may be conducted in the same way as PIQ and VIQ comparisons. In fact, as these scores offer more factorially pure measures of underlying cognitive processes, they are often preferred and may give more accurate findings.

9. Working Memory is a measure of attention and immediate working memory processes. This score should be within 15 points of the FSIQ. In situations involving head injury and most brain disorders, this score will generally stay within the expected range when compared to other IQ scores. A low working memory score, when compared to other indices, often suggests an emotional or motivational process rather than a brain injury, as this score should be less affected by a brain injury than would VIQ or PIQ.

10. Working Memory on the WAIS-III may be compared with Working

Memory on the WMS-III. The two indexes overlap, with the WAIS-III index based on Arithmetic, Digit Span, and Letter Number Sequencing. On the WMS-III, the index is based on Spatial Span and Letter Number Sequencing. As a result, lower scores on the WAIS-III measure generally suggest problems working with numbers whereas lower scores on the WMS-III measure point to problems with short-term visual–spatial retention.

11. Working Memory is very different from the same measures on the WAIS-R and WMS-R owing to the inclusion of Letter Number Sequencing. This task is akin to Digits Backwards in the demands it places on the client and is very difficult for clients with a wide range of problems. As a result, we would expect the new Working Memory measure to be frequently lower than the old measure by as much as one standard deviation in clients without there being any sign of clinically reliable deterioration from an earlier testing with the WAIS-R or WMS-R. As a consequence, differences over two standard deviations (which are quite unlikely) would be necessary before deterioration could be confirmed.

12. The Perceptual Speed Index (PSI) (made up of Digit Symbol and Symbol Search) is generally impaired across all clinical samples. These tests require speed, sustained attention, memory, and understanding of instructions. They are affected by motor impairment (whether central or peripheral), memory losses, inability to concentrate, problems in understanding instructions, confusion, anxiety, depression, indecision, ambivalence, hyperactivity, frustration tolerance, motivation, fatigue, and compulsivity. As such, a significantly lower (15 point) score when compared to the lower of the Verbal or Performance IQ points to significant difficulties suggestive of a mental or organic disorder but does not specify the nature of that disorder.

13. A frequent goal has been to compare IQ scores to premorbid levels of function. Many methods have been developed for such predictions. The most popular include measures taken from within the WAIS-III itself and those based on demographic measures.

14. Measures from within the WAIS-III that best predict premorbid IQ include Information, Comprehension, Vocabulary, and Picture Arrangement. This is based on the assumption that these are "hold" tests, measures that theoretically "hold" their scores even after a brain injury or other disorder. Although such scores do work in individual cases, there are many circumstances in which they do not. First, individuals with language problems as a result of an injury will often have lower scores on these measures. Second, visual problems will interfere with performance on Picture Arrangement (although the pictures on the

WAIS-III are much easier to see than in previous versions of the WAIS).

15. Individuals differ on which of these four measures are used in predicting performance IQ. When predicting against premorbid Verbal IQ, a combination of Information, Comprehension, and Vocabulary is best used. This is completed by adding up the age-adjusted scale scores for the three subtests and multiplying by two. The result can then be translated into a Verbal IQ score by using the Verbal IQ table in the WAIS-III manual.

16. In cases where the prediction is against Full Scale IQ, all four subtest scores (Comprehension, Vocabulary, Information, and Picture Arrangement) should be summed. The score is then divided by four (to get an average) and multiplied by 11 (to project the score to a full 11 subtest full scale IQ). This can be translated to a Full Scale IQ by using the Full Scale IQ table in the WAIS-III manual.

17. In no case should the tests used to predict premorbid IQ be picked on the basis of the client's highest scores. Such a procedure will most often lead to an overestimation of premorbid IQ and inflate any apparent deterioration.

18. After brain injury or a mental disorder, the Verbal IQ and Verbal Comprehension Index (VCI) are usually more stable than Full Scale or Performance IQ. Significant changes from premorbid VIQ or VCIQ (scores more than 10 points lower than premorbid estimates) are often associated with serious brain injury, but rarely seen in mild or even moderate head injuries.

19. Declines of more than 10 points in Full Scale IQ are indicative of a disorder, but the nature of the disorder is less clear. Such declines may be due to depression, anxiety, brain injury, attentional problems, and fatigue/motivation. Such declines are seen both in more severe and milder brain injuries, but they cannot be interpreted as clearly because of the additional factors that may cause the lowering of the results.

20. Premorbid IQ can also be estimated on the basis of demographic information. This is a very attractive alternative as it dos not require any cooperation or performance from the client that could be impacted by a brain injury or other disorder. Such formulas typically use such information as education, occupation, place of residence, gender, and ethnic group as variables in predicting IQ.

21. While such demographic approaches work well in estimating the IQ of large groups of people, they have serious limitations when applied to individuals in clinical settings. These include but are not limited to: (1) serious problems in estimating IQ more than 1.5 standard deviations above or below the mean; (2) biases toward minority groups and certain

geographical regions that are not meaningful for individuals; (3) inaccuracies introduced simply by a nomothetic approach that ignores individual differences; (4) margins of error that exceed one standard deviation in scores; (5) limitations of coding methods for such variables as occupation or geographical region; and (6) tendency for such scores to lead to diagnostic and interpretive errors. As a result of these problems, none of these approaches can be endorsed as adequate in clinical settings.

22. Because the Full Scale IQ serves as a general measure of an individual's average skills, it is expected that other scores will be close to this score. This is often used as a measure of "expected performance" such that scores below FSIQ are interpreted as representing "weaknesses" and scores higher as representing "strengths." This pattern of strengths and weaknesses can then be interpreted as indicating patterns indicative of specific brain disorders or specific locations of brain injuries.

23. The use of the FSIQ as a baseline for other scores is subject to several limitations. First, FSIQ itself may be affected by brain injury which in turn lowers the expected baseline and minimizes the degree of problems that may exist. Second, some skills that are less cognitive in nature have little relevance to FSIQ. These include motor and sensory skills, which are essentially unrelated to IQ. Thus, a high IQ does not predict good motor coordination nor does a low IQ rule out superior motor or sensory performance. Third, in some cases peripheral injuries affect specific tests or testing procedures but not Full Scale IQ as much. Finally, in cases where VIQ and PIQ differ by more than 15 points, FSIQ should be not used as a general baseline. In such situations, VIQ and PIQ (or preferably, VCIQ and POIQ) may be used as a substitute baseline for verbal and nonverbal tests, respectively.

24. In interpreting deviations from an IQ baseline, it must be remembered that two thirds of all scores will naturally fall one standard deviation below or above the baseline (assuming that the normative populations are comparable as discussed in Chapter 2). Scores more than one standard deviation below the mean may be regarded as weaknesses, but it must be recognized that in normals without any brain injury up to 16% of all scores will fall in this range. As a consequence, a low score does not "prove" the existence of a brain injury. In all cases, the pattern of weaknesses must be examined to see if the scores follow a pattern associated with a known injury location or a known pathological process. Only when both conditions are met can one reliably conclude that there is a consistent cognitive deficit from a set of test results. However, even in such a case, this conclusion is not possible without a clear history of the actual origin of the deficit.

25. In cases a very high IQ, more scores than expected will be below the

baseline. When IQ is above 130, scores need to be at least two standard deviations below the baseline before a deficit can be reliably identified on another test.

26. In cases a very low IQ, the restriction of range on many tests makes interpretation a problem. For many tests, scores will bottom out at two to three standard deviations below the mean, making it impossible for the score to fall more than one standard deviation or less below the IQ baseline even when an injury is present.

27. The WAIS-III IQ scores have an essential floor of three standard deviations below the mean. As a result, individuals whose scores may actually fall four to six standard deviations below the mean will demonstrate IQ scores about three standard deviations below normal. When this baseline is compared to neuropsychological tests with a lower floor, there will be apparent discrepancies that are not meaningful.

References for Wechsler Adult Intelligence Scale-III (WAIS-III)

Boone, D. E. (1998). Specificity of the WAIS-R subtests with psychiatric inpatients. *Assessment, 5,* 123–126.

Campbell, J. M., & McCord, D. M. (1996). The WAIS-R comprehension and picture arrangement subtests as measures of social intelligence: Testing traditional interpretations. *Journal of Psychoeducational Assessment, 14,* 240–249.

Flynn, J. R. (1998). WAIS-III and WISC-III gains in the United States from 1972 to 1995: How to compensate for obsolete norms. *Perceptual and Motor Skills, 86*(3; part 2), 1231–1239.

Golden, C. J., Zillmer, E., & Spiers, M. (1992). *Neuropsychological assessment and intervention.* Springfield, IL: Charles C Thomas.

Hawkins, K. A. (1998). Indicators of brain dysfunction derived from graphic representations of the WAIS-III/WMS-III Technical Manual clinical samples data: A preliminary approach to clinical utility. *Clinical Neuropsychologist, 12*(4), 535–555.

Kramer, J. H. (1990). Guidelines for interpreting the WAIS-R subtest scores. *Psychological Assessment, 2,* 202–205.

Lobello, S. G., Thompson, A. P., & Evani, V. (1998). Supplementary WAIS-III tables for determining subtest strengths and weaknesses. *Journal of Psychoeducational Assessment, 16*(3), 196–200.

Matarazzo, J. D. (1972). *Wechsler's measurement and appraisal of adult intelligence* (5th ed.). New York: Oxford University Press.

Ryan, J. J., Lopez, S. J., & Werth, T. R. (1998). Administration time estimates for WAIS-III subtests, scales, and short forms in a clinical sample. *Journal of Psychoeducational Assessment, 16*(4), 315–323.

Ryan, J. J., & Ward, L. C. (1999). Validity, reliability, and standard errors of measurement for two seven-subtest short forms of the Wechsler Adult Intelligence Scale-III. *Psychological Assessment, 11*(2), 207–211.

Sprandel, H. Z. (1995). *The psychoeducational use and interpretation of the Wechsler Adult Intelligence Scale-Revised* (2nd ed.). Springfield, IL: Charles C Thomas.

Wechsler, D. (1981). *WAIS-R manual.* New York: The Psychological Corporation.

Wechsler, D. (1986). *WAIS-R administration and scoring manual.* San Antonio, TX: The Psychological Corporation.

Wechsler, D. (1997). *WAIS-III administration of scoring manual.* San Antonio, TX: The Psychological Corporation.

PEABODY PICTURE VOCABULARY TEST-REVISED (PPVT-R)

The PPVT-R is a simple test, requiring 10–20 minutes for administration. It is commonly used as a quick screening test for general mental ability and cognitive impairments. The PPVT-R assesses the ability to integrate right hemisphere visual stimuli with left hemisphere word knowledge. Thus, the PPVT-R assesses a complex and multifaceted skill that may be related to basic premorbid ability or in some cases to overall neurological integrity or more specific types of damage (Kaufman, 1990).

Interpretation

1. The PPVT-R assesses receptive vocabulary skills for standard American English. It is a measure of verbal ability, an important aspect of general intelligence. The PPVT-R correlates moderately highly with WAIS-R Verbal and Full Scale IQs. The PPVT is closest to the WAIS Vocabulary test, which is the best single method of estimating general intelligence on the Wechsler adult tests.
2. In many cases, the PPVT-R and WAIS Vocabulary tests yield similar scores. In such cases, these can be considered good estimates of premorbid intellectual ability, except when aphasia is present, which tends to decrease both scores.
3. In cases where Vocabulary yields a higher estimate of functioning than the PPVT-R, the client often has difficulty with visual analysis and discrimination, which should be reflected in other verbal tests. When present these deficits usually occur in the posterior right hemisphere.
4. In some cases where Vocabulary is higher than the PPVT-R score, the client does poorly because of perseverative responding on the PPVT-R's multiple-choice format, most often choosing the first or last answer repetitively. This is most often associated with left frontal or bilateral frontal disorders.
5. In cases where the PPVT-R score is higher than Vocabulary, the first possible cause is an expressive language problem as Vocabulary relies heavily on expressive skills. In cases of significant dysfluency, the client may be unable to communicate his or her answer verbally. Such dysfluency suggests injury to the anterior left hemisphere. In addition, posterior lesions may lead to circumlocution in which the client talks around the answer but never gives a good 2-point response.
6. In cases where the PPVT-R is suspected of overestimating IQ, you will usually see a pattern in which the client consistently missed four or five out of every eight items rather than the six of eight required for discontinuation of the test. In such cases, it is useful to use the first time the client missed five of eight as an artificial ceiling level to assess the

impact on IQ. The true IQ is usually between this value and the value indicated using the six of eight cutoff.

7. Visual agnosia should be considered when the client cannot decipher the pictures or describe them accurately. Visual neglect may also be evident as the client ignores the choices on one side (i.e., the right or left sides) of the response page. This will generally show up on tests such as the Rey, Block Design, and the Bender, as well.

8. Although the PPVT-R has often been used as a measure of dominant hemisphere functioning, performance on the PPVT-R represents a complex integration of visual–spatial stimuli and linguistic knowledge. It can offer valuable clues for interpreting score fluctuations on other instruments or depressed scores on other measures of verbal ability. In addition, the PPVT-R has been used as an estimate of premorbid intellectual functioning as well as a measure of residual vocabulary and fund of information.

9. Like the WAIS-III, the PPVT IQ can be used as a baseline to compare all other tests as described in the WAIS-III section. However, as this score is less general than the WAIS-III Full Scale IQ it is not as good a measure. The amount of deviation from a PPVT baseline compared to the FSIQ is equivalent to the deviation of the PPVT from the FSIQ added to the deviations of other tests from the FSIQ. As a consequence, a difference of one standard deviation from the FSIQ baseline is increased to a deviation of 1.5 standard deviations from a PPVT baseline (23 points).

10. Because the PPVT requires no verbal expressive skills, it offers a strong baseline for tests that do require expressive skills. This includes the major verbal tests of the WAIS-III (Vocabulary and Comprehension, and to a lesser degree, Similarities and Information) as well as tests of Verbal fluency and language skills described in this volume. Differences between PPVT scores and verbal expressive deficits point toward oral-expressive difficulties most often seen in anterior left hemisphere injuries.

11. The PPVT also offers a strong comparison to tests such as the Boston Naming Test which requires subjects to name specific objects. As no naming is done on the PPVT, good performance on the PPVT combined with poor performance on the Boston Naming Test (or similar exam) suggests a specific naming problem rather than a visual identification problem or intellectual deficit. Poor performance on both tests may indicate visual or intellectual problems rather than naming problems per se. In such cases, comparison to Vocabulary and Similarities on the WAIS-III is useful as these tests have a verbal expressive component but no visual component. If these are performed well, then the problems are more likely visual rather than language based.

12. In cases where the PPVT deficit is believed to be due to visual limitations, comparison to visual–spatial tests are useful. Picture Completion requires more attention to visual details than the PPVT, so good performance on Picture Completion rules out a visual deficit for the PPVT. Similarly, good performance on Picture Arrangement also generally rules out the visual component of the PPVT as the source of error.

13. In some cases, error on the PPVT is due to perseveration or impulsivity. In such cases, the client will pick the same picture location repeatedly, leading to a poor score. This can be ruled out by looking at the pattern of answers that is generated. This specific deficit may co-exist with good performances on naming tests (such as the Boston) and on Picture Completion (less often on Picture Arrangement). It may be accompanied by a similar performance on other multiple choice tests (such as the Peabody Individual Achievement Test) but not on more open answer tests (such as the Wide Range Achievement Test) and poor performance on frontal lobe tests like the Category Test, Wisconsin Card Sort Test, and Stroop Color and Word Test.

References for Peabody Picture Vocabulary Test-Revised (PPVT-R)

Altepeter, T. S., & Johnson, K. A. (1989). Use of the PPVT-R for intellectual screening with adults: A caution. *Journal of Psychoeducational Assessment, 7*, 39–45.

Craig, R. J., & Olson, R. E. (1991). Relationship between Wechsler scales and Peabody Picture Vocabulary Test-Revised scores among disability applicants. *Journal of Clinical Psychology, 47*(3), 420–429.

Dunn, L. M., & Dunn, L. M. (1981). *Peabody Picture Vocabulary Test-Revised: Manual for Forms L and M*. Circle Pines, MN: American Guidance Service.

Kaufman, A. S. (1990). *Assessing adult and adolescent intelligence*. Boston: Allyn and Bacon.

Ingram, F., Caroselli, J., Robinson, H., Hetzel, R. D., Reed, K., & Masel, B. E. (1998). The PPVT-R: Validity as a quick screen of intelligence in a postacute rehabilitation setting for brain-injured adults. *Journal of Clinical Psychology, 54*(7), 877–884.

Lamport-Hughes, N. (1995). Learning potential and other predictors of rehabilitation. *Journal of Cognitive Rehabilitation, 13*(4) 16–21.

Morgan, A. W., Sullivan, S. A., Darden, C., & Gregg, N. (1997). Measuring the intelligence of college students with learning disabilities: A comparison of results obtained on the WAIS-R and the KAIT. *Journal of Learning Disabilities, 30*(5), 560–565.

SECTION II: VISUAL–SPATIAL TESTS

BLOCK DESIGN SUBTEST (WAIS-III)

The Block Design subtest is one of the six performance subtests on the WAIS-III. It assesses the ability to perceive and analyze designs by breaking down the whole into its parts. It involves visual–constructive skills and nonverbal reasoning. In its original form, it was conceived as a basic abstract measure that would be sensitive to many forms of brain dysfunction.

Interpretation

1. The client's problem-solving approach should be observed. Excessive fumbling of the blocks or failure to check the finished product could suggest anxiety. Failure to check could also suggest impulsivity, reflecting frontal or subcortical disorders.

2. If the examinee twists his or her body to get a better view, or if space is left between the blocks in the design, it could suggest visual–perceptual problems which would indicate posterior lesions. Such clients may use trial-and-error approaches rather than analyzing the design.

3. When basic designs are severely distorted so as to be unrecognizable, perhaps losing even the 2 × 2 or 3 × 3 structure of the squares, this is generally indicative of a right posterior problem. Unilateral neglect may also be present in these cases.

4. Slowness in performance combined with slow motor skills may simply indicate that the motor demand of the task is too high. This is most often seen in motor lesions of the dominant hemisphere, as well as with some subcortical and peripheral motor problems. In cases where the problem appears limited to motor skills, additional time may be allowed to see if the client can generate the correct answer (although performance after time limits is never scored on any of the WAIS-III subtests).

5. If poor right hemisphere based spatial skills are present, the Block Design score should be depressed, as well as the Matrices subtest of the WAIS-III and other visual–motor tests, such as the Bender. Poor scores on Block Design only when drawing tests are intact may reflect problems with the abstract nature of the designs versus the more concrete drawing tests.

6. Block Design can be performed at an average level using verbal mediation strategies. It appears more susceptible to these strategies than are the complex drawing tests. Thus, performance on Block Design, especially in intelligent clients with right posterior injuries, may be better than on these other construction tasks. This pattern of using verbal mediation generally includes good Block Design performance, good Matrices Performance, and good reproduction of simple drawings but poor reproduction of complex drawings (such as the Rey) and poor performance on measures of facial memory and other tasks that are not easily encodable. This is also accompanied by strong performance on verbal tests in general.

7. Slowness or errors on the initial designs suggest serious cognitive impairment, mental retardation, an inability to understand instructions, or severely compromised motor skills. Time should be taken as allowed in the manual to make certain that the client understands the task. Occasionally, a client will make the task nearly impossible by believing that he or she must match the sides as well as the top of the blocks.

8. Scores tend to be decreased in the presence of any kind of brain injury, so decreased performance cannot immediately be related to one area of the brain unless qualitative aspects are assessed, as suggested previously. In general, however, performance is most affected when it is associated with lateralized lesions involving the posterior parietal areas and areas on the right side. This performance is generally marked not only by slowness but also by distortion and confusion over the spatial pattern of the blocks.

9. In clients with left parietal damage, test-taking behavior is dominated by confusion, simplification, and concreteness when handling the designs. These clients are likely to exhibit an orderly approach to problem-solving tasks, and they usually work from left to right. The general shape of the design square is usually preserved. Clients will often have the most difficulty placing the last block in place (as it tends to be on the right side). Time constraints often contribute to lower scores. Errors usually involve rotation of one or two blocks rather than gross distortions seen in right parietal injuries.

10. Clients with right hemisphere damage tend to work from the right to the left side of the design. These clients tend to be disoriented, distort the designs, have difficulty preserving the square shape of the designs, and exhibit misperceptions.

11. In clients with severe frontal lobe damage, carelessness, concreteness, and a lack of logical analysis predominates. These individuals will often approach the design in a random manner and may often fail to correct their answers. Concreteness may be manifested by the problem-solving approach the client takes. He or she may attempt to replicate the design by looking at the top as well as the sides. Designs may be finished in an impulsive manner. Milder frontal injuries will likely not affect performance at all, especially when the predominant damage is on the left side.

12. Block Design may be affected early on by dementia, especially of the Alzheimer's type. Such clients may be impulsive and have difficulty following the instructions. In addition, they may ignore important aspects of the blocks (such as the angle of the line dividing red from white on the mixed squares) or their attempts may be haphazard.

13. Inappropriate rotation (more than 30 degrees) of the designs (except for

the last two) may indicate posterior right hemisphere problems.

14. Good performance on Block Design but poor performance on the WAIS-III Matrices will often indicate problems with organizing the internal abstract designs of the figures, especially in later designs when there are no clear demarcations of where blocks begin and end. This may suggest a mild right hemisphere disorder, which is partially compensated. It may also reflect the greater organizational demands of the Matrices' items which require more active analysis and organization of the material presented than does Block Design.

15. Poor performance on Block Design but good performance on WAIS-III Matrices may reflect two possibilities. First, Matrices (as well as Raven's Matrices) is not timed. Thus, clients who have accurate but slow performance will be penalized on Block Design but not on Matrices or many of the drawing tasks. This can reflect brain injury but may also reflect compulsive attention to detail. Such an impairment will be reflected in poor Coding scores, but not necessarily poor Picture Arrangement scores (which is timed but the time limits are very generous). Second, Block Design is, as noted earlier, a more abstract spatial task. The clients may not be able to see the patterns in Block Design necessary to solve the designs within the time limit. Interestingly, such clients will improve rapidly if shown how to analyze the patterns in an organized manner.

16. Poor performance on drawing tests such as the Bender or Clock Drawing Test, with good performance on Block Design, generally reflects problems with fine motor control. While Block Design is a timed motor task, it requires much less fine coordination than more complex drawing or construction tasks. Coding will also be slow in these cases, but Symbol Search performance will be normal. Tests of simple motor speed such as Finger Tapping may be intact in some cases, although more complex tasks such as the Grooved Pegboard and the Tactual Performance Test will show slowness.

17. Good performance on the Tactual Performance Test (TPT) combined with poor performance on Block Design suggests intact spatial skills but impaired visual or visual motor skills. Good performance on the TPT is inconsistent with either impaired spatial or motor skills. In such cases, poor performance may also be seen on complex drawing tasks and tests requiring good visual analysis such as Matrices and Picture Arrangement. The dissociation between the TPT and these visual tests is an important marker that the performance tests may not be interpreted in traditional ways.

18. Poor performance on Block Design along with poor motor performance on basic tasks such as Finger Tapping suggests motor impairment as a

major cause of the poor performance. In such cases, allowing additional time will show that the client can complete the figures. Performance will also be slow on all timed visual–motor tasks although scores will vary depending on how much time is used as a scoring variable. In cases where motor performance is severely compromised, Block Design is likely invalid and should not be interpreted.

19. Poor Block Design performance combined with poor Line Orientation suggests an impairment of spatial skills. In such a case, all tests dependent on spatial skills that are not easily mediated by alternative verbal strategies will show impairment.

20. Inability to understand instructions secondary to language impairment can have a profound effect on performance, as the test relies on extensive verbal instructions. Repetition of the demonstration items beyond the single repetition in the manual and rephrasing of instructions may allow the client to comprehend the task. In cases where this fails, interpretation of the test is limited neuropsychologically.

21. Poor performance on Block Design combined with good performance on drawing tests, such as the Bender, indicates problems with the abstract nature of the designs.

22. Poor performance on the Clock Drawing Test combined with good performance on Block Design points to problems in visual–motor or motor skills rather than deficits in visual–spatial skills although organizational skills may be impaired as well. When visual–motor skills are implicated, deficits will be evident on the Bender and Benton Visual Retention Test. Normal performance would be expected on Matrix tasks and other nonmotor visual tasks.

23. Poor performance on the VFDT, despite good performance on Block Design, may reflect problems with perseveration. These would usually show up on TPT as well. Thus, if VFDT and TPT are impaired while Block Design, BVRT, and the Bender are intact, the possibility of frontal/executive disorders should be considered. This would typically be reflected in poor performance on the Raven's or WAIS-III Matrices, as well as frontal lobe tests such as Category, WCST, or Part B of the Trail Making Test.

24. Poor performance on Block Design despite good performance on the VFDT suggests that basic visual processes are intact, pointing to either the timed aspect of Block Design or the more analytic spatial component as the cause of the deficit. If the problem is time alone, then untimed tests (Matrices, Raven's, Bender, BVRT) should be performed adequately. If spatial problems are present, we would expect problems on these untimed tests as well.

25. Performance of Picture Arrangement should be compared directly to

the average scaled score performance of the purer visual–spatial tests (Block Design, Matrices, Picture Completion). If Picture Arrangement is more than 3 points below these scores, a defect in verbal or executive/sequencing skill should be considered.

26. When the Hooper is normal, but Block Design or other construction tasks show spatial problems, visual–motor problems should be considered.

27. When the Hooper is abnormal along with Block Design, a general spatial deficit may be present.

References for Block Design Subtest (WAIS-III)

Boone, D. E. (1998). Specificity of the WAIS-R subtests with psychiatric inpatients. *Assessment, 5,* 123–126.

Campbell, J. M., & McCord, D. M. (1996). The WAIS-R comprehension and picture arrangement subtests as measures of social intelligence: Testing traditional interpretations. *Journal of Psychoeducational Assessment, 14,* 240–249.

Golden, C. J., Zillmer, E., & Spiers, M. (1992). *Neuropsychological assessment and intervention.* Springfield, IL: Charles C Thomas.

Hawkins, K. A. (1998). Indicators of brain dysfunction derived from graphic representations of the WAIS-III/WMS-III Technical Manual clinical samples data: A preliminary approach to clinical utility. *Clinical Neuropsychologist, 12*(4), 535–555.

Kramer, J. H. (1990). Guidelines for interpreting the WAIS-R subtest scores. *Psychological Assessment, 2,* 202–205.

Lobello, S. G., Thompson, A. P., & Evani, V. (1998). Supplementary WAIS-III tables for determining subtest strengths and weaknesses. *Journal of Psychoeducational Assessment, 16*(3), 196–200.

Matarazzo, J. D. (1972). *Wechsler's measurement and appraisal of adult intelligence* (5th ed.). New York: Oxford University Press.

Ryan, J. J., Lopez, S. J., & Werth, T. R. (1998). Administration time estimates for WAIS-III subtests, scales, and short forms in a clinical sample. *Journal of Psychoeducational Assessment, 16*(4), 315–323.

Sprandel, H. Z. (1995). *The psychoeducational use and interpretation of the Wechsler Adult Intelligence Scale-Revised* (2nd ed.). Springfield, IL: Charles C Thomas.

Wechsler, D. (1981). *WAIS-R manual.* New York: The Psychological Corporation.

Wechsler, D. (1986). *WAIS-R administration and scoring manual.* San Antonio, TX: The Psychological Corporation.

Wechsler, D. (1997). *WAIS-III administration and scoring manual.* San Antonio, TX: The Psychological Corporation.

BENDER-VISUAL MOTOR GESTALT TEST (BENDER)

The Bender is a relatively simple test: it does not necessitate time limits, memory components, or precise, restrictive instructions that might increase a client's anxiety. For many clients, this test, which was originally created to test the development of gestalt function in children, is a safe one with which to begin owing to its apparent simplicity. It does not overwhelm the client as may a Rey figure or similar, very complex and dense designs. Although the use of the Bender for screening for brain injury in general has been discredited, it remains a good and quick test of relatively complex visual–motor–constructive skills. It is also a purer test of these functions, as it does not demand the complex organizational skills as required by other tests.

Interpretation

1. The Bender is not sensitive enough to detect all cerebral lesions, for example, those affecting the left frontal lobe. Nevertheless, the test may prove helpful in honing in on a parietal impairment, particularly on the right (Crawford et al., 1992). Clients with left parietal impairment (especially after a destructive lesion such as a stroke) may also show impairment on the test. Good performance on the Bender would be strong evidence against a parietal insult, although it alone cannot completely rule out such a possibility.

2. Individuals with Alzheimer's disease (AD) tend to produce excessive errors on the Bender, so a poor performance on the test would support a suspicion of AD. Because of the posterior focus of AD, there are more likely to be deficits arising from early AD than from more frontal dementias, such as Pick's disease.

3. Although test protocol does not necessitate time keeping, paying attention to the haste or delay with which the client copies the figures can help to discern etiology. Persons who spend an inordinate amount of time replicating the figures may be experiencing some cognitive slowing down. Alternatively, those who hurry through their copying may have frontal lobe impulsiveness.

4. Research suggests that the Bender is a better discriminator of organicity in individuals with lower IQs. Higher intelligence appears to render the test less effective in detecting brain damage, so individuals with IQ scores above 110 and with known brain lesions tend to be identified as normal. Conversely, low intelligence scores lead to a relatively high number of false-positive diagnoses, such that individuals with IQs below 79 and with no cerebral insult may execute sufficient errors to meet the criteria for having an organic disorder.

5. While education itself is not necessary for Bender performance, there is a strong correlation between education and intelligence, which does, in turn, influence performance on the test.

6. A comparison with visual–motor tests that require no motor component (such as Line Orientation) is necessary to separate spatial skills from visual–motor and motor skills. In general, clients with true spatial disabilities will produce very distorted versions of the items, while

those with only motor disorders will simply be slow in reproduction. Qualitative observation of how the client performs can give valuable information in this regard. However, in some cases, basic spatial tasks, such as Line Orientation, will be performed poorly, although the Bender is performed well. In such cases, a focal lesion that is generally compensated for is suggested which allows the client to perform the more complex Bender despite the lesion.

7. When paralysis or substantial motor impairment is evident (as seen on tests such as Finger Tapping), interpretation must be limited to the motor aspects of the performance. Performance with the nondominant hand cannot be interpreted in terms of spatial skills.

8. Aphasia has only a minor effect on the Bender, as long as the client understands the instructions. In any case in which the client does not seem to understand, we strongly suggest readministration after the instructions are repeated, along with demonstrations, if necessary. Demonstrations may even use the actual items, as such exposure does not seem to alter performance. Such a procedure allows the examiner to test visual–motor skills while minimizing the role of verbal skills that can contaminate many of the visual–motor tests. However, this practice is ineffective if the language impairment is accompanied by dominant hand motor impairment.

9. Inability to reproduce the figures at all, in the absence of paralysis, suggests dementia, which can be global or may reflect inertia and apathy, as seen in clients with bilateral frontal involvement.

10. Inability to reproduce or recognize the left side of figures or write on the left side of the page may indicate a neglect syndrome that is most characteristic of right posterior lesions.

11. Poor performance on the Bender with good performance on Block Design and Matrices generally reflects problems with fine motor control. While Block Design is a timed motor task, it requires much less fine coordination than the Bender. Coding will also be slow in these cases, but Symbol Search performance will be normal. Tests of simple motor speed such as Finger Tapping may be intact in some cases, although more complex tasks such as the Grooved Pegboard and the Tactual Performance Test will show slowness. In some cases, however, this pattern will point to a problem with abstract items, which may be supported by poor performance on frontal lobe procedures.

12. Good performance on the Bender but poor performance on the copying phase of complex drawing tests, such as the Rey Figure, may indicate intact visual–motor skills but poor organizational skills and mild impairment of complex spatial skills. This pattern may suggest more anterior rather than posterior lesions.

13. Good performance on the Bender accompanied by poor motor perfor-

mance on tasks such as Finger Tapping or Purdue Pegboard indicates intact visual–motor skills and intact basic visual–spatial skills but impairment of motor speed. As the Bender is untimed, it is not affected by lesions or conditions that slow motor speed but do not affect basic coordination. These may include mild brain injuries as well as conditions such as depression, fatigue, or the effects of medication.

14. All drawings should be inspected for the presence of motor tremors.

15. If the Bender is performed well, but Clock Drawing is not, the deficit is likely to be in the planning and organization of the clock rather than in basic visual–motor skills.

16. Poor performance on the Bender combined with a good Clock Drawing is a very unusual finding. This profile may suggest problems with motivation or with understanding the basic task on the Bender.

17. Good performance on the Bender with poor performance on the Benton Visual Retention Test (BVRT) copy phase may indicate problems dealing with details or the possible presence of neglect. In general, these tasks are of similar difficulty in terms of the motor skills required. Poor performance on the memory phase alone, however, points to memory and organizational problems rather than visual–motor problems.

18. Poor performance on the Bender along with good performance on the BVRT copy phase reflects inconsistent performance. This is unusual and may reflect fluctuations in motivation or in comprehension of task demands.

19. Poor performance on the Bender, despite good performance on the VFDT, suggests that basic visual processes are intact, pointing to the motor aspect of the Bender as the cause of the deficit. If the problem is motor, then nonmotor tests (Matrices, Raven's) should be performed adequately while other construction tests (BVRT, Block Design) would show impairment.

20. Good performance on the Bender despite poor performance on the VFDT suggests either the presence of neglect or problems with the multiple-choice format of the VFDT. If neglect is present, an analysis of the client's errors should show omission of the peripheral figures rather than misidentification of the major figures. On the Bender, the client will tend to use only one side of the drawing page, rarely crossing the midline. In addition, similar deficits will be seen on the Raven's or WAIS-III Matrices and on the BVRT. If the multiple-choice format is responsible, these errors are generally perseverative or impulsive and would be seen on Raven's or the WAIS-III Matrices. Such errors usually point to deficits in frontal/executive skills.

21. Motor skills play only a minor role in Picture Arrangement, so high scores on Picture Arrangement, Matrices, and Picture Completion rela-

tive to the Bender, Digit Symbol, and Block Design should suggest analysis of more basic motor measures, including loss of basic motor skills in the dominant hand as measured by Finger Tapping or Purdue Pegboard. Impairment on other Visual–Motor tasks such as the Benton and the Tactual Performance Test should also be examined.

22. When the Hooper is normal, but the Bender, Block Design, or other construction tasks show spatial problems, visual–motor problems should be considered.

23. When the Hooper is abnormal, along with Bender, Block Design, and VFDT, a general spatial deficit may be present.

References for Bender-Visual Motor Gestalt Test (Bender)

Canter, A. (1996). The Bender-Gestalt test. In C. Newmark (Ed.), *Major psychological assessment instruments* (pp. 400–430). Needham Heights, MA: Allyn & Bacon.

Crawford, J. R., Parker, D. M., & McKinlay, W. (1992). *A handbook of neuropsychological assessment.* East Sussex, UK: Lawrence Erlbaum Associates.

Dunn, L. M., & Dunn, L. M. (1981). *Peabody Picture Vocabulary Test-Revised: Manual for Forms L and M.* Circle Pines, MN: American Guidance Service.

Grant, I., & Adams, K. M. (Eds.) (1986). *Neuropsychological assessment of neuropsychiatric disorders.* New York: Oxford University Press.

Hain, J. D. (1963). Scoring system for the Bender Gestalt test (Project No. 7785). Washington, D. C.: American Documentation Institute.

Hain, J. D. (1964). The Bender-Gestalt test: A scoring method for identifying brain damage. *Journal of Consulting Psychology, 28,* 34–40.

Hellkamp, D. T., & Hogan, M. E. (1985). Differentiation of organics from functional psychiatric patients across various IQ ranges using the Bender-Gestalt and Hutt Scoring System. *Journal of Clinical Psychology, 41*(2), 259–264.

Lezak, M. (1995). *Neuropsychological assessment* (3rd ed.). New York: Oxford University Press.

Walsh, W. B., & Betz, N. E. (1995). Projective and behavioral personality assessment. In *Tests and assessment* (3rd ed.). Englewood Cliffs, NJ: Prentice-Hall.

RAVEN'S MATRICES

In 1938, Raven introduced the initial series of the Standard Progressive Matrices (SPM). Designed as a measure of Spearman's "g," the main goal of this paper-and-pencil test was to provide reliable and valid information regarding nonverbal general reasoning capacities of persons of all ages in a wide array of settings. The original series was followed in 1947 by the Colored Progressive Matrices (CPM) and the Advanced Progressive Matrices (APM), extending the lower and upper range of the scale. Since then, the Raven Matrices have undergone several standardizations and received widespread use internationally as both individual and group tests in clinical, educational, and research settings.

Interpretation

1. Many alternate norm sets exist for this test, yet none clearly dominates. It is very important that the characteristics of the norm set employed be considered when making comparisons to other tests. Caution must also be taken in interpreting normative scores (other than raw scores) unless the basis of the normative sample is known.

2. The Raven's is not a measure of the presence or absence of brain injury (as it has been used in some settings) but rather a measure of specific aspects of visual–spatial functioning and the identification of logical patterns and progressions. It is often used as a general measure of intellectual functioning and can serve as a baseline for comparison of other tests. However, it is sensitive to brain injuries and cannot be considered a measure of premorbid intelligence in clients with visual–spatial impairment. It can be used as a premorbid estimate in cases of verbal loss if the client fully understands the instructions. However, the correlation with verbal intelligence, while significant, would require differences of 25 standard score points from this estimate before one could reliably conclude that deterioration in verbal skills had occurred.

3. The new WAIS-III includes a Raven's-like measure called Matrices. Comparison of performances on both tests can yield useful information about the consistency of a client's performance. However, the scoring systems and underlying normative groups for these tests differ considerably. Research as yet is inadequate to precisely define the relationships between these tests.

4. Performance on the Raven's can be compared against performance on tests that require both visual–spatial and motor skills (such as Block Design and drawing tests). However, it is recommended that these comparisons be better made with the WAIS-III Matrices subtest because of its better normative sample.

5. Better performance on the Raven's than on visual–motor tests such as Block Design or the Bender suggests good spatial analysis skills but poor visual–motor skills. In such cases, measures of purer motor skills (such as Finger Tapping) should be administered as well. If the motor measures are found to be intact, then the problem may be in visual–motor coordination. If the motor measures are poor, then no conclusion can be reached about visual–motor abilities. The attainment of a good Raven's score suggests that right posterior areas of the brain are performing well.

6. Poor performance on the Raven's, combined with good performance on drawing and other visual–motor tests, suggests that it is the pattern analysis and logical progression analyses rather than spatial skills that

are impaired. These are associated more with frontal injuries (on either side of the brain).

7. Poor performance on the Raven's and other tests of visual skills point to a right posterior lesion. This is especially true in the presence of neglect and poor construction skills and in the absence of dominant side motor problems.

8. In cases of unilateral neglect, clients will fail to respond to the alternatives on the left side of the page and thus make many errors when the answer is on the left. They may also neglect the left side of the stimulus field itself, creating similar errors. When neglect is suspected, asking the client to describe what he or she sees is often useful.

9. Frontal patients may perseverate, usually selecting the answer in the same position and ignoring alternatives. Item response patterns should be carefully reviewed in cases where this is a possibility.

10. In cases of clients with dominant hemisphere lesions, the Raven's may yield very different scores from tests that require motor coordination or speed. Along with other "motor free" and untimed visual–spatial tasks, a better estimate of true visual–spatial skills can be derived by combining results from such tasks that are in a test battery.

11. Visual attention and visual neglect issues should always be ruled out in cases of poor Raven's performance. These deficits will severely affect performance even though spatial skills may be intact. In some cases, this will be seen by good performance on the Tactual Performance Test which will effectively rule out spatial deficits.

12. Good Raven's performance in the presence of language deficits points to unilateral lesions of the left hemisphere when there is a history of previous normal verbal performance. In other cases, the differences may reflect poor education and language training (including poor mastery of English) rather than brain injury. In such cases, the Raven's may reflect intellectual potential more effectively than the verbal measures.

13. Poor Raven's performance in the absence of aphasia is less specific and may reflect anterior damage of either hemisphere or posterior damage of the right hemisphere. When combined with generally poor Block Design and drawing test performance, these deficits likely reflect right posterior lesions. However, when only Raven's Matrices is impaired, this most likely reflects an anterior lesion or even a preexisting intellectual deficit.

14. Poor Raven's performance with aphasia may reflect a left hemisphere lesion or a more generalized disorder but does not always imply the involvement of the right hemisphere.

15. Good performance on Block Design but poor performance on the Raven's will often indicate problems with organizing the internal ab-

stract designs of the figures, especially in later designs when there are no clear demarcations of where blocks begin and end. This may suggest a mild right hemisphere disorder which is partially compensated. It may also reflect the greater organizational demands of the Raven's items which require more active analysis and organization of the material presented than does Block Design.

16. Poor performance on Block Design but good performance on Raven's Matrices may reflect two possibilities. First, Raven's Matrices is not timed. Thus, clients who have accurate but slow performance will be penalized on Block Design but not on Matrices or many of the drawing tasks. This can reflect brain injury but may also reflect compulsive attention to detail. Such an impairment will be reflected in poor Coding scores, but not necessarily poor Picture Arrangement scores (which is timed but the time limits are very generous). Second, Block Design is, as noted earlier, a more abstract spatial task (although a less complex organizational task). The clients may not be able to see the patterns in Block Design necessary to solve the designs within the time limit. Interestingly, such clients will improve rapidly if shown how to analyze the patterns in an organized manner.

17. Good performance on the Tactual Performance Test (TPT) combined with poor performance on Raven's Matrices and Block Design suggests intact spatial skills but impaired visual or visual–motor skills. Good performance on the TPT is inconsistent with either impaired spatial or motor skills. In such cases, poor performance may also be seen on complex drawing tasks. The dissociation between the TPT and these visual tests is an important marker that the performance tests may not be interpreted in traditional ways.

18. Good performance on Raven's Matrices combined with poor performance on drawing tests (Bender, BVRT, Clock Drawing) generally reflects problems with fine motor control. Coding will also be slow in these cases, but Symbol Search performance will be normal. Tests of simple motor speed such as Finger Tapping may be intact in some cases, although more complex tasks such as the Grooved Pegboard and the Tactual Performance Test will show slowness. In some cases, however, this pattern will point to a problem with abstractive items, which can also be seen in poor performance on frontal lobe measures.

19. Good performance on Raven's Matrices combined with poor performance on the Test of Line Orientation points to basic analysis problems with angles and spatial skills that is compensated for on more complex visual–spatial skills where foundational spatial skills are not as important. In such cases, there may be a highly focal lesion whose general impact is minimal. This performance should be compared to drawing tasks in which the inability to distinguish angles may be more obvious.

20. Poor performance on Raven's Matrices combined with good performance on Line Orientation suggests an impairment in the more complex organizational and logical skills demanded by the Raven's rather than the more basic spatial skills measured by Line Orientation.

21. In cases of unilateral neglect, clear deficits are usually visible on the Raven's and Benton Visual Retention Test. Symptoms may show up on any of the visual tests but most of the other tests can be manipulated by the subject more easily to avoid these deficits. In severe cases, however, the neglect will show up across the visual tests and many of the reading tests as well.

22. Problems with the multiple-choice format of the Raven's will also be clear on the VFDT and Line Orientation. In such cases, the errors are generally impulsive or perseverative reflecting frontal/executive deficits. These deficits should be seen on other frontal lobe tests as well (Category, WCST, Stroop, Trail Making Test Part B).

23. Good Performance on the VFDT, Line Orientation, and Raven's usually indicates intact visual analysis and spatial skills as well as the absence of neglect. In such cases, errors on the motor based visual tests likely arise from timing or visual–motor deficits.

References for Raven's Matrices

Alderton, D. L., & Larson, G. E. (1990). Dimensionality of Raven's Advanced Progressive Matrices items. *Educational and Psychological Measurement, 50*(4), 887–890.

Arthur, W., & Woehr, D. J. (1993). A confirmatory factor analytic study examining the dimensionality of the Raven's Advanced Progressive Matrices. *Educational and Psychological Measurement, 53*(2), 471–478.

Backhoff-Escuden, E. (1996). Prueba de Matrices Progresivas de Raven: Normas de Universitarios Mexicanos (Raven's Standard Progressive Matrices: Mexican university students' norms). *Revista Mexicana de Psicologia, 13*(1), 21–28.

Barnabas, J. P., Kapur, M., & Rao, S. (1995). Norm development and reliability of the Coloured Progressive Matrices test. *Journal of Personality and Clinical Studies, 11*(2), 17–22.

Brooks, D. N., & Aughton, M. E. (1979). Cognitive recovery during the first year after severe blunt brain injury. *International Rehabilitation Medicine, 1*, 166–172.

Caplan, B. (1988). Nonstandard neuropsychological assessment: An illustration. *Neuropsychology, 2*, 13–17.

Campbell, D. C., & Oxbury, J. M. (1976). Recovery from unilateral visuospatial neglect. *Cortex, 12*, 303–312.

Christensen, A. L. (1979). *Lurias neuropsychological investigation* (2nd ed.). Copenhagen: Munsgard.

Cocchi, R., & Chiavarini, M. (1997). Raven's colored matrices in alcoholics before and after detoxification. *Italian Journal of Intellective Impairment, 8*(2), 197–201.

Cocchi, R., & Chiavarini, M. (1997). Raven's colored matrices in alcoholics before and after detoxification: A research on 225 subjects. *Italian Journal of Intellective Impairment, 10*(2), 157–160, 213–217.

Costa, L. D., Vaughan, H. G., Jr., Horwitz, M., & Ritter, W. (1969). Patterns of behavioral deficit with visual spatial neglect. *Cortex, 5*, 242–263.

Court, J. H. (1991). Asian applications of Raven's progressive matrices. *Psychologia: An International Journal of Psychology, 34*(2), 75–85.

Drebing, C. E., Takushi, R. Y., Tanzy, K. S., & Murdock, G. A. (1990). Reexamination of CPM performance and neglect in lateralized brain injury. *Cortex, 26*(4), 661–664.

Dubois, B., Pillon, B., & Legault, F. (1988). Slowing of cognitive processing in supranuclear palsy. *Archives of Neuropsychology, 45*, 1194–1199.

Gainotti, G., D'Erme, P., Villa, G., & Caltagirone, C. (1986). Focal brain lesions and intelligence: A study with a new version of Raven's colored matrices. *Journal of Clinical and Experimental Neuropsychology, 1*, 37–50.

Haxby, J. V., Raffaele, K., & Gillette, J. (1992). Individual trajectories of cognitive decline in patients with dementia of the Alzheimer type. *Journal of Clinical and Experimental Neuropsychology, 14*, 575–592.

Hutchinson, L. J., Amler, R. W., Lybarger, J. A., & Chappell, W. (1992). *Neurobehavioral test batteries for use in environmental health field studies.* Atlanta, GA: Agency for Toxic Substances and Disease Registry. Public Health Services.

Lezak, M. D. (1995). *Neuropsychological Assessment* (3rd ed.). New York: Oxford University Press.

Llabre, M. M. (1984). Standard progressive matrices. In D. J. Keyser & R. C. Sweetland (Eds.), *Test critiques*, Vol. I. Kansas City, MO: Test Corporation of America.

Miceli, G., Caltagirone, C., & Gainotti, G. (1977). Gangliosides in the treatment of mental deterioration: A double blind comparison with placebo. *Journal of Clinical Neuropsychology, 3*, 53–63.

Morris, G. L., & Alcorn, M. B. (1995). Raven's progressive matrices and inspection time: P200 slope correlates. *Personality and Individual Differences, 18*, 81–87.

Nakagawa, A. (1996). Attentional balance and intelligence. *Intelligence, 22*(3), 277–290.

Owen, K. (1992). The suitability of Raven's standard progressive matrices for various groups in South Africa. *Personality and Individual Differences, 13*(2), 149–152.

Pfeffer, R. I., Kurosaki, T. T., & Chance, J. M. (1984). Use of the Mental Function Index in older adults: Reliability, validity, and measurement of change over time. *American Journal of Epidemiology, 114*, 515–527.

Pruneti, C., Fenu, A., Freschi, G., & Rota, S. (1996). Aggiornamento della standardizzazione italiana del test delle Matrici Progressive Colorate di Raven. *Bollettino di Psicologia Applicata, 217*, 51–57.

Raven, J. C., Court, J. H., & Raven, J. (1983). *Manual for Raven's progressive matrices and vocabulary scales.* London: H. K. Lewis.

Richards, M., Cote, L. J., & Stern, Y. (1993). Executive function in Parkinson's disease: Set-shifting or set-maintenance? *Journal of Clinical and Experimental Neuropsychology, 15*, 266–279.

Soukup, V. M., Harrel, E. H., & Clark, T. (1994). Right hemispace presentation and left cueing on Raven's coloured progressive matrices among right-brain damaged neglect patients. *Brain Injury, 8*(5), 449–455.

Zhang, H. C., & Wang, X. P. (1989). Standardization research on Raven's standard progressive matrices in China. *Acta Psychologica Sinica, 21*(2), 113–121.

Wogar, M. A., vanderBroek, M. D., Bradshaw, C. M., & Szabadi, E. (1997). A new performance-curve method for the detection of simulated cognitive impairment. *British Journal of Clinical Psychology, 37*(3), 327–339.

TEST OF LINE ORIENTATION

The Test of Line Orientation is a simple test of basic spatial skills, which requires the client to match a line drawn at an angle against a standard sample of lines. This is an excellent test of basic visual–spatial skills, as it does not require motor ability or higher level problem-solving skills. It is used most often as a test of right hemisphere function, but performance can be affected by other injuries as well.

Interpretation

1. Using the appropriate norms, low scores (at least one standard deviation below normal) generally indicate problems in spatial analysis at a basic level. These are seen most often in posterior right hemisphere disorders but may be seen in left hemisphere aphasics because of a disruption in spatial analysis or an inability to understand or retain the instructions. In general, scores in the 15–18 range are considered borderline and scores below 15 are considered abnormal.

2. Comparison with basic spatial tasks, such as Block Design which has a motor component as well, is important. This test is considered a purer measure of basic spatial skills than the other tests which have a motor component. However, the more complex items of Block Design and the more complex drawings involve problem-solving and strategic skills not reflected in this test. Good performance on the Test of Line Orientation and poor performance on Block Design may suggest a motor rather than a spatial problem. Better performance on Block Design and poor performance on this test is more problematic, and may suggest difficulty in attention or impulsivity.

3. Impulsive behavior (where choices are made quickly and are incorrect) or perseverative behavior (choosing the same answer repeatedly) may indicate frontal problems in either or both hemispheres.

4. For clients whose understanding of verbal instructions is questionable, the sample items should be reviewed a second or even third time to ensure comprehension of the task. This is a problem in aphasic clients, and therefore the presence of aphasia should be considered in interpretation of the results. Clients with memory problems may need repetition of the instructions if they seem to lose track of what is being asked of them.

5. Poor eyesight can contribute to problems, but it is possible to make enlargements of the stimulus figures for such individuals.

6. Attempts by the client to rotate the material usually indicates general confusion or confusion about the task itself. Rotation should not be allowed. This can also reflect a severe problem in the spatial nature of the task.

7. In cases where confusion about the task is thought to exist, read-ministration of the test at a later time is strongly recommended. The test

has high test–retest reliability, so such scores can be directly compared for consistency.

8. Dementia clients generally show early deterioration on this test; this is especially pertinent in the case of a disorder such as Alzheimer's, which has a strong posterior focus. The test may be used as part of a screening battery since it is an unusual but simple task that challenges the demented client. There will be declines with age on the test, but these declines will not push normal scores into the abnormal range.

9. Good performance on Raven's Matrices combined with poor performance on the Test of Line Orientation points to basic analysis problems with angles and spatial skills which is compensated for on more complex visual–spatial skills where foundational spatial skills are not as important. In such cases, there may be a highly focal lesion whose general impact is minimal. This performance should be compared to drawing tasks where the inability to distinguish angles may be more obvious.

10. Poor performance on Raven's Matrices combined with good performance on Line Orientation suggests an impairment in the more complex organizational and logical skills demanded by the Raven's rather than the more basic spatial skills measured by Line Orientation.

11. Poor Block Design performance combined with poor performance on Line Orientation suggests an impairment of spatial skills. In such a case, all tests dependent on spatial skills that are not easily mediated by alternative verbal strategies will show impairment.

12. A comparison of Line Orientation with drawing tests is necessary to separate spatial skills from visual–motor and motor skills. In general, clients with true spatial disabilities will produce very distorted versions of drawings, while those with only motor disorders will simply be slow in reproduction. However, in some cases basic spatial tasks such as Line Orientation will be performed poorly although the Bender or other drawing tests are performed well. In such cases, a focal lesion that is generally compensated for is suggested which allows the client to perform the more complex test despite the lesion.

13. In cases where Line Orientation is intact but drawing tests are impaired, an analysis of motor skills is necessary. Impairment in basic motor coordination tasks would point to motor or visual–motor deficits rather than impairment in basic visual skills.

14. Problems with the multiple-choice format of Line Orientation will also be clear on the Raven's, VFDT, or WAIS-III Matrices. In such cases, the errors are generally impulsive or perseverative reflecting frontal/ executive deficits. These deficits should be seen on the frontal lobe tests as well (Category, WCST, Stroop, Trail Making Test Part B).

15. Good performance on both VFDT, Line Orientation, and either Raven's or WAIS-III Matrices usually indicates intact visual analysis and spatial skills as well as the absence of neglect. In such case, errors on the motor-based visual tests likely arise from timing or visual–motor deficits.

References for Test of Line Orientation

Benton, A. L., Hamsher, K., deS., Varney, N. R., & Spreen, O. (1983). *Contributions to neuropsychological assessment.* New York: Oxford University Press.

Benton, A. L., Hannay, H. J., & Varney, N. R. (1975). Visual perception of line direction in patients with unilateral brain disease. *Neurology, 25,* 907–910.

Benton, A. L., Varney, N. R., & Hamsher, K., deS. (1978). Visuospatial judgment: A clinical test. *Archives of Neurology, 364*–367.

Berman, S. M., & Noble, E. P. (1995). The D-sub-2 dopamine receptor (DRD2) gene and family stress: Interactive effects on cognitive functions in children. *Behavior Genetics, 27*(1), 33–43.

Desmond, D. W., Glenwick, D. S., Stern, Y., & Tatemichi, T. K. (1994). Sex differences in the representation of visuospatial functions in the human brain. *Rehabilitation Psychology, 39*(1), 3–14.

Doyon, J., Bourgeois, C., & Bedard, P. (1996). Deficits visuo-spatiaux associes avec la maladie de Parkinson. *Internaitonal Journal of Psychology, 31*(5), 161–175.

Eden, G. F., Stein, J. F., Wood, H. M., & Wood, F. B. (1996). Differences in visuospatial judgment in reading-disabled and normal children. *Perceptual and Motor Skills, 82,* 155–177.

Eslinger, P. J., & Benton, A. L. (1983). Visuoperceptual performances in aging and dementia: Clinical and theoretical implications. *Journal of Clinical Neuropsychology, 5,* 213–220.

Franzen, M. D., Robbins, D. E., Douglas, E., & Sawicki, R. F. (1989). *Reliability and validity in neuropsychological assessment.* New York: Plenum Press.

Gur, R. C., Ragland, J. D., Resnick, S. M., & Skolnick, B. E. (1994). Lateralized increases in cerebral blood flow during performance of verbal and spatial tasks: Relationship with performance level. *Brain and Cognition, 24*(2), 244–258.

Hannay, H. J., Falgout, J. C., & Leli, D. A. (1987). Focal right temporo-occipital blood flow changes associated with judgment of line orientation. *Neuropsychologica, 25,* 755–763.

Hovestad, A., & de Jong, G. J. (1987). Spatial disorientation as an early symptom of Parkinson's disease. *Neurology, 37*(3), 485–487.

Lezak, M. D. (1995). *Neuropsychological assessment* (2nd ed.). New York: Oxford University Press.

Luria, A. R. (1980). *Higher cortical functions in man* (2nd ed.). New York: Consultants Bureau.

Meador, K. J., Moore, E. E., Nichols, M. E., & Abney, O. L. (1993). The role of cholinergic systems in visuospatial processing and memory. *Journal of Clinical & Experimental Psychology, 15*(5), 832–842.

Mittenberg, W., Seidenberg, M., O'Leary, D. S., & DiGiulio, D. V. (1989). Changes in cerebral functioning associated with normal aging. *Journal of Clinical and Experimental Neuropsychology, 11,* 918–932.

Riccio, C. A., & Hynd, G. W. (1992). Validity of Benton's judgment of line orientation test. *Journal of Psychoeducational Assessment, 10,* 210–218.

Said, S. M. A., Yeh, T. L., Greenwood, R. S., & Whitt, J. K. (1996). *Neuroreport: An international journal for the rapid communication of research in neuroscience, 7*(2), 1941–1944.

Trahan, D. E. (1998). Judgment of Line Orientation in patients with unilateral cerebrovascular lesions. *Assessment, 5*(3), 227–235.

Vanderploeg, R. D., Lalone, L. V., Greblo, P., & Schink, J. A. (1997). Odd-even short forms of the judgment of line orientation test. *Applied Neuropsychology, 4*(4), 244–246.

Woodard, J. L., Benedict, R. H. B., Roberts, V. J., Goldstein, F. C., Kinner, K. M., Capruso, D. X., &

Clark, A. (1996). Short-form alternatives to the judgment of line orientation test. *Journal of Clinical & Experimental Neuropsychology, 18*(6), 898–904.

Woodard, J. L., Benedict, R. H. B., Salthouse, T. A., Toth, J. P., Zgaljardic, D. J., & Hancock, H. E. (1998). Normative data for equivalent, parallel forms of the judgment of line orientation test. *Journal of Clinical and Experimental Neuropsychology, 20*(4), 457–462.

York, C.D., & Cermak, S. A. (1995). Visual perceptual and praxis in adults after stroke. *American Journal of Occupational Therapy, 49*(6), 543–549.

TACTUAL PERFORMANCE TEST (TPT)

The TPT is an elegant and extremely useful test first introduced in the Halstead–Reitan Neuropsychological Battery. The test is sensitive to a wide range of brain lesions, as well as many useful signs helpful in the localization of the lesion. While its biggest drawback is an extensive administration time and bulky equipment, its advantages generally outweigh this disadvantage.

The TPT consists of a standard Sequin–Goodard Form Board with spaces for 10 large and simple geometric shapes. Each shape fits into the corresponding hole on the form board. The board is presented at a 45-degree angle by setting it on a hollow pyramidal structure that holds the geometric shapes when they are not in use. The test is administered three times, once using the dominant hand, the nondominant hand, and then both hands. The most basic score is the time to complete each trial of the test. These three scores are summed to yield a Total Time score. Each of these three basic scores is divided by the number of blocks completed on that trial. So, if the client completed six blocks in 10 minutes on the dominant hand, the time per block is 10/6 or 1.67 minutes. In addition, two scores are generated from the drawing phase at the end of the test. The Memory score is the number of shapes correctly drawn from memory, while the Location score is the number drawn in the correct quadrant of the board and in the correct relationship to the other blocks. The total possible on each of these latter scores is 10. Scores may be transformed into T-scores using the norms of Heaton, Grant, and Matthews (1991).

Interpretation

1. The best information from the TPT comes from the comparison of scores within the test, which allows for possible localization of the underlying lesions. These can, in turn, be compared with basic motor measures and other visual–spatial and frontal lobe tests.
2. Performance of the nondominant hand (ND) should be 33% better than performance of the dominant hand (D).
3. Performace of both hands (B) should be 33% better than the ND time and 55% better than the D hand.

4. When the ND/D ratio is greater than .80, this suggests impairment in the nondominant hand.

5. When the ND/D ratio is less than 55%, this suggests impairment in the dominant hand.

6. When the B/D ratio is greater than 55%, this suggests that there has been inadequate learning of the visual–spatial relationships during the test.

7. When the B/ND ratio is greater than 80%, this suggests inadequate learning during the trials.

8. When the B/D ratio is greater than 55% and the B/ND ratio is greater than 80%, this strongly suggests impairment in learning over trials. If only one of these ratios is significant, it is possible that the individual is unable to use both hands in an effective manner because one hand interferes with the other.

9. When impairment in learning takes place in the absence of motor and/or sensory losses on more basic tests, the possibility of prefrontal involvement is strong.

10. Prefrontal involvement may be manifested through inconsistent trial-and-error learning approaches, perseveration by trying to force a block into a space it does not fit, impulsivity, and poor planning.

11. Good performance on Memory with poor performance on Localization suggests poor visual–spatial problems, especially when there is below expected improvement from trial to trial.

12. Poor performance on both Memory and Localization, combined with overall poor performance across trials, suggests brain impairment but is not localizable by itself.

13. In cases where there is evidence of dominant side problems, valuable information may be gained by comparing Finger Tapping (FT) and TPT performance using this formula: (DOM[FT] × DOM[TPT]) divided by (ND[FT] × ND[TPT]), where FT scores are expressed in average taps per 10 seconds and TPT scores in time per block. (Note: In cases where zero blocks are placed on a single trial, we assign an arbitrary score of 10 minutes.)

14. In cases where the D-RATIO defined in no. 13 is between 1.35 and 1.65, there are equal deficits in the dominant hand on the two tests.

15. In cases where the D-RATIO is greater than 1.65, this suggests greater impairment on the TPT dominant hand which indicates more posterior dominant hemisphere involvement.

16. In cases where the D-RATIO is less than 1.35, this suggests greater impairment on the FT dominant hand, which indicates more anterior dominant hemisphere involvement.

17. In cases in which there is evidence of nondominant motor and sensory

problems on FT and TPT, we can use the ND-RATIO to compute whether there is more anterior or posterior involvement. This is the reverse of the D-RATIO and expressed as (ND[TPT] × ND[FT]) divided by (D[TPT] × D[FT]).

18. When the ND-RATIO is between 1.5 and 1.8, then the relative impairment on the tests is equal.

19. When the ND-RATIO is greater than 1.8, then more TPT impairment is indicated, which is suggestive of a more posterior focus.

20. When the ND-RATIO is less than 1.5, then there is more impairment on FT, which is suggestive of a more anterior focus.

21. Good performance on the Tactual Performance Test (TPT) combined with poor performance on Block Design suggests intact spatial skills but impaired visual or visual motor skills. Good performance on the TPT is inconsistent with either impaired spatial or motor skills. In such cases, poor performance may also be seen on complex drawing tasks and tests requiring good visual analysis such as Matrices and Picture Arrangement. The dissociation between the TPT and these visual tests is an important marker that the performance tests may not be interpreted in traditional ways.

22. Poor performance on the TPT along with poor performance on visual–spatial tests (Bender, Block Design, Raven's, etc.) points to a generalized visual–spatial deficit that usually involves the right posterior area of the brain. In these cases, TPT performance is generally depressed across the board with significant impairment on Localization and Memory.

23. In the elderly, performance on the TPT declines rapidly. As a result, standard scores or T-scores may be artificially elevated as a result of the high standard deviations in the normal population. This may make it impossible to reliably identify specific patterns of deficits.

24. In cases of substantial frontal injuries, the TPT may be disrupted even in the presence of normal visual–spatial and visual motor skills. This situation is verified through several indicators: (1) good relative performance on the WAIS-III Performance tests as well as drawing tests such as the Bender and spatial tests such as the Raven's and Test of Line Orientation; (2) performance on motor tests such as Finger Tapping and the sensory examinations inconsistent with the TPT trials, most often with the TPT showing a lateralized dominant hand deficit that does not show up on Finger Tapping or a basic sensory examination; (3) on the TPT, the worst performance is on the first trial; (4) improvement to the second trial is less than expected; (5) improvement on the third trial (both hands) is greater than expected; (6) Memory and Location scores are adequate or better; (7) performance on Category and Wisconsin Card Sort is usually impaired, although in milder cases only one may

show impairment; and (7) impairment on Trails B or the Stroop. Not all of these factors need to be present in any given injury, but most of them should be observable or borderline.

25. When the Clock Drawing and TPT are the major areas of deficit while other visual–spatial–motor tests are performed better, organizational and executive skills are strongly implicated.

26. Profiles in which the WCST is impaired but Category, COWAT, Stroop, TPT, and Trails B are normal points to problems with the client figuring out the intent of the test. (See the WCST interpretation section for more detail.)

27. Profiles in which Category and TPT are impaired but WCST, COWAT, Trails B, and Stroop are normal suggest that the difficulties are with the visual–spatial nature of these tests. While there is a visual component to WCST, there is not a spatial component comparable to Category and TPT for most clients.

28. Profiles in which WCST, COWAT, Stroop, and Trails B are impaired but Category and TPT (frontal signs) are normal point to problems dealing with verbal executive skills, usually reflecting damage to the anterior left (dominant) hemisphere.

29. Profiles in which Category, WCST, and TPT (frontal signs) are impaired but COWAT, Stroop, and Trails B are intact suggest problems with visual executive skills, suggesting lesions in the anterior right (nondominant) hemisphere. In such cases, the client attempts to solve the WCST in a nonverbal manner.

30. Profiles in which the Stroop, COWAT, and Trails B are impaired but Category, WCST, and TPT are normal point to specific verbal analysis problems related to poor flexibility for verbal material.

31. Because of the length and complexity of TPT, it generally demands more sustained attention than do other memory tests. Thus, problems in sustained attention, as reflected in poor IVA or TOVA performance (particularly on visual portions), may correlate with poor performance. In such cases, impairment will also be seen on the WCST, Faces, Category, and the Rey Figure, which also require sustained attention for good performance. Similar tests that require less sustained attention (e.g., BVRT, Stroop, COWAT, Trails B, Working Memory) will generally be normal if this is the primary problem, except in the more severe deficits which can potentially affect any test.

References for Tactual Performance Test (TPT)

Arnold, B. R., Montgomery, G. T., Castaneda, I., & Longoria, R. (1994). Acculturation and performance of Hispanics on selected Halstead–Reitan neuropsychological tests. *Assessment*, *1*(3), 239–248.

Charter, R. A., Walden, D. K., & Hoffman, C. (1998). Interscorer reliabilities for memory and localization scores of the tactual performance test. *Clinical Neuropsychologist, 12*(2), 245–247.

Halstead, W. C. (1947). *Brain and intelligence: A quantitative study of the frontal lobes.* Chicago: University of Chicago Press.

Heaton, R. K., Grant, I., & Matthews, C. G. (1991). *Comprehensive norms for an expanded Halstead–Reitan battery: Demographic corrections, research findings, and clinical applications.* Odessa, FL: Psychological Assessment Resources.

Heilbronner, R. L., Henry, G. K., Buck, P., & Adams, R. L. (1991). Lateralized brain damage and performance on trail making A and B, digit span forward and backward, and TPT memory and location. *Archives of Clinical Neuropsychology, 6*(4), 251–258.

Heilbronner, R. L., & Parsons, O. A. (1989). The clinical utility of the Tactual Performance Test (TPT): Issues of lateralization and cognitive style. *Clinical Neuropsychologist, 3*(3), 250–264.

Searight, H. R., Dunn, E. J., Grisso, T., & Margolis, R. B. (1992). The relation of the Halstead–Reitan neuropsychological battery to ratings of everyday functioning in a geriatric sample: Clarification. *Neuropsychology, 6*(4), 394.

Thompson, L. L., & Heaton, R. K. (1991). Pattern of performance on the tactual performance test. *Clinical Neuropsychologist, 5*(4), 322–328.

Welch, L. W., Cunningham, A. T., Eckardt, M. J., & Martin, P. R. (1997). Fine motor speed deficits in alcoholic Korsakoff's syndrome. *Alcoholism: Clinical & Experimental Research, 21*(1), 134–139.

CLOCK DRAWING TEST (CDT)

The Clock Drawing Test (CDT) is a simple and quick test to administer. It has its beginnings in many earlier neurological examinations and is thought to be sensitive to a wide variety of specific brain injuries, as well as to dementia. The subject is asked to draw a clock, mark in the hours, and then draw the hands to indicate a specified time. The test is cost efficient and nonthreatening. Language, education, and cultural differences do not appear to have a significant influence on performance (Shulman, Gold, Cohen, & Zucchero, 1993). However, the decline in the use of analog clocks, in favor of digital clocks, has made this test inappropriate for some clients.

Interpretation

1. Inability to place the hands on a clock in an individual who was once able to tell time on an analog clock suggests visual–spatial disorders which may occur in the posterior area of either hemisphere, although this deficit is thought to be more specific to the right hemisphere.
2. Inability to comprehend the meaning of a clock or time indicates posterior left hemisphere dysfunction.
3. Stimulus-bound responses include errors in time setting. This may reflect a perseverative tendency (frontal) or visual–spatial problems.
4. In some cases, the subject may perseverate, drawing more than two hands or numbering beyond 12. These observations are strongly suggestive of anterior lesions.

5. The presence of neglect will cause the client to ignore the left side of the clock and is usually associated with right parietal problems.

6. Frontal planning skills may be evident in the drawing of the clock. It should be noted whether the subject begins by spacing the 12, 3, 6, and 9, and then proceeds to fill in the gaps with the remaining numbers, or if the subject begins numbering at 12 and continues consecutively and in a clockwise fashion.

7. Backward orientation of the clock (counting down rather than up in a clockwise direction) suggests visual–spatial disorders characteristic of right hemisphere lesions.

8. Inability to recognize or reproduce numbers suggests a form of acalculia that is most often seen in left posterior dysfunction.

9. Inability to draw a simple circle when asked or to understand what a clock is suggests verbal problems which are suggestive of receptive language problems arising from the left hemisphere. It is useful in such cases to ask the client to copy a circle to see if the problem is visual–motor in nature or exists only in response to a verbal command. Cases in which the client can copy but not draw to command suggest a verbal problem. If the client can draw to command but not copy, the client may have a severe visual–spatial or visual recognition problem.

10. The circle drawings and hands should be inspected for evidence of tremors (either voluntary while drawing or tremors before or after drawing). Resting tremors (before drawing) may suggest subcortical lesions, while voluntary tremors point to lesions of the cortical motor system.

11. If the Bender is performed well, but Clock Drawing is not, the deficit is likely to be in the planning and organization of the clock rather than basic visual–motor skills.

12. Poor performance on the Bender combined with a good clock drawing is a very unusual finding suggesting problems with motivation or understanding the basic task on the Bender, or reflecting inconsistent motivation.

13. Poor performance on the Clock Drawing combined with good performance on Block Design, Raven's, WAIS-III Matrices, Line Orientation, and/or the VFDT points to problems in visual-motor or motor skills rather than deficits in visual–spatial skills, although organizational skills may be impaired as well. When visual–motor skills are implicated, deficits will be evident on the Bender and Benton Visual Retention Test. Normal performance would be expected on Matrix tasks and other nonmotor visual tasks.

14. Poor performance on Clock Drawing alone with the drawing and WAIS-III tasks performed in a normal manner points to frontal problems. There should be evidence of deficits on other executive tests such

as Category, Wisconsin Card Sorting, Stroop, or the Trail Making Test to support this conclusion.

15. When the Clock Drawing and TPT are the major areas of deficit while other visual–spatial–motor tests are performed better, organizational and executive skills are strongly implicated.

16. Impairment in the VFDT along with good clock drawing suggests problems with the multiple-choice format of the VFDT rather than visual–spatial problems.

17. When the Hooper is normal, but Clock Drawing, the Bender, Block Design, or other construction tasks show spatial problems, visual–motor problems should be considered.

18. When the Hooper is abnormal along with Clock Drawing, Bender, Block Design, and VFDT, a general spatial deficit may be present.

References for Clock Drawing Test (CDT)

Agrell, B., & Dehlin, O. (1998). The clock-drawing test. *Age and Ageing, 27*(3), 399–403.

Agrell, B., & Dehlin, O. (1999). Inter-rater reliability of the clock-drawing test—Reply. *Age and Ageing, 28*(3), 327–328.

Brodaty, H., & Moore, C. M. (1997). The Clock Drawing Test for dementia of the Alzheimer's type: A comparison of three scoring methods in a memory disorders clinic. *International Journal of Geriatric Psychiatry, 12*(6), 619–627.

Cahn, D. A., Salmon, D. P., Monsch, A. U., Butters, N., Wiederholt, W. C., Corey-Bloom, J., & Barrett-Connor, E. (1996). Screening for dementia of the Alzheimer type in the community: The utility of the clock drawing test. *Archives of Clinical Neuropsychology, 11*(6), 529–539.

Ferrucci, L., Cecchi, F., Guralnik, J. M., Giampaoli, S., Noce, C. L., Salani, B., Bandinelli, S., & Baroni, A. (1996). Does the clock drawing test predict cognitive decline in older persons independent of the mini-mental state examination? *Journal of the American Geriatrics Society, 44*, 1326–1331.

Gruber, N. P., Varner, R. V., Chen, Y., & Lesser, J. M. (1997). A comparison of the clock drawing test and the Pfeiffer short portable mental status questionnaire in a geropsychiatry clinic. *International Journal of Geriatric Psychiatry, 12*, 526–532.

Libon, D. J., Malamut, B. L., Swenson, R., Sands, L. P., & Cloud, B. S. (1996). Further analysis of clock drawings among demented and nondemented older subjects. *Archives of Clinical Neuropsychology, 11*(3), 193–205.

Libon, D. J., Swenson, R. A., Barnoski, E. J., & Sands, L. P. (1993). Clock drawing as an assessment tool for dementia. *Archives of Clinical Neuropsychology, 8*, 405–415.

Lieberman, D., Galinsky, D., Fried, V., Grinshpun, Y., Mytlis, N., Tylis, R., & Lieberman, D. (1999). Factors affecting the results of the Clock Drawing Test in elderly patients hospitalized for physical rehabilitation. *International Journal of Geriatric Psychiatry, 14*(5), 325–330.

O'Rourke, N., Tuokko, H., Hayden, S., & Beattie, B. L. (1997). Early identification of dementia: Predictive validity of the clock test. *Archives of Clinical Neuropsychology, 12*(3), 257–267.

Rouleau, I., Salmon, D. P., & Butters, N. (1996). Longitudinal analysis of clock drawing in Alzheimer's disease patients. *Brain and Cognition, 31*, 17–34.

Shulman, K. I., Gold, D. P., Cohen, C. A., & Zucchero, C. A. (1993). Clock-drawing and dementia in the community: A longitudinal study. *International Journal of Geriatric Psychiatry, 8*(6), 487–496.

Suhr, J., Grace, J., Allen, J., Nadler, J., & McKenna, M. (1998). Quantitative and qualitative performance of stroke versus normal elderly on six clock drawing systems. *Archives of Clinical Neuropsychology, 13*(6), 495–502.

Sunderland, T., Hill, J. L., Mellow, A. M., et al. (1989). Clock drawing in Alzheimer's disease. *Journal of the American Geriatrics Society, 37*, 725–729.

Tracy, J. I., DeLeon, J., Doonan, R., Musciente, J., Ballas, T., & Josiassen, R. C. (1996). Clock drawing in schizophrenia. *Psychological Reports, 79*, 923–928.

Tuokko, H., Jadjistavropoulos, T., Miller, J. A., & Beattie, B. L. (1992). The clock test: A sensitive measure to differentiate normal elderly from those with Alzheimer disease. *Journal of American Geriatrics Society, 40*, 579–584.

Van Hout, H., & Berkhout, S. (1999). Inter-rater reliability of the clock-drawing test. *Age and Ageing, 28*(3), 327.

Wolf-Klein, G. P., Silverstone, F. A., Levy, A. P., et al. (1989). Screening for Alzheimer's disease by clock drawing. *Journal of the American Geriatrics Society, 37*, 730–734.

BENTON VISUAL RETENTION TEST (BVRT)

The Benton Visual Retention Test (BVRT) is an elegant test of visual memory that is used in neurological screening for the presence of organic brain dysfunction. The test contains three alternate forms, which may be given using four different methods of administration. Each form of the test takes about 5 minutes to administer, and is scored quickly using complex but easily learned scoring guides. This test employs familiar-figure stimuli and measures the ability to perceive and briefly retain familiar and unfamiliar geometric figures. The BVRT assesses nonfrontal lobe functioning and is sensitive to the presence of brain damage, especially to the parietal lobes. The delayed administration is also sensitive to lateralized damage to the right hemisphere. Although the BVRT is a powerful diagnostic tool that differentiates between brain-damaged and normal groups, it is most frequently used within a neuropsychological battery rather than as a single measure.

Interpretation

1. Norms tables for both adults and children are provided in the test manual, and these norms range from age 8 to age 64. On Administration C, the copying task, normal clients have an error score of 4 or less, while brain-injured individuals demonstrated a greater number of distortions, omissions, and rotations.

2. Defective performance on Administration C (copying) is seen in individuals with posterior right hemisphere lesions (with occipital involvement) more often than left hemisphere lesions in general. As this is a relatively simple task, defective performance usually reflects significant injuries, such as those seen after a stroke or with a tumor rather

than a less focal lesion, such as a mild head injury. The major exception to this is a situation in which the deficit arises from a dominant hand motor deficit, which prevents the motor reproduction of the figure. Good performance on copying indicates good visual–motor skills and suggests that other factors (memory, attention, perseveration) are responsible for deficits on the other administrations.

3. Failure on Administration A or B combined with good performance on Administration C excludes visual–constructive deficits and suggests memory functions or attentional functions are involved. Clients with frontal lesions may fail to adequately study the figures and thus be unable to reproduce them. Individuals with temporal lobe or subcortical memory problems may study the designs but be unable to reproduce more than the initial part of the multipart designs.

4. Frontal patients may show perseverations within and between figures. Such clients show an awareness that they have seen and retained the figures, but may reproduce them at the wrong time, showing evidence of proactive and retroactive interference. They are also generally less aware of their problems with the figures (although this is also seen in cases of unilateral neglect).

5. Nonresponsiveness to stimuli in the left or right halves of visual space has been observed, suggesting hemianopsia (loss of one side of the visual field). Unilateral neglect occurs when the client omits the figure on one side (usually the left) even after being alerted to the existence of this figure. In other cases, loss of the visual field can be compensated for by the client if he or she is told of the error. Neglect may show up more dramatically in the memory rather than the copying phases, but the clearest cases will be evident regardless of which administration method is employed.

6. Rotational errors are common in both normal and brain-injured clients. These are often seen in figures that are presented at an angle, but the client draws it on its side in a more stable position. If such errors are the primary problems in the protocol, they are unlikely a reflection of brain injury.

7. Size errors occur when the relative sizes of the figures are reversed (e.g., a smaller object in the design is drawn as the larger object on the response sheet). Such distortions may occur despite an accurate reproduction of the figure itself. These errors are generally suggestive of brain injury. In the presence of accurate reproduction but inaccurate size, there is usually an injury to the dominant hemisphere or to anterior rather than posterior areas (although this is not consistent).

8. Subjects with lesions of the occipital lobes generally perform worse

than clients with parietal injuries. Visual agnosia may cause a client to be able to reproduce only the central dominant figure. Distortions of the figures are associated more with right occipital parietal disorders. Individuals with similar disorders will generally have problems on both copying and memory phases of the test.

9. Left parietal lesions are also reflected on the memory form and the copying form of the test. In severe cases, these clients may be unable to reproduce the figures owing to poor analysis of the figures, as well as sensorimotor problems. Such clients do not usually distort figures but leave out important details and oversimplify.

10. Individuals with right parietal lesions with no occipital involvement perform better than those with left parietal lobe lesions, although still at the subnormal level. Right-lesioned clients frequently demonstrate problems in spatial relationships. Clients with right hemisphere injury make more misplacement errors while those with left hemisphere injury make more motoric distortion errors. However, right parietal clients will show much more distortion on more complex drawing tasks, such as the Rey Figure.

11. Subjects with unilateral cerebral injury demonstrate poor performance and produce more errors when reproducing figures in the contralateral visual field, and have a tendency to draw the designs on the side of the paper of the unaffected visual field (an ipsilateral shift of the entire design). More errors were made when reproducing figures corresponding to the contralateral visual field. The contralateral errors and ipsilateral shift are valuable indicators of the side of the lesion.

12. Schizophrenic patients as a group demonstrate extreme variability on the BVRT, as some perform within normal limits. An "autistic" reproduction reflects no clear relevance to the stimulus.

13. Malingerers tend to perform worse than do brain-injured patients, with more distortion errors and fewer omissions, perseverations, and size errors. They have significantly fewer correct reproductions and often include unusual and bizarre features. Significant age effects have been observed.

14. Poor performance on the BVRT, Bender, and Clock Drawing combined with good performance on Raven's, Matrices, or Block Design points to problems in visual–motor or motor skills rather than deficits in visual–spatial skills although organizational skills may be impaired as well. When visual–motor skills are implicated, deficits will be evident on the Bender and Benton Visual Retention Test. Normal performance would be expected on Matrix tasks and other nonmotor visual tasks.

15. In cases of unilateral neglect, clear deficits are usually visible on the

Raven's and Benton Visual Retention Test. Symptoms may show up on any of the visual tests but most of the other tests can be manipulated by the subject more easily to avoid these deficits. In severe cases, however, the neglect will show up across the visual tests and many of the reading tests as well.

16. Good performance on the BVRT is inconsistent with poor performance on the Bender. In such cases, motivational issues or understanding of the instructions must be raised.

17. Good performance on the Bender with poor performance on the BVRT is most often associated with unilateral neglect or with the memory components of the BVRT. Rarely does such a pattern point to visual–motor deficits.

18. Poor performance on the BVRT despite good performance on the VFDT suggests that basic visual processes are intact, pointing to the motor aspect of the Benton as the cause of the deficit. If the problem is motor, then nonmotor tests (Matrices, Raven's) should be performed adequately while other construction tests (Bender, Block Design) should show impairment.

19. Good performance on the Benton despite poor performance on the VFDT suggests problems with the multiple-choice format of the VFDT. If this is the case, similar errors will usually be seen on the Raven's or WAIS-III Matrices. In general, such errors arise from impulsivity or perseveration, suggesting executive deficits.

20. If both the BVRT and VFDT are intact, it is unlikely that the client has difficulties with visual neglect. However, if both are impaired, neglect should be considered. If neglect is present, an analysis of the client's errors should show omission of the peripheral figures rather than mis-identification of the major figures. On the Bender, the client will tend to use only one side of the drawing page, rarely crossing the midline. In addition, similar deficits will be seen on the Raven's or WAIS-III Matrices.

21. Motor skills play a minor role in Picture Arrangement, so high scores on Picture Arrangement, Matrices, and Picture Completion relevant to Digit Symbol, the BVRT, and Block Design should lead to analysis of more basic motor measures. This should include loss of basic motor skills as measure by Finger Tapping or Purdue Pegboard in the dominant hand and impairment on Visual–Motor tasks such as the Bender as well as the Tactual Performance Test.

22. When the Hooper is normal, but the Benton, Block Design, or other construction tasks show spatial problems, visual–motor problems should be considered.

23. When the Hooper is abnormal along with Benton, Block Design, and VFDT, a general spatial deficit may be present.

References for Benton Visual Retention Test (BVRT)

Benton, A. L. (1974). *Revised Visual Retention Test manual* (4th ed.). New York: The Psychological Corporation.

Bowers, T. G., Washburn, S. E., & Livesay, J. R. (1986). Predicting neuropsychological impairment by screening instruments and intellectual evaluation indices: Implications for the meaning of Kaufman's factor III. *Psychological Reports, 59*, 487–493.

Crockett, D. J., Clark, C., Browning, J., & MacDonald, J. (1983). An application of the background interference procedure to the Benton visual retention test. *Journal of Clinical Neuropsychology, 5*(2), 181–185.

Hakola, H. P. A. (1998). Benton's Visual Retention Test in patients with polycystic lipomembranous dysplasia with sclerosing leukoencephalopathy. *Dementia and Geriatric Cognitive Disorders, 9*(1), 39–43.

Lannoo, E., & Vingerhoets, G. (1997). Flemish normative data on common neuropsychological tests: Influence of age, education, and gender. *Psychologica Belgica, 37*(3), 141–155.

Larabee, G. J., Kane, R. L., Schuck, J. R., & Francis, D. J. (1985). Construct validity of various memory testing procedures. *Journal of Clinical and Experimental Neuropsychology, 7*(3), 239–250.

LaRue, A. (1984). Neuropsychological testing. *Psychiatric Annals, 14*(3), 201–204.

Lezak, M. D. (1995). *Neuropsychological Assessment* (3rd ed.). New York: Oxford University Press.

Marsh, G. G., & Hirsch, S. H. (1982). Effectiveness of two tests of visual retention. *Journal of Clinical Psychology, 38*(1), 115–118.

Morrison-Stewart, S. L., Williamson, P. C., Corning, W. C., Kutcher, S. P., Snow, W. G., & Merskey, H. (1992). Frontal and non-frontal lobe neuropsychological test performance and clinical symptomatology in schizophrenia. *Psychological Medicine, 22*, 353–359.

Tamkin, A. S., & Kunce, J. T. (1985). A comparison of three neuropsychological tests: The Weigl, Hooper, and Benton. *Journal of Clinical Psychology, 41*(5), 660–664.

Vakil, E., Blachstein, H., Sheleff, P., & Grossman, S. (1989). BVRT-Scoring system and time delay in the differentiation of lateralized hemispheric damage. *International Journal of Clinical Neuropsychology, XI*(3), 125–128.

MATRICES (WAIS-III)

This is a relatively new test, introduced in 1997 as part of the WAIS-III. It appears to be an adaptation of Raven's Matrices but with a bigger emphasis on pattern analysis that can be done either visually or with verbal mediation. It also requires close attention and analysis of verbal details, especially at higher levels. While it shares a strong spatial component with Block Design, the absence of a time limit or time bonuses on this test may result in differential scores between these tests. In normals, these issues may be minor, but they may turn out to be more important in general neuropsychological populations. As there is a paucity of research owing to the newness of this measure, changes in interpretive strategies will likely take place over time.

Interpretation

1. A Matrix Reasoning score of more than 3 points below the Performance mean score suggests deficits in spatial pattern analysis. If both Block Design and Matrices are more than 3 points below the Performance mean score, then there is likely a general visual–spatial deficit without any basic visual deficit.
2. Normal scores on Matrix Reasoning can rule out severe visual–spatial processing problems, but because the test can be verbally mediated, milder disorders may be missed. When Matrix Reasoning is more poorly performed, the possibility of an analytic deficit should be considered.
3. Matrices can be performed at an average level using verbal mediation strategies. It appears more susceptible to these strategies than are the complex drawing tests. Thus, performance on Matrices, especially in intelligent clients, may be better than on these other construction tasks. This pattern of using verbal mediation generally includes good Block Design performance, good Raven's Matrices Performance, and good reproduction of simple drawings put poor reproduction of complex drawings (such as the Rey) and poor performance on measures of facial memory and other tasks that are not easily encodable. This is also accompanied by strong performance on verbal tests in general.
4. Good performance on Block Design but poor performance on the WAIS-III Matrices will often indicate problems with organizing the internal abstract designs of the figures, especially in later designs when there are no clear demarcations of where blocks begin and end. This may suggest a mild right hemisphere that is partially compensated. It may also reflect the greater organizational demands of the Matrice's items which require more active analysis and organization of the material presented than does Block Design.
5. Poor performance on Block Design but good performance on WAIS-III Matrices may reflect two possibilities. First, Matrices (as well as Raven's Matrices) is not timed. Thus, clients who have accurate but slow performance will be penalized on Block Design but not on Matrices or many of the drawing tasks. This can reflect brain injury but may also reflect compulsive attention to detail. Such an impairment will be reflected in poor Coding scores, but not necessarily poor Picture Arrangement scores (which is timed but the time limits are very generous). Second, Block Design is, as noted earlier, a more abstract spatial task. The clients may not be able to see the patterns in Block Design necessary to solve the designs within the time limit. Interestingly, such clients will improve rapidly if shown how to analyze the patterns in an organized manner.

6. Poor performance on the drawing tests (Bender, BVRT, Clock Drawing) with good performance on Block Design and Matrices generally reflects problems with fine motor control. While Block Design is a timed motor task, it requires much less fine coordination than the Bender. Coding will also be slow in these cases, but Symbol Search performance will be normal. Tests of simple motor speed such as Finger Tapping may be intact in some cases, although more complex tasks such as the Grooved Pegboard and the Tactual Performance Test will show slowness. In some cases, however, this pattern will point to a problem with abstractive items which can also be seen in poor performance on frontal lobe procedures.

7. Matrices and the Raven's Matrices are clearly similar tests. However, there is no adequate research on the actual relationships between the tests. Comparison of performance on both tests can yield useful information about the consistency of a client's performance. Scores on Matrix Reasoning and the Raven's Matrices should generally be within one standard deviation of each other when scores are converted to standard scores. However, the scoring systems and underlying normative groups for these tests differ considerably.

8. Better performance on Matrices than on visual–motor tests such as the Bender, Benton, or Clock Drawing suggests good spatial analysis skills but poor visual–motor skills. In such cases, measures of purer motor skills (such as Finger Tapping) should be administered as well. If the motor measures are found to be intact, then the problem may be in visual–motor coordination. If the motor measures are poor, then no conclusion can be reached about visual–motor abilities. The attainment of a good Matrices score suggests that right posterior areas of the brain are functioning.

9. Poor performance on Matrices, combined with good performance on drawing and other visual–motor tests, suggests that it is the pattern analysis and logical progression analyses rather than spatial skills that are impaired. These are more associated with frontal injuries (on either side of the brain).

10. Poor performance on Matrices and other tests of visual skills point to a right posterior lesion. This is especially true in the presence of neglect and poor construction skills and in the absence of dominant side motor problems.

11. In cases of unilateral neglect, clients will fail to respond to the alternatives on the left side of the page and thus make many errors when the answer is on the left. They may also neglect the left side of the stimulus field itself, creating similar errors. When neglect is suspected, asking the client to describe what he or she sees is often useful.

12. Frontal patients may perseverate, usually selecting the answer in the same position and ignoring alternatives. Item response patterns should be carefully reviewed in cases where this is a possibility.

13. In cases of clients with dominant hemisphere lesions, Matrices may yield very different scores from tests that require motor coordination or speed. Along with other "motor free" and untimed visual–spatial tasks, a better estimate of true visual–spatial skills can be derived by combining results from such tasks that are in a test battery.

14. Visual attention and visual neglect issues should always be ruled out in cases of poor Matrices performance. These deficits will severally affect performance even though spatial skills may be intact. In some cases, this will be seen by good performance on the Tactual Performance Test, which will effectively rule out spatial deficits.

15. Good Matrices performance in the presence of language deficits points to unilateral lesions of the left hemisphere when there is a history of previous normal verbal performance. In other cases, the differences may reflect poor education and language training (including poor mastery of English) rather than brain injury. In such cases, Matrices may reflect intellectual potential more effectively than the verbal measures.

16. Poor Matrices performance in the absence of aphasia is less specific and may reflect anterior damage of either hemisphere or posterior damage of the right hemisphere. When combined with generally poor Block Design and drawing test performance, these deficits likely reflect right posterior lesions. However, when only Matrices is impaired, this most likely reflects an anterior lesion or even a preexisting intellectual deficit.

17. Poor Matrices performance with aphasia may reflect a left hemisphere lesion or a more generalized disorder but does not always imply the involvement of the right hemisphere.

18. Good performance on the Tactual Performance Test (TPT) combined with poor performance on Matrices and Block Design suggests intact spatial skills but impaired visual or visual motor skills. Good performance on the TPT is inconsistent with either impaired spatial or motor skills. In such cases, poor performance may also be seen on complex drawing tasks. The dissociation between the TPT and these visual tests is an important marker that the performance tests may not be interpreted in traditional ways.

19. Good performance on Matrices combined with poor performance on drawing tests (Bender, BVRT, Clock Drawing) generally reflects problems with fine motor control. Coding will also be slow in these cases, but Symbol Search performance will be normal. Tests of simple motor speed such as Finger Tapping may be intact in some cases, although

more complex tasks such as the Grooved Pegboard and the Tactual Performance Test will show slowness. In some cases, however, this pattern will point to a problem with abstractive items which can also be seen in poor performance on frontal lobe procedures.

20. Good performance on Matrices combined with poor performance on the Test of Line Orientation points to basic analysis problems with angles and spatial skills which is compensated for on more complex visual–spatial skills where foundational spatial skills are not as important. In such cases, there may be a highly focal lesion whose general impact is minimal. This performance should be compared to drawing tasks in which the inability to distinguish angles may be more obvious.

21. Poor performance on Matrices combined with good performance on Line Orientation suggests an impairment in the more complex organizational and logical skills demanded by the Raven's rather than the more basic spatial skills measured by Line Orientation.

22. In cases of unilateral neglect, clear deficits are usually visible on Matrices, the Raven's, Clock Drawing, and Benton Visual Retention Test. Symptoms may show up on any of the visual tests but most of the other tests can be manipulated by the subject more easily to avoid these deficits. In severe cases, however, the neglect will show up across the visual tests and many of the reading tests as well.

23. Problems with the multiple-choice format of Matrices will also be clear on the Raven's Line Orientation, or VFDT. In such cases, the errors are generally impulsive or perseverative, reflecting frontal/executive deficits. These deficits should be seen on the frontal lobe tests as well (Category, WCST, Stroop, Trail Making Test Part B).

24. Good performance on VFDT, Line Orientation, and Matrices usually indicates intact visual analysis and spatial skills as well as the absence of neglect. In such case, errors on the motor-based visual tests likely arise from timing or visual–motor deficits.

References for Matrices (WAIS-III)

Boone, D. E. (1998). Specificity of the WAIS-R subtests with psychiatric inpatients. *Assessment, 5,* 123–126.

Campbell, J. M., & McCord, D. M. (1996). The WAIS-R comprehension and picture arrangement subtests as measures of social intelligence: Testing traditional interpretations. *Journal of Psychoeducational Assessment, 14,* 240–249.

Golden, C. J., Zillmer, E., & Spiers, M. (1992). *Neuropsychological assessment and intervention.* Springfield, IL: Charles C Thomas.

Hawkins, K. A. (1998). Indicators of brain dysfunction derived from graphic representations of the WAIS-III/WMS-III Technical Manual clinical samples data: A preliminary approach to clinical utility. *Clinical Neuropsychologist, 12*(4), 535–555.

Kramer, J. H. (1990). Guidelines for interpreting the WAIS-R subtest scores. *Psychological Assessment, 2,* 202–205.

Matarazzo, J. D. (1972). *Wechsler's Measurement and Appraisal of Adult Intelligence* (5th ed.). New York: Oxford University Press.

Ryan, J. J., Lopez, S. J., & Werth, T. R. (1998). Administration of time estimates for WAIS-III subtests, scales, and short forms in a clinical sample. *Journal of Psychoeducational Assessment, 16*(4), 315–323.

Sprandel, H. Z. (1995). *The psychoeducational use and interpretation of the Wechsler Adult Intelligence Scale-Revised* (2nd ed.). Springfield, IL: Charles C Thomas.

Wechsler, D. (1981). *WAIS-R manual.* New York: The Psychological Corporation.

Wechsler, D. (1986). *WAIS-R administration and scoring manual.* San Antonio, TX: The Psychological Corporation.

Wechsler, D. (1997). *WAIS-III administration and scoring manual.* San Antonio, TX: The Psychological Corporation.

VISUAL FORM DISCRIMINATION TEST (VFDT)

The Visual Form Discrimination Test (VFDT) is a 16-item multiple-choice test of visual recognition for one-dimensional designs (Lezak, 1995). Each item consists of one card with a target figure, presented to the patient at a 45-degree angle, and a multiple-choice card containing four figures, lying flat on the table below the target. On the target item, a peripheral design appears to the right of the two major figures on eight items and to the left of the major figures on the other eight items. Each multiple-choice item contains the correct design and three incorrect designs containing either a displacement or rotation of the peripheral figure, a rotation of one of the major figures, or a distortion of the other major figure (Benton, Sivan, Hamsher, Varney, & Spreen, 1994).

Interpretation

1. To carry out the VFDT, patients must be awake, alert, and able to attend to and concentrate on the task. Attention and concentration play a significant role in VFDT performance (Benton et al., 1994), so comparison of scores to tests such as the TOVA or Digit Span and Digit symbol is important.

2. The manner in which the patient will attend to the task can be viewed as either "bottom-up" processing or "top-down" processing (Kolb & Whishaw, 1996). Bottom-up processing is more automatic and driven by stimulus and environment cues. In contrast, top-down processing is more conceptually driven. For instance, while attempting to find the correct design from the multiple-choice card, the patient will attend to specific features of the stimuli and not others and then disengage from the first feature and shift attention to the next feature, based on inte-

grated information from memory and even his or her expectations of the task.

3. The types of errors made by clients are important. In cases of severe visual analysis problems, they may not be able to even match simple figures, their errors representing gross distortions of one of the major figures. Such deficits are accompanied by significant losses on such tests as Block Design or the Tactual Performance Test. These are generally associated with occipital or parietal–occipital injuries and may also be reflected in naming problems to visual stimuli but not to auditory descriptions.

4. Clients may show unilateral neglect by missing minor figures to the left of the major figure. This will also be evident across tests of drawing, writing, and reading where the left side will be neglected. These deficits are most often associated with right posterior injuries after a cerebrovascular disorder or similar destructive lesion. Neglect will especially result in poor performance on the BVRT.

5. Errors in which the figures are rotated suggest visual–spatial problems most often associated with right hemisphere lesions. This should also be seen in rotations of drawings and rotations in other constructional tasks.

6. Good performance on this test but poor performance on motor-based construction tasks (Block Design, Bender, BVRT, etc.) suggests intact visual–spatial skills but poor visual–motor skills. This may suggest impairment in the motor area opposite the dominant hand or in the connections leading to this area.

7. Poor performance on this test despite good performance on Block Design and TPT or similar tests suggests either substantial motivational or attentional inconsistency in performance or a misunderstanding of what was required. In such cases, a readministration of the task may be useful in fully understanding what is happening. In some cases, such errors may reflect perseveration problems but these would usually show up on TPT as well. However, if VFDT and TPT are impaired while Block Design, BVRT, and the Bender are intact, the possibility of frontal/executive disorders should be considered. This would typically be reflected in poor performance on the Raven's or WAIS-III Matrices, as well as frontal lobe tests such as Category, WCST, or Part B of the Trail Making Test. In some cases, Clock Drawing will be impaired as well, especially in clients whose abilities to read analog clocks were weak prior to their injury.

8. Good performance on this test combined with poor performance on Raven's or WAIS-III Matrices rules out impulsive/perseverative responding as a likely cause of the errors. In such cases, visual discrimi-

nation or neglect is also unlikely, suggesting that the higher analytic processes tapped by these tests are more likely the cause of the deficits.

9. Poor performance on Block Design despite good performance on the VFDT suggests that basic visual processes are intact, pointing to either the timed aspect of Block Design or the more analytic spatial component as the cause of the deficit. If the problem is time alone, then untimed tests (Matrices, Raven's, Bender, BVRT) should be performed adequately. If spatial problems are present, we would expect problems on these untimed tests as well.

10. Poor performance on the Bender or BVRT, despite good performance on the VFDT, suggests that basic visual processes are intact, pointing to the motor aspect of the Bender as the cause of the deficit. If the problem is motor, then nonmotor tests (Matrices, Raven's) should be performed adequately while other construction tests (Block Design) should show impairment.

11. Good performance on the Bender despite poor performance on the VFDT suggests the presence of either neglect or problems with the multiple-choice format of the VFDT. If neglect is present, an analysis of the client's errors should show omission of the peripheral figures rather than misidentification of the major figures. On the Bender, the client will tend to use only one side of the drawing page, rarely crossing the midline. In addition, similar deficits will be seen on the Raven's or WAIS-III Matrices and on the BVRT.

12. Problems with the multiple-choice format of the VFDT will also be clear on the Raven's, Line Orientation, or WAIS-III Matrices. In such cases, the errors are generally impulsive or perseverative reflecting frontal/executive deficits. These deficits should be seen on the frontal lobe tests as well (Category, WCST, Stroop, Trail Making Test Part B).

13. Good performance on both VFDT, Line Orientation, and either Raven's or WAIS-III Matrices usually indicates intact visual analysis and spatial skills as well as the absence of neglect. In such case, errors on the motor-based visual tests likely arise from timing or visual–motor deficits.

14. When the Hooper is abnormal, but the VFDT is not, the role of naming in the poor Hooper performance should be considered. In such cases, it is helpful to have the client describe rather than name the object.

References for Visual Form Discrimination Test (VFDT)

Benton, A. L., Sivan, A. B., Hamsher, K., Varney, N. R., & Spreen, O. (1994). *Contributions to neuropsychological assessment: A clinical manual* (2nd ed.). New York: Oxford University Press.
Caplan, B., & Scultheis, M. T. (1998). An interpretive table for the visual form discrimination test. *Perceptual and Motor Skills, 87*(3; part 2), 1203–1207.

Iverson, G. L., Slick, D., & Seemiller, L. S. (1997). Screening for visual–perceptual deficits following closed head injury: A short form of the Visual Form Discrimination Test. *Brain Injury, 11*(2), 125–128.

Kolb, B., & Wishaw, I. O. (1996). *Fundamentals of human neuropsychology.* New York: W. H. Freeman & Company.

Lezak, M. D. (1995). *Neuropsychological assessment* (2nd ed.). New York: Oxford University Press.

HOOPER VISUAL ORGANIZATION TEST (HVOT)

The Hooper Visual Organization Test (HVOT) was developed to identify patients in mental hospitals with organic brain conditions (Hooper, 1958). The test consists of 30 pictures of readily recognizable objects on 4″ × 4″ cards. Each object has been cut up into two or more parts and rearranged. The examinee is instructed to name the object as if it were put together in one piece. The examinee can either name the object verbally (if given individually) or write the object's name in spaces provided in the test booklet (if given in a group format). All 30 of the items are administered. However, Wetzel and Murphy (1991) found that discontinuing the test after five consecutive failures does not significantly change the scoring of this test. Scoring ranges from 0 to 30. The time required for administration is approximately 10–15 minutes.

Norms were first published by Hooper in 1958. Cognitively intact persons generally fail no more than six HVOT items. A score of 26 corresponds to a T-score of 50 (average), a score of 21 to a T-score of 60 (1 SD below average), and a score of 16 to a T-score of 70 (2 SD below average). Spreen and Strauss (1998) published more recent norms and found that persons who obtain a score 23–19 comprise a group that includes emotionally disturbed or psychotic patients, as well as those with mild to moderate brain disorders. Furthermore, more than 11 failures usually indicates organic brain pathology.

Interpretation

1. The HVOT is used to assess visual organization skills. According to Lezak (1998), the face validity of the test lies in its demand on perceptual differentiation and conceptual reorganization (including metal rotation) of the fragmented objects.
2. The presence of unilateral neglect will cause severe impairment in performance as the client will fail to see all the pieces.
3. When the Hooper is normal, but Block Design or other construction tasks show spatial problems, visual–motor problems should be considered.
4. When the Hooper is abnormal, but the VFDT is not, the role of naming in the poor Hooper performance should be considered. In such cases, it is helpful to have the client describe rather than name the object.

5. When the Hooper is abnormal along with Block Design, a general spatial deficit may be present.

6. When naming problems are suspected as the cause of the Hooper deficit, a comparison should be made to the Boston Naming Test or similar measure of naming disorders.

7. When the Hooper is abnormal, but Block Design is not, naming or frontal disorders should be considered.

8. Clients with frontal lobe damage usually have much trouble on the HVOT because they cannot conceptualize, or at least identify, the finished product in order to mentally assemble it. These patients are often concrete and thus have difficulty comprehending the abstract design of fragmented pictures. In addition, problems in starting appear in decreased spontaneity, decreased productivity, decreased rate at which the behavior is emitted, or decreased loss of initiative. A lesion in this area can cause extreme dissociation between words and deeds which is pathological inertia. With this type of disorder the patient may be able to describe the correct response to the test with cueing or guidance, but has difficulty acting it out.

9. According to Lezak (1995) several of the HVOT items are particularly effective in eliciting the kind of perceptual fragmentation that is most likely associated with lesions of the right frontal lobe. Patients with right frontal lobe lesions are more likely to do poorly on the HVOT as a result of their approach to the task rather than from a lack of knowledge or from perceptual or language incapacities. These patients demonstrate accurate perception and accuracy in naming or writing, but they have trouble in carrying out all of the intentional performance; hence their responses may be perseverative. They may be unable to change cognitive sets with each picture but rather focus on one aspect of one card. Such patients who exhibit this phenomenon will often be able to identify most of the items correctly, thus demonstrating that they understand the organizational demand of the instructions.

10. Frontal patients may focus on only one picture fragment. They have a tendency to view their world in a fragmented manner and will interpret that one piece without attending to any others in the item (Lezak, 1995).

11. Lesions in the portion of the motor association area (left frontal lobe) that mediates the motor organization and patterning of speech may result in disruption of speech production, interfering with answering the Hooper. If given a multiple-choice format the individual is likely to perform adequately.

12. Visual agnosia may result in poor performance and an inability to simultaneously see and integrate fragments. Visual agnosias are most likely to occur with bilateral occipital lesions. In apperceptive visual

agnosia, patients cannot synthesize what they see. They may indicate awareness of discrete parts of a word or phase, or recognize elements of an object without organizing the discrete percepts into a perceptual whole.

13. Patients with associative visual agnosia (or visual object agnosia) can perceive the whole of a visual stimulus, such as a familiar object or a personal possession, but cannot recognize it. Hence, on the Hooper the patient will be able to synthesize the percepts but will not be able to recognize the completed object.

14. Since the right parietal lobe is involved in visual–spatial integration, patients with a lesion in this area may not be able to perceptually differentiate and reorganize fragmented objects on the HVOT. The HVOT is thought to be most sensitive to detecting this type of lesion.

15. Visual–spatial disturbances associated with right parietal lesions include impairment of topographical or spatial thought and memory. On the HVOT, an individual may name bits and pieces of the card, but would be unable to organize the discrete features into recognizable objects. For example, on card one, the patient may say, "This is an eye, this is a gill," but not recognize that these pieces compose parts of a fish.

References for Hooper Visual Organization Test

Hooper, H. E. (1993). *The Hooper Visual Organization Test manual*. Beverly Hills, CA: Western Psychological Services.

Johnston, B., & Wilhelm, K. L. (1997). The construct validity of the Hooper Visual Organization Test. *Assessment, 4*(3), 243–248.

Lezak, M. D. (1995). *Neuropsychological assessment* (2nd ed.). New York: Oxford University Press.

Spreen, O., & Strauss, E. (1998). *A compendium of neuropsychological tests: Administration, norms, & commentary* (2nd ed.). New York: Oxford University Press.

Wetzel, L., & Murphy, S. G. (1991). Validity of the use if a discontinue rule and evaluation of discriminability of the Hooper Visual Organization Test. *Neuropsychology, 5*, 119–122.

SECTION III: VERBAL TESTS

REITAN APHASIA EXAMINATION

The aphasia examination consists of a series of short commands and tasks designed to screen for basic language deficits. The tasks include: (1) naming simple objects and shapes; (2) reading simple words; (3) spelling; (4) following simple commands; (5) following complex commands; (5) simple word fluency (pronouncing words and sentences correctly); (6) construction skills (drawing a cross and a key); (7) following instructions involving the identification of right and left; (8) demonstrating the use of an object; and (9) arithmetic. It is intended as a screening tool rather than an extensive aphasia examination.

Interpretation

1. While a scoring system for this test exists (see Heaton, Grant, & Matthews, 1993), qualitative interpretation is generally more useful, although more difficult. The scoring system allows for a general conclusion on whether there are problems, but it does poorly when one tries to relate it to other tests in a detailed pattern analysis. The norms for the scoring system do not allow for interpretation of specific problems, but instead allow for the interpretation of overall performance. The strength of the test is as a screening device that can quickly indicate the need for more detailed testing in specific areas.

2. Most of the deficits identified on the test are associated with the function of the dominant left hemisphere. The absence of any errors suggests that the basic language areas of the brain are relatively intact and argues against a current destructive etiology involving the language areas.

3. The exception to the language dominance of the test is the drawing of four figures: square, triangle, Greek cross, and a key. Errors in drawing these figures generally reflect visual–motor problems which are relatively severe as these figures are simple. Such errors should indicate the need for additional tests such as the Benton, Bender, or the Clock Drawing. Spatial distortion is rarely seen on the simpler fingers (square and triangle) but may be very apparent in the Greek cross and key. Any reproductions of the key that distort the key or the Greek cross so that it is no longer recognizable are most associated with right posterior lesions.

4. Reproductions of the key in which the shape of the key is intact but the details are missing are most associated with left posterior injuries. In general, the other items do not reflect serious problems in the absence of motor or sensory impairment from such an injury. In cases where there are tremors or marked difficulty with drawing or paralysis, interpretation must be based on the performance of the motor tests (such as Finger Tapping) or sensory tests. Generally, only dominant hemisphere motor or sensory losses affect the ability to draw directly.

5. Drawn reproductions of the key or the cross that show tremors, inconsistent control of the pencil, and poor line quality, despite intact spatial reproduction, suggest dominant hemisphere motor or sensory impairment.

6. Spatial distortion of the Greek cross is a sensitive measure of posterior

nondominant hemisphere function, especially when spatially simpler figures and writing are intact.

7. Disorders of arithmetic and spelling must be compared to premorbid levels. In many populations, these deficits are educationally related. Errors that reflect a failure to understand basic phonemics or basic arithmetic processes are most likely to be associated with actual brain injury. In such cases, posterior left hemisphere lesions are implicated. Use of a more comprehensive achievement test (such as the Peabody) or a step-by-step analysis of skills through the LNNB Writing or Arithmetic scales can confirm the specific details of the errors and the underlying lesion.

8. When the constellation of errors on spelling and arithmetic reflect problems in sequencing letters and with the spatial aspects of math (such as carrying from one column to another), while there is an intact understanding of letters, numbers, basic language, and phonemics, the pattern may reflect a posterior right (nondominant) hemisphere lesion. Specific analysis of these deficits may be achieved through the step-by-step procedures of the LNNB Writing and Arithmetic scales.

9. Dysarthria—the inability to pronounce words fluently—is most associated with the frontal motor areas. Good performance on all of these items generally rules out the presence of significant fluency problems, but errors require follow-up with more detailed evaluations such as the LNNB Expressive Language scales. The Aphasia Screening Examination can identify fluency problems when the client is repeating a word, naming an object, or in free speech in response to a question. Non-scored fluency errors can of course be noted simply during this test and other tests that require a verbal response (such as Information or Comprehension), although these tests do not score for fluency directly. The absence of fluency errors when a left hemisphere lesion is suspected points to lesions that are very anterior (pre frontal) or posterior (parietal). The presence of fluency errors points to lesions in the posterior frontal areas or in some subcortical pathways involved in motor speech.

10. Naming problems (dysnomia) in the absence of fluency difficulties may reflect posterior dominant hemisphere language dysfunction if visual matching tasks are intact. In such cases, the client can often describe the function, use, or other aspect of the object despite the inability to name it. This screen is a gross indicator of naming and any errors should be followed up with a more comprehensive evaluation of naming such as the Boston Naming Test.

11. Naming problems in the presence of fluency problems may reflect anterior dominant hemisphere expressive language problems. As noted

previously, this screen is a gross indicator of naming and any errors should be followed up with a more comprehensive evaluation of naming such as the Boston Naming Test.

12. Reading difficulties are often an expression of premorbid levels in low-education clients. However, the inability to phonemically decode words in an approximate manner in a person previously able to read is associated with significant insults to the posterior temporal–occipital areas of the dominant hemisphere. Reading deficits on this test should be followed up by detailed achievement testing or by a more detailed analysis of underlying reading skills as provided by the LNNB Reading scale.

13. Reading problems that are due to spatial difficulties in scanning or maintaining position on a page may not show up on this test owing to the simplicity of the items. In cases where such problems are suspected, primarily when there are signs of visual–spatial disorders and complaints about reading problems, then a more detailed analysis with a test that looks at paragraph level reading (such as the LNNB Reading scale) is necessary.

14. Difficulty naming, along with significant spatial distortions of the key and cross, may indicate a lesion of the posterior nondominant hemisphere. In such cases, the problem lies not with naming but with the visual recognition process. In such cases, Picture Completion is usually performed poorly as are the Performance tests of the WAIS-III in general. However, good performance on Picture Completion generally rules out such a deficit. When this deficit exists, clients will do well on tests of naming by description (e.g., LNNB Expressive Language Scale), tests requiring verbal explanations without pictures (e.g., Comprehension, Information, Vocabulary, and Similarities on the WAIS-III) as well as on tests of verbal fluency (such as the Controlled Word Association Test).

15. The inability to follow simple commands suggests receptive language problems most often associated with a stroke or tumor if the person previously functioned at a higher level. Any errors on these items must be followed up in more detail. An error involving the inability to draw a given figure, such as the triangle, can be an error in comprehension or an inability to draw. In such a case, performance on this task should be compared to performance on a copying task (Greek Cross or key). If copying tasks are performed well, then receptive language issues must be considered. More detailed analysis can be achieved using the LNNB Receptive Language Scale. In addition, peripheral or central hearing losses must be ruled out before a language deficit is inferred. In more significant cases, receptive language problems will also be reflected in

performance on Comprehension and Vocabulary, but not in more subtle disorders.

16. Peripheral motor deficits will result in poor drawings on this instrument, but will not be accompanied by deficits on tests of nonmotor visual skills (such as Raven's Matrices or Visual Form Discrimination Test).

17. As a screening test, the Reitan Aphasia Examination test is rarely administered after a deficit has already been identified by another test or procedure, as it does not provide a detailed analysis of most of these conditions although it serves as a very successful short screening examination.

References for Reitan Aphasia Examination

Brooks, J., Fos, L. A., Greve, K. W., & Hammond, J. S. (1999). Assessment of executive function in patients with mild traumatic brain injury. *Journal of Trauma-Injury Infection and Critical Care*, 46(1), 159–163.

Heaton, R. K., Grant, I., & Matthews, C. G. (1991). *Comprehensive norms for an expanded Halstead-Reitan battery: Demographic corrections, research findings, and clinical applications*. Odessa, FL: Psychological Assessment Resources.

Jacobs, D. M., Sano, M., Albert, S., Schofiel, P., Dooneief, G., & Stern, Y. (1997). Cross-cultural neuropsychological assessment: A comparison of randomly selected, demographically matched cohorts of English- and Spanish-speaking older adults. *Journal of Clinical and Experimental Neuropsychology*, 19(3), 331–339.

Lezak, M. (1995). *Neuropsychological assessment* (3rd ed.). New York: Oxford University Press.

Reitan, R. M., & Wolfson, D. (1993). *The Halstead–Reitan neuropsychological test battery: Theory and clinical interpretation* (2nd ed.). S. Tucson, AZ: Neuropsychology Press.

Snyder, P. J., & Nussbaum, P. D. (1998). *Clinical neuropsychology: A pocket handbook for assessment*. Washington, D.C.: American Psychological Association.

Williams, J. M., & Shane, B. (1986). The Reitan–Indiana aphasia screening test: Scoring and factor analysis. *Journal of Clinical Psychology*, 42(1), 156–160.

INFORMATION (WAIS-III)

Information is one of the subtests of the Wechsler Adult Intelligence Scale. It is one of the simpler tests, asking the client basic questions that reflect things one learns primarily in the school setting. It is not widely used to detect neuropsychological abnormalities, but may be useful in establishing premorbid levels of functioning.

Interpretation

1. Information correlates highly with VIQ but is more related to educational experience than are such tests as Vocabulary and Comprehension.

2. An Information score that is significantly lower than Vocabulary and Comprehension scores suggests poor school achievement that is below the intellectual potential of the client. This pattern is rarely a sign of brain injury but rather reflects someone whose learning was outside of a traditional school context or attendance at a poorly functioning school.

3. In the absence of language deficits, Information may be averaged with Vocabulary and Comprehension to form a premorbid estimate of verbal functioning (see section on WAIS-III IQ).

4. When Information is four or more scale scores below Comprehension and Vocabulary, only Vocabulary and Comprehension should be used to estimate premorbid IQ.

5. When Information is more than four scale scores above Comprehension and Vocabulary, this suggests a possible problem in expressive language. Answers for Information items are shorter and generally require fewer expressive skills and less internal language analysis; thus, Information may be spared when there are mild to moderate language problems. These are frequently problems in "word finding" that interfere with the more language-based answers demanded by Vocabulary and Comprehension. However, more impaired naming will affect information as well. Poor performance on this subtest should be compared to performance on a naming test (such as the Boston Naming Test). If naming is poor, scores should not be interpreted as reflecting premorbid skills as they will likely underestimate premorbid functioning.

6. Low scores on Information, Vocabulary, and Comprehension, in comparison to other scores, are more consistent with early childhood brain injury than with adult-onset problems.

7. The WAIS-III Information subtest and the General Information subtest from the PIAT-R should be highly related to one another. Discrepancies of more than 15 standard score points may indicate fluctuating attention or motivation.

8. High scores on Information combined with low scores on Reading or Spelling may indicate specific learning disabilities (or other school-related problems) if the problems have been life long. If the problems are new, these patterns may reflect lesions of the dominant temporal–occipital areas of the brain which are often limited in scope, as more massive lesions will affect performance on Information as well.

9. Significantly lower Information scores than Reading scores in the presence of fluency deficits may suggest word finding difficulties which should be further evaluated with naming tasks. In some cases, this may reflect someone who has memorized word sounds using strong rote memory skills despite lower overall intellectual scores. This can be confirmed by the presence of poor Reading Comprehension scores, as well as poor performance on Vocabulary and Comprehension subtests.

10. Significantly lower Information than Spelling scores (which is rare) suggests an individual who has memorized word sounds using strong rote memory skills despite lower overall intellectual scores. This can be confirmed by poor scores on Reading Comprehension, Vocabulary, and Comprehension.

References for Information (WAIS-III)

Boone, D. E. (1998). Specificity of the WAIS-R subtests with psychiatric inpatients. *Assessment, 5*, 123–126.

Campbell, J. M., & McCord, D. M. (1996). The WAIS-R comprehension and picture arrangement subtests as measures of social intelligence: Testing traditional interpretations. *Journal of Psychoeducational Assessment, 14*, 240–249.

Golden, C. J., Zillmer, E., & Spiers, M. (1992). *Neuropsychological assessment and intervention.* Springfield, IL: Charles C Thomas.

Hawkins, K. A. (1998). Indicators of brain dysfunction derived from graphic representations of the WAIS-III/WMS-III Technical Manual clinical samples data: A preliminary approach to clinical utility. *Clinical Neuropsychologist, 12*(4), 535–555.

Kramer, J. H. (1990). Guidelines for interpreting the WAIS-R subtest scores. *Psychological Assessment, 2*, 202–205.

Matarazzo, J. D. (1972). *Wechsler's measurement and appraisal of adult intelligence* (5th ed.). New York: Oxford University Press.

Ryan, J. J., Lopez, S. J., & Werth, T. R. (1998). Administration time estimates for WAIS-III subtests, scales, and short forms in a clinical sample. *Journal of Psychoeducational Assessment, 16*(4), 315–323.

Sprandel, H. Z. (1995). *The psychoeducational use and interpretation of the Wechsler Adult Intelligence Scale-Revised* (2nd ed.). Springfield, IL: Charles C Thomas.

Wechsler, D. (1986). *WAIS-R administration and scoring manual.* San Antonio, TX: The Psychological Corporation.

Wechsler, D. (1997). *WAIS-III administration and scoring manual.* San Antonio, TX: The Psychological Corporation.

Wechsler, D. (1981). *WAIS-R manual.* New York: The Psychological Corporation.

COMPREHENSION (WAIS-III)

The Comprehension subtest is one of the six verbal subtests of the WAIS-III. It assesses the understanding of social convention or practical knowledge, as well as remote memory. In addition, this is a test of verbal reasoning and abstract logic. Comprehension includes 18 verbal items, which are orally presented. This task requires clients to respond verbally to a series of questions about everyday problems.

Interpretation

1. An inability to understand the orally presented questions is associated with receptive aphasia or severe intellectual impairment. In cases of auditory agnosia (inability to understand spoken speech), the client

may do better if the questions are presented visually (although such a procedure cannot be scored on the WAIS-III). Aphasic disorders of this type are usually associated with posterior left hemisphere lesions. However, disorders of auditory and reading problems may easily coexist. In such cases, deficits will be present across a wide range of verbal tests.

2. An inability to respond orally to a question may involve expressive language disorders. This may exist in the context of general problems with fluency which can be seen on the LNNB Expressive Language Test and similar procedures. In some cases, the test may elicit stuttering, slurring, and other signs of dysfluency that are not present in everyday conversation, as the client has more difficulty speaking properly when he has to focus on thinking at the same time. In most cases, expressive language (fluency) disorders are associated with left anterior or left subcortical lesions. However, some peripheral disorders also can cause expressive language problems.

3. Naming disorders may be evidenced in attempts by the client to use circumlocution (speaking around the words that cannot be found). In some cases, circumlocution may be misidentified as tangentiality. Suspected naming disorders should be verified on a test such as the Boston Naming Test. Naming disorders may reflect anterior or posterior lesions of the dominant hemisphere dependent on whether the general speech is fluent (posterior) or dysfluent (anterior). Because Comprehension uses no visual images, naming disorders seen on this test do not arise from visual agnosia or other possible causes of naming disorders.

4. In the absence of an expressive or receptive language disorder. Comprehension is considered, along with Information and Vocabulary, as a good "hold" test that is relatively insensitive to right hemisphere lesions and such etiologies as head trauma. The average of the age-corrected scaled scores of these subtests yields a baseline for comparing other age-corrected scale scores. Theoretically, other scores should be within 3 points (higher or lower) of this average. If other scores are consistently lower, then the presence of intellectual loss is suggested which may be seen in dementia, head trauma, and other conditions. A simple comparison of the average of Arithmetic, Digit Span, and Similarities can reveal whether these are 3 or more points lower than the baseline average. In cases where the baseline average is below the other scores, it is likely that any deficits go back to the client's early life rather than reflecting a recent injury.

5. Comprehension is a good measure of remote memory if it can be established that the material was previously learned. It is substantially affected by cultural factors, and therefore great care should be taken

when administering this test to someone who is not from the mainstream cultural or ethnic group (i.e., individual who is not born or raised in the United States, whose culture differs significantly from the normative group, or whose first language is not English). Although not reflected in the WAIS-III manual, answers from clients from other cultures should be considered for adequacy based on whether they are good or bad answers for the client's cultural background rather than being based simply on American norms and answers.

6. Clients with poor verbal memory may need repetition of the questions. This is especially a problem in clients with Verbal Memory Quotients (Immediate) of less than 80 on a test such as the WMS-III. Errors when the client forgets the question cannot be interpreted as reflecting the actual knowledge of the client.

7. Frontal clients may generate answers that are tangential or impulsive. Repetition of the question and focusing of the client is helpful in understanding the client's actual level of comprehension. This occurs most frequently in clients who show a high level of perseveration on the WCST or Category Test.

8. High-intelligence clients for whom this material is overlearned will show the least effects from a nonaphasic injury. However, lower IQ clients (with an original score that may have been below a scaled score of 6) are likely to show more loss from generalized brain injuries even in the absence of language problems. In such clients, these skills are less overlearned and more subject to disruption by diffuse injuries.

9. The Comprehension score is relatively insensitive to the effects of normal aging (with many improving with age), so losses with age more likely reflect a pathological process of some kind.

10. Comprehension correlates highly with VIQ. It is influenced by education but is less related to educational experience than the Information subtest, reflecting in many cases more general life experiences.

11. A Comprehension score that is significantly lower than Vocabulary and Information suggests problems with expressive speech or possible confusion that may have a neurological or psychological etiology. This pattern may be a sign of brain injury when there is evidence of dysfluency or substantial problems with memory testing.

12. In the absence of language deficits, Information may be averaged with Vocabulary and Comprehension to form a premorbid estimate of verbal functioning (see section on WAIS-III IQ).

13. When Comprehension is four or more scale scores below Information and Vocabulary, only Vocabulary and Information should be used to estimate premorbid IQ.

14. When Comprehension is more than four scale scores above Informa-

tion and Vocabulary, this suggests a possible problem in the educational experience. This can be the result of poor schooling, motivation, or attendance or it can reflect an inability to take advantage of school learning owing to early brain injury, retardation, or language barriers.

15. Low scores on Information, Vocabulary, and Comprehension, in comparison to other scores, are more consistent with early childhood brain injury than adult-onset problems.

16. Low scores on Picture Arrangement, along with low scores on Comprehension, may reflect poor awareness of societal norms and expectations. This can be associated with diffuse cognitive impairment or with significant mental illness. Both of these scores should be at least 3 points below the respective Verbal and Performance scale score means before this can be identified as a focal weakness (as opposed to simply reflecting lower overall cognitive skills).

References for Comprehension (WAIS-III)

Boone, D. E. (1998). Specificity of the WAIS-R subtests with psychiatric inpatients. *Assessment, 5,* 123–126.

Campbell, J. M., & McCord, D. M. (1996). The WAIS-R comprehension and picture arrangement subtests as measures of social intelligence: Testing traditional interpretations. *Journal of Psychoeducational Assessment, 14,* 240–249.

Golden, C. J., Zillmer, E., & Spiers, M. (1992). *Neuropsychological assessment and intervention.* Springfield, IL: Charles C Thomas

Hawkins, K. A. (1998). Indicators of brain dysfunction derived from graphic representations of the WAIS-III/WMS-III Technical Manual clinical samples data: A preliminary approach to clinical utility. *Clinical Neuropsychologist, 12*(4), 535–555.

Kramer, J. H. (1990). Guidelines for interpreting the WAIS-R subtest scores. *Psychological Assessment, 2,* 202–205.

Matarazzo, J. D. (1972). *Wechsler's measurement and appraisal of adult intelligence* (5th ed.). New York: Oxford University Press.

Ryan, J. J., Lopez, S. J., & Werth, T. R. (1998). Administration time estimates for WAIS-III subtests, scales, and short forms in a clinical sample. *Journal of Psychoeducational Assessment, 16*(4), 315–323.

Sprandel, H. Z. (1995). *The psychoeducational use and interpretation of the Wechsler Adult Intelligence Scale-Revised* (2nd ed.). Springfield, IL: Charles C Thomas.

Wechsler, D. (1981). *WAIS-R manual.* New York: The Psychological Corporation.

Wechsler, D. (1986). *WAIS-R administration and scoring manual.* San Antonio, TX: The Psychological Corporation.

Wechsler, D. (1997). *WAIS-III administration and scoring manual.* San Antonio, TX: The Psychological Corporation.

BOSTON NAMING TEST (BNT)

The Boston Naming Test (BNT) provides a detailed analysis of naming skills. Several neuropsychological conditions must be satisfied for a client to adequately perform the tasks required by the BNT. First, obviously, he or she must be awake, alert, and able to sustain attention and concentration. The client must be able to hear well enough to perceive the instructions and cues and to understand speech so that the test makes sense. Next, the client must demonstrate a sufficiently acute level of visual perception and the ability to integrate the individual percepts of the picture into an integrated whole. After perceiving the stimuli, the client is required to generate the correct name from a lexicon of possibilities and suppress all irrelevant and incorrect alternatives. Also, the client must have the ability to use expressive speech to give the answers.

Interpretation

1. One essential prerequisite for successful performance on the BNT is sufficiently clear visual perception. This can be established through performance on nonmotor visual tests such as the Visual Form Discrimination Test and Picture Completion. The presence of visual problems will invalidate the BNT. Naming is then best evaluated through description items (such as on the LNNB Expressive Language scale) and general verbal performance on the WAIS-III.

2. If only one hemisphere is affected, the client may suffer from loss of part of one of the visual fields (scotoma, quadrantanopia, or hemianopsia). In most cases, this partial loss of the visual field will not have an impact on the client's BNT performance. Typically, such defects are well compensated for by functional adaptations of the retina and movements of the eyes and head.

3. Lesions in the visual pathway of the right hemisphere, including the primary visual cortex, my result in unilateral neglect in which the client does not notice defects of the visual field and does not compensate for them with eye or head movements. As a result, the client can see only the right side of the stimulus pictures. The client may be unable to recognize the item because he can see only half of it, and will likely attribute his difficulties to presumed defects in the material presented. This will show up on numerous tests including the Benton, VFDT, and Matrices. In some cases, the BNT may be given if the stimulus is placed so that it is entirely within the right visual field.

4. Lesions of the secondary occipital regions are associated with visual agnosia, the inability to recognize complete objects or their pictorial representations. These clients have a disturbance of the synthesizing or integration function of visual percepts. Although they are able to see individual features, and sometimes even individual parts of the depicted objects, they cannot combine these individual features into a complete form. The client with a lesion of the secondary visual cortex will perceive only fragmented parts and will then attempt to deduce the

meaning of the entire image from those parts. Thus, when presented with a picture of a harmonica, the client will not know what it is and will examine it closely. He will then start to guess, perhaps saying "There is a square and another square and some lines, maybe walls, is it a building?" In cases of more localized lesions, these signs are less overt and become evident only when the client is shown more complex pictures. Thus, in less severe cases the client may be able to recognize and name the tree but not the abacus. In some clients with right hemisphere lesions, object naming may be intact but a basic defect in the attribution of ownership may be present. Thus, such a client may be able to identify the picture of the trellis but may recognize it as the one in his own yard. This deficit will be reflected in performance on Picture Completion as well as Picture Arrangement.

5. Poor performance on the BNT, when compared to other verbal identification tasks that do not require visual identification (such as Vocabulary, Similarities, and Comprehension), may indicate that the visual identification is a primary issue in the defect on the test.

6. Lesions involving the motor expression of speech will have an extremely disruptive effect on the test. In such cases the client may be able to demonstrate the use of an object or even describe its use but not be able to identify the specific name of the object. In such cases, speech will usually be dysfluent on any test of articulation. Such individuals will often produce impoverished general speech as well. Scores on most verbal measures will show significant impairment.

7. Massive lesions of the dominant hemisphere may result in global aphasia in which both receptive and expressive speech are impaired. Such cases do not benefit from the use of cues and show widespread problems throughout all tests of language, regardless of how they are presented. Such lesions are accompanied by right-sided motor and sensory deficits along with extremely poor performance on all tests with verbal content.

8. Clients with some frontal lesions may fail to scan the visual field, focusing on small segments, which leads to incorrect identifications. Such clients can do better when encouraged to look at the whole field as they have no problems in visual analysis per se, but rather are perseverative and show behavioral inertia. Clients with visual agnosia—who may present in the same way on the surface—will typically not benefit from such scanning or from encouragement. Again, these deficits will be seen on other picture identification tasks without a verbal or a motor component (Benton, VFDT, Picture Completion).

9. When a normal individual is asked to view and name an object, he perceives it visually and then attaches a verbal label to it. The label is, in

essence, a code, which considers the essential features of the object and places it into a semantic category. However, in a client with a parietal–occipital lesion of the dominant hemisphere, the integrity of the simultaneously existing semantic schemes is disturbed. Thus, when presented with a picture of an object, the amnestic (anomic) aphasic client may be able to determine the object's general classification, yet be unable to match it with its name. The anomic aphasic will be not be aided by the presentation of the semantic cue. He already is able to discern the basic classification in which the object belongs. He is unable to find the precise word within that system and match it with the picture. Therefore, when he is presented with the phonemic cue, the client will often be able to recall the correct name. Such individuals generally show fluent speech (although content may be effected) but have trouble with measures of Receptive Language (such as the LNNB Receptive Language scale). The performance on pure nonverbal and left-sided motor and sensory tasks are usually indicated as long as the client is able to understand the basic intent of each question and in the absence of motor impairment in the dominant hand.

10. Difficulties on the BNT, as they reflect basic language processes, may cause a lowering of scores across all verbal tests. This may invalidate interpretation of verbal tests of intelligence and executive skills.

References for Boston Naming Test (BNT)

Brooks, J., Fos, L. A., Greve, K. W., & Hammond, J. S. (1999). Assessment of executive function in patients with mild traumatic brain injury. *Journal of Trauma-Injury Infection and Critical Care*, *46*(1), 159–163.

Coen, R. F., Kidd, N., Denihan, A., Cunningham, C., Bruce, I., Buggy, F., O'Neill, D., Walsh, J. B., Coakley, D., & Lawlor, B. A. (1999). The utility of naming tests in the diagnosis of Alzheimer's disease. *Irish Journal of Psychological Medicine*, *1*(2), 43–46.

Fastenau, P. S. (1998). Validity of regression-based norms: An empirical test of the comprehensive norms with older adults. *Journal of Clinical and Experimental Neuropsychology*, *20*(6), 906–916.

Fastenau, P. S., Denburg, N. L., & Maue, B. A. (1998). Parallel short forms for the Boston Naming Test: Psychometric properties and norms for older adults. *Journal of Clinical and Experimental Neuropsychology*, *20*(6), 828–834.

Ferman, T. J., Ivnik, R. J., & Lucas, J. A. (1998). Boston naming test discontinuation rule: Rigorous versus lenient interpretations. *Assessment*, *5*(1), 13–18.

Goldman, W. P., Baty, J. D., Buckles, V. D., Sahrmann, S., & Morris, J. C. (1998). Cognitive and motor functioning in Parkinson's disease: Subjects with and without questionable dementia. *Archives of Neurology*, *55*(5), 674–680.

Henderson, L. W., Frank, E. M., Pigatt, T., Abramson, R. K., & Houston, M. (1998). Race, gender, and educational level effects on Boston Naming Test scores. *Aphasiology*, *12*(10), 901–911.

Kaplan, E. F., Goodglass, H., & Weintraub, S. (1983). *The Boston Naming Test* (2nd ed.). Philadelphia, PA: Lea & Febiger.

Kohnert, K. J., Hernandez, A. E., & Bates, E. (1998). Bilingual performance on the Boston Naming Test: Preliminary norms in Spanish and English. *Brain and Language, 65*(3), 422–440.

Larrain, C. M., & Cimino, C. R. (1998). Alternate forms of the Boston Naming Test in Alzheimer's disease. *Clinical Neuropsychologist, 12*(4), 525–530.

Lezak, M. D. (1995). *Neuropsychological assessment* (3rd ed.). New York: Oxford University Press.

Lukatel, K., Malloy, P., Jenkins, M., & Cohen, R. (1998). The naming deficit in early Alzheimer's and vascular dementia. *Neuropsychology, 12*(4), 565–572.

Ross, T. P., & Lichtenberg, P. A. (1998). Expanded normative data for the Boston Naming Test for use with urban, elderly medical patients. *Clinical Neuropsychologist, 12*(4), 475–481.

Snyder, P. J., & Nussbaum, P. D. (1998). *Clinical neuropsychology: A pocket handbook for assessment.* Washington, D.C.: American Psychological Association.

SIMILARITIES (WAIS-III)

This is a subtest of the Wechsler Adult Intelligence Scale. The original idea was adapted from similar procedures used as part of mental status examinations. The test attempts to tap into abstract verbal skills thought to theoretically reflect higher cortical functions of the brain.

Interpretation

1. Similarities offers a good estimate of general intelligence in normal populations, but is more scattered in brain–injured patients and is not considered to be a good estimate of premorbid functions because of its partial sensitivity to a variety of injuries and its lower correlation with general intelligence than tests such as Vocabulary.

2. Very low scores on Similarities, defined as profiles in which it is the lowest Wechsler verbal score by 3 or more points (not including Arithmetic), suggests impairment in verbal abstract skills. Such clients usually show very concrete responding, giving a large number of 1 point responses after the initial simple items. This can be a reflection of prefrontal injuries which can be identified through deficits in such verbal tests as the Stroop, Trails B, and Controlled Word Association and nonverbal tests such as WCST and Category. The interpretation of a localized prefrontal injury is strengthened if these scores occur in the absence of language, motor, or sensory problems.

3. If the low Similarities score is accompanied by fluent expressive language but impairment in general language problems (such as BNT, Aphasia Screen, LNNB Receptive Language), injury to the parietal lobe around the angular gyrus should be considered.

4. If a low Similarities score is attained along with a poor BNT score, then the impairment may be less a restriction of abstract thought and reflect word-finding problems.

5. A Similarities score that is 5 or more points higher than Matrix Reasoning may indicate a specific problem in nonverbal reasoning that may reflect nondominant hemisphere or subcortical injuries. Block Design is usually depressed in these cases as well, along with Category and the WCST. Performance on Controlled Word Association and the Stroop will typically be in the normal range in individuals with this disorder.

6. When Similarities is 5 or more points lower than Matrix Reasoning, this may indicate a specific problem in verbal reasoning. This can be seen in the impairment of executive tests that are primarily verbal (Controlled Word Association, Stroop, Trail Making Test) while the nonverbal executive tests (Category, WCST) are intact.

7. At scale scores below 10, Similarities may measure less abstractive skills. As a result, the lack of change after a brain injury in a low IQ client may not indicate that abstract skills have remained intact. Similarly, more intelligent individuals may experience the task as too simple and overlearned, again failing to show any evidence of abstract problems. These weaknesses make the subtest unreliable in identifying abstractive deficits.

8. Although sometimes offered as a measure of temporal lobe function on the dominant side, the sensitivity appears to be related as often to problems in language or impulsivity rather than the abstractive nature of the task. This relationship to temporal functioning is inconsistent in the literature and should be considered unreliable.

References for Similarities (WAIS-III)

Boone, D. E. (1998). Specificity of the WAIS-R subtests with psychiatric inpatients. *Assessment, 5,* 123–126.

Campbell, J. M., & McCord, D. M. (1996). The WAIS-R comprehension and picture arrangement subtests as measures of social intelligence: Testing traditional interpretations. *Journal of Psychoeducational Assessment, 14,* 240–249.

Golden, C. J., Zillmer, E., & Spiers, M. (1992). *Neuropsychological assessment and intervention.* Springfield, IL: Charles C Thomas.

Hawkins, K. A. (1998). Indicators of brain dysfunction derived from graphic representations of the WAIS-III/WMS-III Technical Manual clinical samples data: A preliminary approach to clinical utility. *Clinical Neuropsychologist, 12*(4), 535–555.

Kramer, J. H. (1990). Guidelines for interpreting the WAIS-R subtest scores. *Psychological Assessment, 2,* 202–205.

Matarazzo, J. D. (1972). *Wechsler's measurement and appraisal of adult intelligence* (5th ed.). New York: Oxford University Press.

Ryan, J. J., Lopez, S. J., & Werth, T. R. (1998). Administration time estimates for WAIS-III subtests, scales, and short forms in a clinical sample. *Journal of Psychoeducational Assessment, 16*(4), 315–323.

Sprandel, H. Z. (1995). *The psychoeducational use and interpretation of the Wechsler Adult Intelligence Scale-Revised* (2nd ed.). Springfield, IL: Charles C Thomas.

Wechsler, D. (1981). *WAIS-R manual*. New York: The Psychological Corporation.
Wechsler, D. (1986). *WAIS-R administration and scoring manual*. San Antonio, TX: The Psychological Corporation.
Wechsler, D. (1997). *WAIS-III administration and scoring manual*. San Antonio, TX: The Psychological Corporation.

SPEECH–SOUNDS PERCEPTION TEST (SSPT)

A component of the Halstead–Reitan Neuropsychological Battery, the Speech–Sounds Perception Test (SSPT) measures not only auditory perception, but also attention/concentration. In general, this test is a sensitive indicator of brain damage, measuring a wide variety of skills including attention, concentration, receptive language, spelling, reading, and decision making. Halstead originally conceived of the test as a measure of frontal skills, but later work has identified a broader role for the test.

Interpretation

1. The score on the SSPT reflects the number of pseudowords misidentified on the answer sheet. This score is often compared to the results of the Seashore Rhythm Test (SRT), which has a greater attention and concentration component. Thus, if scores on the SSPT are worse, this suggests that the language components are more likely the cause of the problem (implicating the left hemisphere). If the SRT scores are worse, this suggests that the attention/concentration or nonverbal aspects of the stimuli are responsible, indicating a right hemisphere or subcortical focus. While the SSPT can be compared to other tests requiring concentration, the SRT is almost a perfect comparison test because it uses similar skills and procedures to those of the SSPT.
2. Scores should be compared with achievement test scores in reading and spelling. If significant spelling or reading problems exist, the SSPT cannot be interpreted beyond suggesting the presence of reading or spelling problems.
3. Scores should also be compared to tests of language comprehension (aphasia exams). The presence of phonemic deficits invalidates the other aspects of this test. Receptive aphasia can also be tested by having the client repeat the words on the test rather than identify their spelling. In the absence of an expressive language (fluency) deficit, the inability to repeat the words would point to a receptive language or hearing deficit.
4. Clients who tend to pick the same answer every time (usually the first or last answer) may be showing frontal perseverative problems. This may

also be reflected in perseverative performance on tests such as Category and WCST.

5. Clients who consistently miss only the ending consonant or beginning consonant may be exhibiting receptive language problems, whereby the speed of processing phonemes is impaired. Such individuals may not present with deficits in conversation or when hearing familiar or over-learned words. More detailed analysis of phonemic skills is appropriate in such cases, such as the analysis on the LNNB Receptive Language Scale.

6. The test should not be used with illiterate clients or clients whose primary language is not English, as the norms are inappropriate.

7. Good performance on SSPT rules out the presence of a significant phonemic deficit and establishes the presence of adequate short-term attentional and concentration skills. Such clients also tend to show few signs of impulsiveness or perseveration that are neurologically based.

8. In cases where attentional tests are impaired, SSPT scores may simply reflect attentional inconsistency. Administration of the test one item at a time will usually yield vastly improved scores.

References for Speech–Sounds Perception Test

Charter, R. A., & Dobbs, S. M. (1998). Long and short forms of the speech-sounds perception test: Item analysis and age and education corrections. *Clinical Neuropsychologist, 12*(2), 213–216.

Charter, R. A., & Dutra, R. L. (1998). Speech–Sounds Perception Test: Analysis of a randomized answer form. *Perceptual and Motor Skills, 87*(1), 64–66.

Charter, R. A., Dutra, R. L., & Lopez, M. N. (1997). Speech–Sounds Perception Test: Analysis of error types in normal and diffusely brain damaged patients. *Perceptual and Motor Skills, 84*, 1507–1510.

Golden, C. J., & Anderson, S. M. (1977). Short form of the Speech–Sounds Perception Test. *Perceptual and Motor Skills, 45*, 485–486.

Keyser, D. J., & Sweetland, R. C. (1984). The Halstead–Reitan Neuropsychological Battery and Allied Procedures. In *Test Critiques*, Vol. I. Kansas City, MO: Test Corporation of America.

Lezak, M. (1995). Perception. In *Neuropsychological Assessment* (3rd ed.). New York: Oxford University Press.

Ryan, J. J., & Larsen, J. (1983). Comparison of three Speech Sounds Perception Test short forms. *Clinical Neuropsychology, 5*(4), 173–175.

Stringer, A. Y., & Green, R. C. (1996). Stimulus Imperception. In *A guide to adult neuropsychological diagnosis*. Philadelphia, PA: F. A. Davis.

EXPRESSIVE SPEECH SCALE (C6, LNNB)

The Expressive Speech Scale is a subtest of the Luria–Nebraska Neuropsychological Battery (LNNB) designed for the purpose of evaluating the client's ability to repeat simple sounds and words and to produce automatic as well as more complex verbal statements. This scale is not intended to assess the meaningfulness of the client's statements but rather the fluency and articulatory skills of the client. In general, this scale detects injuries in the left hemisphere, especially in the temporal–frontal area and parietal lobe. However, individual sections of the scale can be analyzed independently for further, more specific interpretations. The entire test may be given or portions to select specific functions (naming, articulation, repetition, automatic speech, and expressive–intellectual skills) may be administered as a result of observations in other test procedures.

Interpretation

1. Elevated scores overall on the Expressive Speech Scale, especially those above 70T, generally indicate left hemisphere injury. Usually, this injury involves the temporal–frontal area, especially the posterior part of the frontal lobe. Such deficits are characterized by poor expressive fluency and poor performance on the WAIS-III verbal tests and the Boston Naming Test.
2. In cases where the client's deficits do not involve fluency and scores exceed a T-score of 70, the damage is most likely to the parietal lobe. This is usually accompanied by impaired scores on the Boston Naming Test, measures of verbal intelligence, and achievement deficits.
3. When scores are impaired but less than a T-score of 70, injury to prefrontal or right hemisphere lesions must be considered. Right hemisphere injuries will generally not affect any of the basic items on the test, although injuries that result in paralysis of the left side of the face and tongue can cause slurring or slowing of oral motor processes and speech. Right hemisphere injuries can also affect items on the second half of the scale representing backwards sequencing (items 161 and 163), picture interpretation (164–165), identification of pictures (157–158), and incomplete or mixed up sentences (170–174). Prefrontal injuries (anterior to the motor areas as measured by intact performance on Motor tests) will produce problems on the same items, but because of problems with impulsivity, inflexibility, and perseveration.
4. The first and second sections of the scale require the client to repeat sounds and words after reading (145–153) or hearing them (133–144). If a client is able to pass either one of these sections, he or she does not have significant basic expressive speech deficits. These items are a good section to administer when performance on the Aphasia Screen or elsewhere suggests the possibility of fluency problems.
5. In cases where reading items results in normal speech but auditory presentation does not, this suggests a problem in receptive language or repetition rather than in fluency. This should be evaluated through a

more detailed receptive language evaluation with the LNNB Receptive Language Scale as well as the Speech–Sounds Perception Test.

6. In cases where repeating items results in normal speech but reading does not, a reading decoding or visual decoding problem is suggested. This can be evaluated through any of the achievement tests.

7. In profiles where only repetition is impaired across the scale, a disconnection disorder between the receptive and expressive language areas should be investigated. If an injury is limited to this deficit, other verbal tests may be performed normally as comprehension typically is not affected.

8. If the client is unable to produce speech spontaneously after looking at a picture, hearing a story, or being given a discussion topic (items 164–169), but seems to have no difficulty performing other items of the scale, there is the possibility of low intelligence and/or frontal lobe damage. Cases of low intelligence will be seen on the WAIS-III or PPVT. In prefrontal injuries, intelligence will generally be normal while executive tests such as Category, Trails B, or the WCST will be performed in an abnormal manner.

9. If elevated scores are limited to the more complex items of the battery, such as items 170–174, then the damage is located in the prefrontal area of the brain rather than the more posterior areas.

10. Naming disorders from visual images (157–158) and description (159) are tested. These evaluate basic naming problems but not to the extent of the Boston Naming Test. Problems with just the visual presentation suggest a visual rather than a naming problem, while problems with just the description items suggest a receptive comprehension problem speech rather than a basic naming disorder.

11. Items 160 and 162 require naming the days of the week and counting forward, while items 161 and 163 require this information backwards. In some cases of milder expressive disorder, the additional stress of repeating backwards will cause a deterioration in speech performance. In such cases, it is assumed that normal speech is the result of extensive effort on the client's part. This effort is disturbed by the demands of the intellectual task, causing the reappearance of the expressive problems. This may be seen after mild disorders or in clients who have recovered from more serious injuries with the deficits representing residual problems. Such deficits will occur only in verbal tasks that are challenging to the client. The level of difficulty needed for such a challenge to occur is dependent on intelligence. These subtle deficits are often seen in individuals who suffered a serious injury but now appear to be recovered. In such cases these represent mild residual deficits of the more serious earlier problems.

12. All the items after 157 require an intellectual as well as motor speech component. It is essential to note the nature of errors in these items. Motor speech/fluency problems on these items are consistent with injuries to Broca's area while other errors are attributed to the interaction of cognitive and motor speech functions. These errors should be classified as precisely as possible through qualitative observation of the client's performance. In general, those deficits due to motor speech alone will not affect other tests that do not penalize for speech problems except in cases where the problem is so severe as to limit communication. In such cases, tests such as the PPVT and other verbal tests that do not require an oral response are useful to investigate cognitive deficits, as well as allowing the client to write answers (when there is no writing disorder present).

References for Expressive Speech Scale (C6, LNNB)

Chelune, G. J. (1982). A reexamination of the relationship between the Luria–Nebraska and Halstead-Reitan batteries: Overlap with the WAIS. *Journal of Consulting and Clinical Psychology, 59,* 578–580.

Golden, C. J., & Grier, C. A. (1998). Detecting malingering on the Luria–Nebraska Neuropsychological Battery (pp. 133–162). *Detection of malingering during head injury litigation.* New York: Plenum Press.

Golden, C. J., Purisch, A. D., & Hammeke, T. A. (1985). *Luria–Nebraska Neuropsychological Battery: Forms I and II Manual.* Los Angeles: Western Psychological Services.

Mayes, A. R. (1995). The assessment of memory disorders. In A. D. Baddeley, B. A. Wilson, et al. (Eds.), *Handbook of memory disorders* (pp. 367–391). Chichester, England: John Wiley & Sons.

McKinzey, R. K., Roecker, C. E., Puente, A. E., & Rogers, E. B. (1998). Performance of normal adults on the Luria–Nebraska Neuropsychological Battery, Form I. *Archives of Clinical Neuropsychology, 13*(4), 397–413.

Moses, J. A., & Pritchard, D. A. (1999). Performance scales for the Luria–Nebraska Neuropsychological Battery-Form I. *Archives of Clinical Neuropsychology, 14*(5), 285–302.

Moses, J. A., & Purisch, A. D. (1997). The evolution of the Luria–Nebraska Neuropsychological Battery-Form I (pp. 131–170). *Contemporary approaches to neuropsychological assessment.* New York: Plenum Press.

RECEPTIVE SPEECH (C5, LNNB)

Scale C5 of the Luria–Nebraska Neuropsychological Battery (LNNB) is a simple test that is used to screen for deficits in the functional system of receptive speech. Consistent with conventional views about the specific brain anatomy thought to be correlated with receptive speech, C5 is generally used as a means by which to detect damage to the left hemisphere and the left temporal lobe in particular, given the subject is right-handed and his or her brain functions are lateralized in a typical manner. However, many items on C5 tap abilities that extend beyond the left temporal lobe to include the widespread anatomical sites involved in various levels of receptive speech. As with the other LNNB scales discussed in this volume, the scale may be given as a whole to screen for a wide range of problems or specific sections may be administered to follow up on findings from other parts of a test battery.

Interpretation

1. Elevated T-scores for scale C5 indicate that the examinee is impaired with respect to receptive speech. Damage to the left hemisphere is strongly suspected, particularly to the left temporal lobe, although damage to other areas of the brain cannot be completely ruled out without first conducting an item analysis. Scores above 70T are strongly suggestive of impairment to the dominant hemisphere, while lower elevations may be seen in nondominant hemisphere injuries.

2. For items 100 through 105, the examinee hears simple phonemes and then must repeat or write them. The examiner is to note whether the examinee is able to say them, write them, or both. The ability to repeat phonemes but not to write them suggests impairment in the left angular gyrus. The ability to write phonemes but not to say them suggests a disorder of repetition rather than receptive speech, consistent with damage to the inferior divisions of the premotor (Broca's) area or damage to areas connecting these divisions to the temporal lobe. If the client is unable to respond correctly in either written or verbal form, a deficit in phonemic discrimination is suspected, consistent with damage to the left superior temporal lobe. Items 100–107 act as a good screen for potential phonemic hearing deficits which may be suggested by Speech–Sounds or in misunderstanding of verbal material anywhere in the test battery.

3. Item 106 requires the examinee to discriminate phonemes by appropriately raising the right or left hand rather than via verbal response. Left temporal lobe damage and, in some cases, interhemispheric damage can affect performance on this item. If the client can perform these items, but not repeat phonemes or write them, the possibility of a general motor problem must be considered. This can be done using other language tests that do not require a verbal response (such as PPVT).

4. Item 107 tests the ability to understand phonemes spoken at different levels of pitch. Damage to the right temporal lobe may affect performance on this item. When seen alone, it is most significant when there is a context of poor performance on nonverbal tests such as Rhythm, Block Design, Matrices, and the Benton Test of Line Orientation in the absence of specific problems on verbal tests. These deficits may lead to individuals who have trouble understanding the nonverbal (e.g., emotional)

aspects of speech and those who speak languages in which tone is an inherent part of the communication (such as Chinese).

5. Items 108 through 122 involve the understanding of simple words, sentences, and instructions. The examinee performs relatively simple tasks of naming, pointing, identification, following simple directions, and defining simple words. The intent is to determine if the client is hearing properly and correctly interpreting what is said to him or her. Impairment on these items indicates the need for caution in interpreting all other tests, as clients may not understand instructions. Paraphrasing and simplification of instructions may be necessary to allow the other tests to be meaningfully interpreted. Damage to the left temporal lobe or the left temporal–occipital region (angular gyrus) may affect performance on these items.

6. Items 118 through 132 can also be affected by damage to the right hemisphere as they require a degree of logical/spatial orientation on the part of the examinee. If the examinee appears to understand the sentence, but shows spatial difficulty, right hemisphere damage is suspected. Items that require comparisons (e.g., 121, 122, and 125 through 131) are also sensitive to left parietal–occipital damage, although they may also be affected by lack of examinee understanding due to damage to the left temporal lobe or the angular gyrus. Impairment on these procedures in the presence of intact performance on the earlier items will usually be accompanied by a pattern of spatial deficits on such tests as the Bender, Benton Test of Line Orientation, Block Design, and Matrices.

7. Impairment on the latter items has implications for the understanding of more complex instructions typically seen on tests of executive function, such as Category and WCST. In cases where a language problem exists, the potential role of the language deficit must be considered in analyzing any impaired performance on the executive tests.

8. Performance on the more complex items from 122 to 132 may be affected by severe memory disorders as well. When this is suspected, asking the client to repeat items is a good way to see if he or she have adequately retained the information for analysis. If he or she is unable to repeat the items, then the level of cognitive analysis cannot be determined.

References for Receptive Speech (C5, LNNB)

Chelune, G. J. (1982). A reexamination of the relationship between the Luria–Nebraska and Halstead–Reitan batteries: Overlap with the WAIS. *Journal of Consulting and Clinical Psychology, 50,* 578–580.

Golden, C. J., Purisch, A. D., & Hammeke, T. A. (1985). *Luria–Nebraska Neuropsychological Battery: Forms I and II Manual.* Los Angeles: Western Psychological Services.

Mayes, A. R. (1995). The assessment of memory disorders. In A. D. Baddeley, B. A. Wilson, et al. (Eds.), *Handbook of memory disorders* (pp. 367–391). Chichester, England: John Wiley & Sons.

SECTION IV: NONVERBAL TESTS

PICTURE ARRANGEMENT (WAIS-III)

The Picture Arrangement subtest of the WAIS-III consists of 11 sets of comic-strip-like picture cards. The cards are presented to the examinee in a standard mixed-up order and the examinee rearranges the cards to create a logical story within the specified time limit (Wechsler, 1997). According to Matarazzo (1972), the Picture Arrangement subtest is the type of test that "effectively measures a subject's ability to comprehend and size up a total situation." It requires the ability to perceive the whole or "gestalt" of a situation. In addition, it is believed to require the skills of perceptual organization, sequencing, verbal comprehension, planning ability, and social knowledge.

Interpretation

1. While Picture Arrangement is included among the Performance tests on the WAIS-III, it shares a great deal of variance with the Verbal tests. While the attention and analysis of visual detail is crucial to the test, verbal skills are necessary for constructing an appropriate story and detecting the logic and pattern of the details. As a result, the test can be sensitive to lesions of both hemispheres.

2. Performance of Picture Arrangement should be compared directly to the average scaled score performance of the purer visual–spatial tests (Block Design, Matrices, Picture Completion). If Picture Arrangement is more than 3 points below these scores, a defect in verbal or executive/sequencing skill should be considered.

3. When a sequencing deficit is suspected, it is best identified through looking at the difference between Digit Span Forward and Backwards as well as Spatial Span Forward and Backwards. In cases where Picture Arrangement is more than 3 points below the Picture Completion, Block Design and Matrices average and either Digits Backwards or Spatial Span Backwards is impaired (more than 4 raw score points below the respective Forward score), a sequencing deficit can be strongly inferred.

4. If both Digits Backwards and Spatial Span Backwards are impaired relative to the forward scores along with Picture Arrangement relative

to the Performance scores, a generalized sequencing deficit can be inferred. If only Digits Backwards is impaired along with Picture Arrangement, then a more specific verbal sequencing deficit should be considered. Conversely, if only Spatial Span Backwards and Picture Arrangement are impaired, then a specific visual sequencing deficit can be inferred.

5. If neither Spatial Span Backwards or Digit Span Backwards is impaired while Picture Arrangement is down relative to the spatial scores, a verbal deficit in the Picture Arrangement should be considered. In such cases, VIQ will generally be at least 12 points below PIQ or VCIQ will be 12 points below POIQ.

6. If there is no evidence of sequencing or verbal problems, the role of executive/frontal dysfunction in Picture Arrangement should be considered when it is depressed compared to Block Design, Picture Completion, and Matrices. In such cases, verbal and performance IQs should be within normal limits, while there is impairment in tests of executive function such as the WCST, Category, and Trail Making Part B.

7. When Picture Arrangement is the lowest score in a WAIS-III profile, the possibility of a right anterior lesion should be considered. In such cases, basic posterior skills (verbal and spatial) are intact, while the nonverbal sequencing/analysis skills are impaired. This may arise from some left anterior lesions as well. The absence of such a deficit, however, does not rule out an anterior lesion.

8. Analysis of how a client performs is important. This can be achieved after the test is over by asking the client to describe the pictures and to tell the story he or she used. This allows the examiner to determine if the visual details were seen properly and the logic of the story employed.

9. In cases of unilateral neglect arising from right posterior lesions, the client may ignore the cards on the left side of the line of cards or the left side of individual cards. When one determines this is occurring, it helps to shift all the cards to the right so that other aspects of the test may be examined. This will also be evident on the construction tasks (such as the Benton), visual–spatial tasks (such as Visual Form Discrimination), and the WAIS-III Matrices and Raven's Matrices tasks.

10. In cases of visual agnosia, the client will be unable to focus on the picture as a whole and will see only one object or section of the picture. He or she is unable to perceive the remainder even when prompted. This finding is indicative of a posterior lesion. Generally, there is significant impairment in Picture Completion and visual naming tasks, such as the Boston Naming test.

11. Aphasic clients who are unable to communicate well but can verbally reason may show good Picture Arrangement scores. This is suggestive of verbal skills being stronger than they appear, as well as the clients having intact visual skills.

12. Clients with significant frontal lesions may focus on one part of the pictures and confabulate the remainder. They are, however, able to recognize other aspects of the picture when cued.

13. Poor scores on Picture Arrangement, along with poor scores on Comprehension, may reflect poor awareness of societal norms and expectations. This can be associated with diffuse cognitive impairment or with significant mental illness. These scores should both be at least 3 points below the respective Verbal and Performance scale score means before this is identified as a focal weakness (as opposed to simply reflecting lower overall cognitive skills).

14. Clients who attempt to solve the sets of pictures on a trial-and-error basis, that is, arranging them in various sequences to see if they make sense, are demonstrating a lower level of perceptual organization. In the absence of visual deficits, this suggests a frontal lesion. Other scores should reflect a frontal pattern as described previously.

15. Some clients with left frontal lesions may be unable to use speech internally to organize the information in the pictures. Such clients will spontaneously describe the picture out loud to themselves in order to use language comprehension skills to analyze rather than use their more internalized frontal skills. This will usually be associated both with verbal comprehension deficits and frontal executive signs.

16. Motor skills play a minor role in Picture Arrangement, so high scores on Picture Arrangement, Matrices, and Picture Completion relevant to Digit Symbol and Block Design should lead to analysis of more basic motor measures. This should include loss of basic motor skills as measured by Finger Tapping or Purdue Pegboard in the dominant hand and impairment on Visual–Motor tasks such as the Benton and Bender, as well as the Tactual Performance Test.

17. Impaired scores primarily on the Seashore Rhythm Test, Rey Figure (or other complex drawing test), Picture Arrangement, and Digits Backwards may suggest an anterior right hemisphere injury.

References for Picture Arrangement (WAIS-III)

Boone, D. E. (1998). Specificity of the WAIS-R subtests with psychiatric inpatients. *Assessment, 5,* 123–126.

Campbell, J. M., & McCord, D. M. (1996). The WAIS-R comprehension and picture arrangement subtests as measures of social intelligence: Testing traditional interpretations. *Journal of Psychoeducational Assessment, 14,* 240–249.

Golden, C. J., Zillmer, E., & Spiers, M. (1992). *Neuropsychological assessment and intervention*. Springfield, IL: Charles C Thomas.

Kramer, J. H. (1990). Guidelines for interpreting the WAIS-R subtest scores. *Psychological Assessment, 2*, 202–205.

Matarazzo, J. D. (1972). *Wechsler's measurement and appraisal of adult intelligence* (5th ed.). New York: Oxford University Press.

Sprandel, H. Z. (1995). *The psychoeducational use and interpretation of the Wechsler Adult Intelligence Scale-Revised* (2nd ed.). Springfield, IL: Charles C Thomas.

Wechsler, D. (1981). *WAIS-R manual*. New York: The Psychological Corporation.

Wechsler, D. (1986). *WAIS-R administration and scoring manual*. San Antonio, TX: The Psychological Corporation.

Wechsler, D. (1997). *WAIS-III administration and scoring manual*. San Antonio, TX: The Psychological Corporation.

DIGIT SYMBOL (WAIS-III)

Digit Symbol is a subtest of the Wechsler Adult Intelligence Scale. It is a complex, timed, fine motor test, which makes it sensitive to a wide array of brain injuries and also to psychiatric, motivational, and other non-neurological problems. It is a useful test but must be analyzed carefully before any conclusions are reached.

Interpretation

1. Digit Symbol measures fine motor control, speed, memory, stress tolerance, and sustained attention, making it a highly sensitive test to a wide range of neurological and psychiatric disorders. It acts as an excellent screening test for pathology in general but cannot be used to pinpoint etiology.

2. When evaluating the Digit Symbol score, many factors within the test need to be separated. Performance should be compared to purer measures of motor function, such as Finger Tapping (FT). In cases where FT is depressed in the dominant writing hand, Digit Symbol most likely is affected even when performed with an intact nondominant hand.

3. Since motor skills play a minor role in Picture Arrangement, Matrices, and Picture Completion, higher scores relevant to Digit Symbol and Block Design should also lead to analysis of more basic motor measures. This should include loss of basic motor skills as measured by Finger Tapping or Purdue Pegboard in the dominant hand and impairment on Visual–Motor tasks such as the Benton and Bender as well as the Tactual Performance Test.

4. The WAIS-III contains a copying task using the Digit Symbol symbols as stimuli (optional). If this is performed at normal speed, motor speed

concerns can be eliminated. This should be associated with normal performance on other copying tasks such as the Bender and Benton as well.

5. The role of memory in Digit Symbol is also important. In cases in which immediate memory or working memory are implanted, deficits on Digit Symbol are expected as well.

6. If Digit Symbol is significantly better (by 4 or more scale points) than Digit Span, the role of numerical memory or emotional reactions to "math" may be involved in the Digit Span performance. This will be associated with poor performance on the Arithmetic subtest on the WAIS-III and achievement tests as well (e.g., PIAT-R, WRAT-3, LNNB).

7. If Digit Span and Number–Letter Memory are better than Digit Symbol by 4 or more points, motor problems or visual problems are more likely the cause of the deficit. If visual skills are impaired sufficiently to affect Digit Symbol, deficits would also be seen on basic visual tasks such as Visual Form Discrimination and Picture Completion, as well as basic copying tasks (such as the Bender). If such visual signs are missing and there is no evidence of a motor speed problem, a relatively low Digit Symbol score may reflect problems with stress tolerance.

8. Digit Symbol on the WAIS-III offers an optional incidental learning scale to help rule out memory problems. Poor performance on this optional part of the test implies a memory component to any deficit. Good performance on this task likely rules out a significant role for memory in the client's problem. A poor performance should be reflected in poor immediate visual memory scores, impairment in Spatial Span scores, and poor performance on the Benton short memory tasks relative to copying.

9. Good performance on the optional copying phase rules out visual impairment as the cause of the performance deficit.

References for Digit Symbol (WAIS-III)

Boone, D. E. (1998). Specificity of the WAIS-R subtests with psychiatric inpatients. *Assessment, 5,* 123–126.

Campbell, J. M., & McCord, D. M. (1996). The WAIS-R comprehension and picture arrangement subtests as measures of social intelligence: Testing traditional interpretations. *Journal of Psychoeducational Assessment, 14,* 240–249.

Golden, C. J., Zillmer, E., & Spiers, M. (1992). *Neuropsychological assessment and intervention.* Springfield, IL: Charles C Thomas.

Kramer, J. H. (1990). Guidelines for interpreting the WAIS-R subtest scores. *Psychological Assessment, 2,* 202–205.

Matarazzo, J. D. (1972). *Wechsler's measurement and appraisal of adult intelligence* (5th ed.). New York: Oxford University Press.

Sprandel, H. Z. (1995). *The psychoeducational use and interpretation of the Wechsler Adult Intelligence Scale-Revised* (2nd ed.). Springfield, IL: Charles C Thomas.

Wechsler, D. (1981). *WAIS-R manual*. New York: The Psychological Corporation.
Wechsler, D. (1986). *WAIS-R administration and scoring manual*. San Antonio, TX: The Psychological Corporation.
Wechsler, D. (1997). *WAIS-III administration and scoring manual*. San Antonio, TX: The Psychological Corporation.

PICTURE COMPLETION SUBTEST (WAIS-III)

Picture Completion is a simple test that requires the client to identify verbally or nonverbally what essential detail is missing in a drawing. As it is included in the Wechsler Adult Intelligence Scale, it is a frequently given test in neuropsychological evaluations, although it is not considered particularly sensitive to the presence of brain damage.

Interpretation

1. In the WAIS-R, Picture Completion was the best estimator of premorbid Performance IQ. This is likely to be true on the WAIS-III as well. The absence of a significant motor, spatial, or speed component makes it the least sensitive of the WAIS-III performance tests to brain injury.
2. In the WAIS-III, preliminary evidence suggests that Picture Completion and Matrix Reasoning are the best two estimators of premorbid intelligence. In the WAIS-R, Picture Completion and Object Assembly were considered to provide the two best estimates of premorbid intelligence.
3. Measures from within the WAIS-III that best predict premorbid IQ include Information, Comprehension, Vocabulary, and Picture Arrangement. This is based on the assumption that these are "hold" tests, which theoretically "hold" their scores even after a brain injury or other disorder. While such scores do work in individual cases, there are many circumstances in which they do not. First, individuals with language problems as a result of an injury will often have lower scores on these measures. Second, visual problems will interfere with performance on Picture Arrangement (although the pictures on the WAIS-III are much easier to see than in previous versions of the WAIS).
4. In cases where the prediction is against Full Scale IQ, all four subtest scores (Comprehension, Vocabulary, Information, and Picture Arrangement) should be summed. The score is then divided by 4 (to get an average) and multiplied by 11 (to project the score to a full 11 subtest Full Scale IQ). This can be translated to a Full Scale IQ by using the Full Scale IQ table in the WAIS-III manual.

5. Impaired performance on Picture Completion compared to the other performance tests (the lowest performance by 2 or more scale points and more than 3 points below the average of Performance scale scores) is rare. While poor performance can be based on attention, understanding of instructions, visual agnosia, poor eyesight, or lack of motivation, such factors should affect the other tests as well, such that profiles with Picture Completion 4 or more points below the Performance Mean are difficult to interpret and may suggest malingering or a lack of effort. Readministration of the test is often useful in these circumstances.

6. Profiles with low Picture Completion scores that have many "I don't know" answers may be misleading and reflect a lack of effort. The examiner should strongly encourage the client to make guesses.

7. Frontal clients may show a tendency to focus on a single part of the stimulus and disregard the rest, making the task nearly impossible. Such clients should be encouraged to look at and describe the whole picture. A perseveration on one aspect, with an inability to break away, is a strong sign of frontal disorders. Such clients may accurately identify missing but irrelevant parts and should be pushed to look for the relevant detail. This may be observed in psychotic patients as well.

8. Clients with visual agnosia may be unable to interpret or describe what is seen when asked to do so. However, good performance on this subtest rules out substantial basic visual discrimination problems and can be used as a marker for other visual tests as well as visual naming tasks such as the Boston Naming Test.

9. Clients who are unable to name the missing object may be showing symptoms of dominant hemisphere parietal damage if their speech is otherwise fluent. This should be reflected in poor performance on tests of naming. In the absence of verbal fluency, frontal disorders should be strongly considered. This should be reflected in poor performance on frontal tests such as Category and Wisconsin Card Sorting.

10. Both frontal and psychiatric clients may perseverate on irrelevant aspects of the stimulus. Sometimes skipping a card and returning to it later is useful in breaking a perseverative response, although this will not be the case in more moderate to severe disorders.

11. Severe attentional problems, which are easily observed at this level, may not allow the client to complete the test in an adequate fashion. Therefore, attempts should be made to refocus the clients. An inability to focus on Picture completion generally indicates very severe attentional problems that will be obvious across almost all neuropsychological tests.

12. Clients with frontal and subcortical problems may answer quickly and impulsively without surveying the entire stimulus. Such clients typ-

ically show much better performance if the testing situation is structured to push for more extended study of the stimulus picture.

References for Picture Completion Subtest (WAIS-III)

Boone, D. E. (1998). Specificity of the WAIS-R subtests with psychiatric inpatients. *Assessment, 5,* 123–126.

Campbell, J. M., & McCord, D. M. (1996). The WAIS-R comprehension and picture arrangement subtests as measures of social intelligence: Testing traditional interpretations. *Journal of Psychoeducational Assessment, 14,* 240–249.

Golden, C. J., Zillmer, E., & Spiers, M. (1992). *Neuropsychological assessment and intervention.* Springfield, IL: Charles C Thomas.

Kramer, J. H. (1990). Guidelines for interpreting the WAIS-R subtest scores. *Psychological Assessment, 2,* 202–205.

Matarazzo, J. D. (1972). *Wechsler's measurement and appraisal of adult intelligence* (5th ed.). New York: Oxford University Press.

Sprandel H. Z. (1995). *The psychoeducational use and interpretation of the Wechsler Adult Intelligence Scale-Revised* (2nd ed.). Springfield, IL: Charles C Thomas.

Wechsler, D. (1981). *WAIS-R manual.* New York: The Psychological Corporation.

Wechsler, D. (1986). *WAIS-R administration and scoring manual.* San Antonio, TX: The Psychological Corporation.

Wechsler, D. (1997). *WAIS-III administration and scoring manual.* San Antonio, TX: The Psychological Corporation.

SEASHORE RHYTHM TEST

The Seashore Rhythm Test was originally conceived as part of a battery of tests to identify musical talent, but was later incorporated by Halstead into what is now called the Halstead–Reitan Neuropsychological Battery (Reitan & Wolfson, 1993). It is used to measure nonverbal auditory perception and is administered using a standardized cassette tape recording that is approximately 5 minutes in duration. This test measures the ability to discriminate between pairs of rhythmical patterns. In addition, it requires sustained attention in order to follow along with the tape presentation and record answers on the response form.

Interpretation

1. Those with brain damage (i.e., left, right, and generalized) averaged between 18 and 22 correct (8 and 12 errors) (Reitan & Wolfson, 1989).
2. As the test is a simple forced-choice exam, scores around 13–17 suggest random performance, while scores below 13 may indicate deliberate errors. This does not apply when clients fail to answer questions at all due to confusion or refusal.
3. Clients will get confused within a series as to which item they are on. Such cases may arise from an inability to separate out the rhythmic

stimuli, general confusion, or attentional problems. Clients should be urged to answer all questions despite this, to avoid the appearance of malingering or refusal. Such performance reveals problems with sustained attention, but may not reflect any specific form of brain injury.

4. The results of the SRT can be compared with the Speech–Sounds Perception Test (SSPT). If the SSPT is normal, but there is impairment on SRT, this suggests problems in attentional and nonverbal processing associated with the right hemisphere or subcortical areas.

5. If the SRT is normal and the SSPT is abnormal, then this suggests impairment in speech processes (receptive language, reading, and/or spelling) which indicates a left hemisphere process.

6. If both SRT and SSPT are abnormal, then this suggests left hemisphere or bilateral dysfunction.

7. In mild to moderate head injury, impairment on the SSPT without impairment on the SRT suggests a preexisting disorder or possible malingering.

8. Good scores on the SRT with impaired performance on the Category, Trail Making, or Wisconsin Card Sorting Test (WCST) may indicate a relatively static or old disorder, or may suggest mild frontal problems.

9. Impaired scores primarily on the SRT, Rey Figure (or other complex drawing test), Picture Arrangement, and Digits Backwards may suggest an anterior right hemisphere injury.

10. Although the SRT is very sensitive to attentional deficits and problems with sustained concentration, it is not highly related to the performance of other neuropsychological tests which generally do not require the intense sustained attention as does the SRT. As noted earlier, it shares some of these characteristics with the SSPT, but even that test is attentionally less demanding. Only the continuous performance tests such as the TOVA demand a similar level of focusing. As a consequence, correlations with other test performance is generally low.

References for Seashore Rhythm Test

Charter, R. A., & Webster, J. S. (1997). Psychometric structure of the Seashore Rhythm Test. *The Clinical Neuropsychologist, 11*(2), 167–173.

Gfeller, J. D., & Cradock, M. M. (1998). Detecting feigned neuropsychological impairment with the Seashore Rhythm Test. *Journal of Clinical Psychology, 54*(4), 431–443.

Reitan, R. M., & Wolfson, D. (1989). The Seashore Rhythm Test and brain functions. *The Clinical Neuropsychologist, 3*, 70–78.

Reitan, R. M., & Wolfson, D. (1993). *The Halstead–Reitan Neuropsychological Test Battery: Theory and Clinical Interpretation* (2nd ed.). Arizona: Neuropsychology Press.

Young, K. L., & Delay, E. R. (1993). Seashore Rhythm Test: Comparison of signal detection theory and standard scoring procedures. *Archives of Clinical Neuropsychology, 8*, 111–121.

SECTION V: MOTOR AND SENSORY TESTS

FINGER TAPPING TEST (FTT)

The Finger Tapping Test (also referred to as the Finger Oscillation Test), which is part of the Halstead–Reitan Battery, is one of the most widely used measures of motor functioning. It is a simple and quick test that allows for the comparison between performance of motor speed and coordination of the right and left hands. While it is often used in combination with other tests as part of a more comprehensive battery, it can be used on its own to detect differences between motor functioning of both hands. It represents a basic measure of speeded motor function with minimal demands on eye–hand coordination and fine motor skills.

Interpretation

1. Using a level of performance indicator, impairment on the FTT is noted when the dominant hand falls below 50 taps and the nondominant hand falls below 45 taps. Alternately, T-scores corrected for age, gender, and education can be found in Heaton, Grant, and Matthews (1993).
2. Women and men with short fingers generally score some 10% below these norms, lowering cutoff scores to 45 for the dominant hand and 40 for the nondominant hand.
3. Dominant finger tapping should be 10% faster than the nondominant finger tapping score.
4. Dominant finger tapping problems are indicated if the nondominant score is equal to or larger than the raw dominant finger tapping score. This suggests a motor problem arising from the dominant hemisphere or a peripheral problem in the dominant hand.
5. Nondominant finger tapping problems are indicated if the nondominant hand's score is less than 80% of the dominant hand's score. This suggests motor problems arising from the nondominant hemisphere or peripheral problem in the nondominant hand.
6. Central motor problems should not be diagnosed without ruling out peripheral motor problems. The presence of a lateralized motor loss may be due to either cortical or subcortical factors.
7. Impairment on FTT that shows lateralized damage and is worse than performance on the TPT suggests a more anterior focus to the damage.
8. In cases where there is evidence of dominant side problems, valuable information may be gained by comparing Finger Tapping (FT) and TPT performance using this formula: (DOM[FT] × DOM[TPT]) divided by (ND[FT] × ND[TPT]), where FT scores are expressed in average taps per 10 seconds and TPT scores in time per block. (Note: In cases where zero blocks are placed on a single trial, we assign an arbitrary score of 10 minutes or 600 seconds.)

9. In cases where the D-Ratio defined in No. 8 is between 1.35 and 1.65, then there are equal deficits in the dominant hand on the two tests.

10. In cases where the D-RATIO is greater than 1.65, this suggests greater impairment on the TPT dominant hand which indicates more posterior dominant hemisphere involvement.

11. In cases where the D-RATIO is less than 1.35, this suggests greater impairment on the FT dominant hand which indicates more anterior dominant hemisphere involvement.

12. In cases in which there is evidence of nondominant motor and sensory problems on FT and TPT, we can use the ND-RATIO to compute whether there is more anterior or posterior involvement. This is the reverse of the D-RATIO and expressed as (ND[TPT] × ND[FT]) divided by (D[TPT] × D[FT]).

13. When the ND-RATIO is between 1.5 and 1.8, then the relative impairment on the tests is equal.

14. When the ND-RATIO is greater than 1.8, then more TPT impairment is indicated, which is suggestive of a more posterior focus.

15. When the ND-RATIO is less than 1.5, then there is more impairment on FT, which is suggestive of a more anterior focus.

16. Inconsistency in lateralization on FTT, TPT, and sensory tests suggests either attentional and/or subcortical processes. This may be evident in such disorders as multiple sclerosis, depressive disorders, or after diffuse head trauma.

17. Overall poorer performance on Finger Tapping compared to the Purdue Pegboard indicates speed problems without fine motor coordination problems. Overall poorer performance on the Purdue Pegboard compared to Finger Tapping suggests less speed impairment and greater problems in fine motor control. Poorer performance is defined by T-scores for one test that are 10 points or more below the T-scores for the other test.

18. Lateralized deficits on Finger Tapping which are greater than the lateralized deficit on the Purdue Pegboard indicates more speed than fine motor problems in the affected hand. Similarly, greater lateralized deficits on the Purdue Pegboard than on Finger Tapping indicate greater problems with fine motor control as opposed to basic speed.

19. A greater lateralized deficit can be calculated computing the following ratio:

$$\frac{FT\ (DOM)/FT\ (NON\text{-}DOM)}{PP\ (DOM)/PP\ (NON\text{-}DOM)}$$

Finger Tapping (FT) is expressed as average taps per 10 seconds and Purdue Pegboard (PP) is expressed as pegs placed in 30 seconds.

20. In cases where DOM hand scores are higher than NON-DOM scores, a ratio of 1.2 or more indicates more lateralized Finger Tapping Perfor-

mance while a ratio less than .83 indicates more lateralized Purdue Pegboard Performance.

21. In cases where NON-DOM scores are higher than DOM scores for both tests, a ratio of 1.2 indicates more lateralized performance on the Purdue Pegboard while a ratio less than .83 indicates more lateralized performance on the Finger Tapping Test.

22. Lateralized dominant hand deficits on Finger Tapping or generalized slowing will affect all visual–motor tasks in a test battery. Profiles in which there is a motor deficit and on which all deficits are seen on motor-dependent tasks must be interpreted cautiously for deficits other than motor speed.

23. Overall poorer performance on Finger Tapping compared to Grip Strength indicates speed problems with less strength or larger muscle problems. Overall poorer performance on Grip Strength compared to Finger Tapping suggests less speed impairment and greater problems in gross motor strength. Poorer performance is defined by T-scores for one test that are 10 points or more below the T-scores for the other test.

24. Lateralized deficits on Finger Tapping that are greater than the lateralized deficit on Grip Strength indicate more speed than strength problems in the affected hand. Similarly, greater lateralized deficits on Grip Strength than on Finger Tapping indicate greater problems with strength as opposed to basic speed.

25. A greater lateralized deficit can be calculated by computing the following ratio:

$$\frac{\text{FT (DOM)/FT (NON-DOM)}}{\text{GS (DOM)/GS (NON-DOM)}}$$

Finger Tapping (FT) is expressed as average taps per 10 seconds and Grip Strength (GS) is expressed as average strength.

26. In cases where DOM hand scores are higher than NON-DOM scores, a ratio of 1.2 or more indicates more lateralized Finger Tapping Performance while a ratio less than .83 indicates more lateralized Grip Strength Performance.

27. In cases where NON-DOM scores are higher than DOM scores for both tests, a ratio of 1.2 indicates more lateralized performance on Grip Strength while a ratio less than .83 indicates more lateralized performance on the Finger Tapping Test.

References for Finger Tapping Test (FTT)

Arnold, B. R., Montgomery, G. T., Castaneda, I., & Longoria, R. (1994). Acculturation and performance of Hispanics on selected Halstead–Reitan neuropsychological tests. *Assessment, 1*(3), 239–248.

Bigler, E. D., & Tucker, D. M. (1981). Comparison of verbal IQ, tactual performance, seashore rhythm and finger oscillation tests in the blind and brain-damaged. *Journal of Clinical Psychology, 37*(4), 849–851.

Bornstein, R. A. (1983). Relationship of age and education to neuropsychological performance in patients with symptomatic carotid artery disease. *Journal of Clinical Psychology, 39*(4), 470–478.

Bornstein, R. A. (1985). Normative data on selected neuropsychological measures from a nonclinical sample. *Journal of Clinical Psychology, 41*(5), 651–659.

Bornstein, R. A. (1986). Classification rates obtained with "standard" cut-off scores on selected neuropsychological measures. *Journal of Clinical and Experimental Neuropsychology, 8*(4), 413–420.

Cousins, M., Corrow, C., Finn, M., & Salamone, J. D. (1998). Temporal measures of human finger tapping: Effects of age. *Pharmacology, Biochemistry, and Behavior, 59*(2), 445–449.

Haaland, K. Y., & Delaney, H. D. (1981). Motor deficits after left or right hemisphere damage due to stroke or tumor. *Neuropsychologia, 19,* 17–27.

Haaland, K. Y., Temkin, N., Randahl, G., & Dikmen, S. (1994). Recovery of simple motor skills after head injury. *Journal of Clinical and Experimental Neuropsychology, 16*(3), 448–456.

Lezak, M. (1995). *Neuropsychological assessment* (3rd ed.). New York: Oxford University Press.

O'Donnell, J. P. (1983). Lateralized sensorimotor asymmetries in normal learning-disabled and brain-damaged young adults. *Perceptual and Motor Skills, 57,* 227–232.

Prigatono, G. P., & Parsons, O. A. (1976). Relationship of age and education to Halstead test performance in different patient populations. *Journal of Consulting and Clinical Psychology, 44*(4), 527–533.

Reitan, R. M., & Wolfson, D. (1993). The Halstead–Reitan Neuropsychological Test Battery: Theory and clinical interpretations (2nd ed.). S. Tucson, AZ: Neuropsychology Press.

Schear, J. M., & Sato, S. D. (1989). Effects of visual acuity and visual motor speed and dexterity on cognitive test performance. *Archives of Clinical Neuropsychology, 4,* 25–32.

Volkow, N. D., Gu, R. C., Wang, G. J., Fowler, J. S., Moberg, P. J., Ding, Y. S., Hitzemann, R., Smith, G., & Logan, J. (1998). Association between decline in brain dopamine activity with age and cognitive and motor impairment in healthy individuals. *American Journal of Psychiatry, 155*(3), 344–349.

PURDUE PEGBOARD TEST

The Purdue Pegboard Test is a quick and easy to administer test that was originally designed as a measure of manipulative finger dexterity in personnel selection. It is now also used to aid in the assessment of brain damage, specifically for identifying lateralized brain lesions. Although it can provide valuable information when used by itself, it is most commonly used as a part of a battery. The Purdue Pegboard Test is a good method of screening for brain damage owing to its brief administration and because it is unlikely to fatigue the client. It is generally seen as requiring more fine motor control than Finger Tapping.

Interpretation

1. The Purdue Pegboard Test scores reflect an individual's ability to produce rapid, competent, controlled, manipulative handling of small objects with the use of the fingers. They are also reflective of the

individual's capacity to coordinate arm–hand motions in order to ma-
neuver larger objects. In general, individuals perform some 10% better
on the preferred hand trial than on the nonpreferred hand trial. The
Purdue Pegboard is scored as the number of pegs placed in 30 seconds.

2. Patterns of performance in which the dominant hand is slower than the
   nondominant hand suggest clear deficits in the dominant hand.

3. Patterns of performance in which the nondominant hand is less than
   80% of the dominant hand indicate slowness in the nondominant hand.

4. Results should be coordinated with scores from the Finger Tapping Test
   (FTT), the Tactual Performance Test (TPT), Grip Strength, and other
   lateralized motor and sensory examinations. If consistent findings are
   found on one side of the body, then a lesion of the contralateral hemisphere is suggested. Inconsistent findings may suggest a subcortical
   disorder or motivational problems, which must be considered in the
   interpretation.

5. In cases where there is evidence of dominant side problems, valuable
   information may be gained by comparing Purdue Pegboard (PP) and
   TPT performance using this formula: (DOM[PP] × DOM[TPT]) divided by (ND[PP] × ND[TPT]), where PP scores are expressed in total
   pins in 30 seconds and TPT scores in time per block. (Note: In cases
   where zero blocks are placed on a single trial, we assign an arbitrary
   score of 10 minutes.)

6. In cases where the D-RATIO defined in no. 5 is between 1.35 and 1.65,
   then there are equal deficits in the dominant hand on the two tests.

7. In cases where the D-RATIO is greater than 1.65, this suggests greater
   impairment on the TPT dominant hand which indicates more posterior
   dominant hemisphere involvement.

8. In cases where the D-RATIO is less than 1.35, this suggests greater
   impairment on the PP dominant hand which indicates more anterior
   dominant hemisphere involvement.

9. In cases in which there is evidence of nondominant motor and sensory
   problems on PP and TPT, we can use the ND-RATIO to compute
   whether there is more anterior or posterior involvement. This is the
   reverse of the D-RATIO (no. 5) and expressed as (ND[TPT] × ND[PP])
   divided by (D[TPT] × D[PP]).

10. When the ND-RATIO is between 1.5 and 1.8, then the relative impair-
    ment on the tests is equal.

11. When the ND-RATIO is greater than 1.8, then more TPT impairment is
    indicated, which is suggestive of a more posterior focus.

12. When the ND-RATIO is less than 1.5, then there is more impairment on
    PP, which is suggestive of a more anterior focus.

13. Overall poorer performance on Finger Tapping compared to the Purdue
    Pegboard indicates speed problems without fine motor coordination

problems. Overall poorer performance on the Purdue Pegboard compared to Finger Tapping suggests less speed impairment and greater problems in fine motor control. Poorer performance is defined by T-scores for one test that are 10 points or more below the T-scores for the other test.

14. Lateralized deficits on Finger Tapping which are greater than the lateralized deficit on the Purdue Pegboard indicates more speed than fine motor problems in the affected hand. Similarly, greater lateralized deficits on the Purdue Pegboard than on Finger Tapping indicate greater problems with fine motor control as opposed to basic speed.

15. A greater lateralized deficit can be calculated by computing the following ratio:

$$\frac{\text{FT (DOM)/FT (NON-DOM)}}{\text{PP (DOM)/PP (NON-DOM)}}$$

Finger Tapping (FT) is expressed as average taps per 10 seconds and Purdue Pegboard (PP) is expressed as pegs per 30 seconds.

16. In cases where DOM hand scores are higher than NON-DOM scores, a ratio of 1.2 or more indicates more lateralized Finger Tapping Performance while a ratio less than .83 indicates more lateralized Purdue Pegboard Performance.

17. In cases where NON-DOM scores are higher than DOM scores for both tests, a ratio of 1.2 indicates more lateralized performance on the Purdue Pegboard while a ratio less than .83 indicates more lateralized performance on the Finger Tapping Test.

18. Lateralized dominant hand deficits on Purdue Pegboard (and Finger Tapping) or generalized slowing will affect all visual–motor tasks in a test battery. Profiles in which there is a motor deficit and on which all deficits are seen on motor-dependent tasks must be interpreted cautiously for deficits other than motor speed.

19. The degree of impairment on this measure and sensory measures must be compared. If there are greater sensory than motor deficits, a lesion of the sensory system is suggested, while greater deficits on the Pegboard suggest a focus in the motor system.

20. In all cases, peripheral motor and other peripheral causes for any deficits must be considered. In some cases, clients with heavily callused hands may have trouble picking up the small pegs, as will clients with arthritis or peripheral neuropathies.

21. Overall poorer performance on Finger Tapping compared to the Purdue Pegboard indicates speed problems without fine motor coordination problems. Overall poorer performance on the Purdue Pegboard compared to Finger Tapping suggests less speed impairment and greater problems in fine motor control. Poorer performance is defined by

T-scores for one test that are 10 points or more below the T-scores for the other test.

22. Lateralized deficits on Finger Tapping which are greater than the lateralized deficit on the Purdue Pegboard indicates more speed than fine motor problems in the affected hand. Similarly, greater lateralized deficits on the Purdue Pegboard than on Finger Tapping indicates greater problems with fine motor control as opposed to basic speed.

23. A greater lateralized deficit can be calculated by computing the following ratio:

$$\frac{\text{FT (DOM)/FT (NON-DOM)}}{\text{PP (DOM)/PP (NON-DOM)}}$$

Finger Tapping (FT) is expressed as average taps per 10 seconds and Purdue Pegboard (PP) is expressed as pegs placed in 30 seconds.

24. In cases where DOM hand scores are higher than NON-DOM scores, a ratio of 1.2 or more indicates more lateralized Finger Tapping Performance while a ratio less than .83 indicates more lateralized Purdue Pegboard Performance.

25. In cases where NON-DOM scores are higher than DOM scores for both tests, a ratio of 1.2 indicates more lateralized performance on the Purdue Pegboard while a ratio less than .83 indicates more lateralized performance on the Finger Tapping Test.

26. Lateralized dominant hand deficits on Finger Tapping or generalized slowing will affect all visual–motor tasks in a test battery. Profiles in which there is a motor deficit and on which all deficits are seen on motor-dependent tasks must be interpreted cautiously for deficits other than motor speed.

27. Impairments on two-hand scores, as well as impairments on scores of both single-hand trials, are indicative of nonlateralized, more diffuse brain damage. Studies have shown that individuals with cerebellar disease, Parkinson's disease, and Huntington's disease have difficulty producing two-hand movements on the Purdue Pegboard.

28. Overall poorer performance on the Purdue Pegboard compared to Grip Strength indicates speed or fine motor problems without strength or larger muscle problems. Overall poorer performance on Grip Strength compared to Purdue Pegboard suggests less speed or fine motor impairment and greater problems in gross motor strength. Poorer performance is defined by T-scores for one test that are 10 points or more below the T-scores for the other test.

29. Lateralized deficits on the Purdue Pegboard that are greater than the lateralized deficit on Grip Strength indicate more speed or fine motor than strength problems in the affected hand. Similarly, greater lateralized deficits on Grip Strength than on Purdue Pegboard Tapping

indicate greater problems with strength as opposed to basic speed or coordination.

30. A greater lateralized deficit can be calculated by computing the following ratio:

$$\frac{\text{PP (DOM)/PP (NON-DOM)}}{\text{GS (DOM)/GS (NON-DOM)}}$$

Purdue Pegboard (PP) is expressed as average taps per 10 seconds and Grip Strength (GS) is expressed as average strength.

31. In cases where DOM hand scores are higher than NON-DOM scores, a ratio of 1.2 or more indicates more lateralized Purdue Pegboard Performance while a ratio less than .83 indicates more lateralized Grip Strength Performance.

32. In cases where NON-DOM scores are higher than DOM scores for both tests, a ratio of 1.2 indicates more lateralized performance on Grip Strength while a ratio less than .83 indicates more lateralized performance on the Purdue Pegboard.

References for Purdue Pegboard Test

Axelrod, B. N., & Milner, I. B. (1997). Neuropsychological findings in a sample of operation desert storm veterans. *Journal of Neuropsychiatry, 9*, 23–28.

Brown, R. G., & Jahanshahi, M. (1998). An unusual enhancement of motor performance during bimanual movement in Parkinson's disease. *Journal of Neurology, Neurosurgery, and Psychiatry, 64*(6), 813–816.

Jodar, M., & Junque, C. (1998). Frontal functions in normal aging and the performance in Purdue Pegboard test. *Research and Practice in Alzheimer's Disease 1998*, 151–162.

Lezak, M. D. (1995). *Neuropsychological assessment* (2nd ed.). New York: Oxford University Press.

McCaffrey, R. J., Ortega, A., & Haase, R. F. (1993). Effects of repeated neuropsychological assessments. *Archives of Clinical Neuropsychology, 8*, 519–524.

Reddon, J. R., Gill, D. M., Gauk, S. E., & Maerz, M. D. (1988). Purdue pegboard: Test–retest estimates. *Perceptual and Motor Skills, 66*, 503–506.

Spreen, O., & Strauss, E. (1998). *A compendium of neuropsychological tests: Administration, norms, and commentary* (2nd ed.). New York: Oxford University Press.

Verdino, M., & Dingman, S. (1998). Two measures of laterality in handedness: The Edinburgh Handedness Inventory and the Purdue Pegboard test of manual dexterity. *Perceptual and Motor Skills, 86*(2), 476–478.

Yeudall, L. T., Fromm, D., Reddon, J. R., & Stefanyk, W. O. (1986). Normative data stratified by age and sex for 12 neuropsychological tests. *Journal of Clinical Psychology, 42*(6), 918–946.

GRIP STRENGTH TEST

The Grip Strength Test, which is a part of many standard neurological exams as well as the Halstead–Reitan Neuropsychological Battery, is used as a measure of voluntary motor strength. It allows for the measurement of the strength of each of the patient's upper extremities. While it is often used in combination with other tests as part of a more comprehensive battery, it can be used on its own to detect differences between the strength of the right and left hands. It is used with the assumption that lateralized brain damage may affect the strength of the contra-lateral hand (Lezak, 1995).

Interpretation

1. Interpretation of the Grip Strength Test focuses on whether or not there is a disparity between the dominant and nondominant hands. Neuro-logically healthy individuals are expected to obtain higher scores with their dominant hand. Because strength varies widely in the normal population as well as within and between gender groups, it is generally recommended that comparisons of the left and right hands be empha-sized more than "level of performance," except in cases where scores are at least two standard deviations below the norms.

2. Overall poorer performance on the Purdue Pegboard compared to Grip Strength indicates speed or fine motor problems without strength or larger muscle problems. Overall poorer performance on Grip Strength compared to Purdue Pegboard suggests less speed or fine motor impair-ment and greater problems in gross motor strength. Poorer performance is defined by T-scores for one test being 10 points or more below the T-scores for the other test.

3. Lateralized deficits on the Purdue Pegboard that are greater than the lateralized deficit on Grip Strength indicate more speed or fine motor problems than strength problems in the affected hand. Similarly, greater lateralized deficits on Grip Strength than on Purdue Pegboard Tapping indicate greater problems with strength as opposed to basic speed or coordination.

4. A greater lateralized deficit can be calculated by computing the follow-ing ratio:

$$\frac{PP\ (DOM)/PP\ (NON\text{-}DOM)}{GS\ (DOM)/GS\ (NON\text{-}DOM)}$$

Purdue Pegboard (PP) is expressed as average taps per 10 seconds and Grip Strength (GS) is expressed as average strength.

5. In cases where DOM hand scores are higher than NON-DOM scores, a ratio of 1.2 or more indicates more lateralized Purdue Pegboard Perfor-mance while a ratio less than .83 indicates more lateralized Grip Strength Performance.

6. In cases where NON-DOM scores are higher than DOM scores for both tests, a ratio of 1.2 indicates more lateralized performance on Grip

Strength while a ratio less than .83 indicates more lateralized performance on the Purdue Pegboard.

7. The dominant hand is expected to be 10% stronger than the nondominant hand. Cases in which the nondominant hand is equal to or greater than the dominant hand suggests impairment of the dominant hand.

8. The nondominant hand should be 90% of the dominant hand. Cases in which the nondominant hand is less than 80% of the dominant hand suggest impairment to the nondominant hand.

9. When deficits occur in Grip Strength, peripheral disorders of the muscles or bones or skin must be considered as possible peripheral causes. In addition, such deficits frequently arise from injuries to the spinal cord or the associated nerve roots. In cases where clients show chronic lateralized strength differences, one should also be able to observe gross muscle atrophy of the affected arm compared to the intact arm.

10. Overall poorer performance on Finger Tapping compared to Grip Strength indicates speed problems without gross motor or larger muscle problems. Overall poorer performance on Grip strength compared to Finger Tapping suggests less speed impairment and greater problems in gross motor strength. Poorer performance is defined by T-scores for one test being 10 points or more below the T-scores for the other test.

11. Lateralized deficits on Finger Tapping that are greater than the lateralized deficit on Grip Strength indicate more speed than strength problems in the affected hand. Similarly, greater lateralized deficits on Grip strength than on Finger Tapping indicate greater problems with strength as opposed to basic speed.

12. A greater lateralized deficit can be calculated by computing the following ratio:

$$\frac{\text{FT (DOM)/FT (NON-DOM)}}{\text{GS (DOM)/GS (NON-DOM)}}$$

Finger Tapping (FT) is expressed as average taps per 10 seconds and Grip Strength (GS) is expressed as average strength.

13. In cases where DOM hand scores are higher than NON-DOM scores, a ratio of 1.2 or more indicates more lateralized Finger Tapping Performance while a ratio less than .83 indicates more lateralized Grip Strength Performance.

14. In cases where NON-DOM scores are higher than DOM scores for both tests, a ratio of 1.2 indicates more lateralized performance on Grip Strength while a ratio less than .83 indicates more lateralized performance on the Finger Tapping Test.

15. Overall poorer performance on the Purdue Pegboard compared to Grip Strength indicates speed or fine motor problems without strength or

larger muscle problems. Overall poorer performance on Grip Strength compared to Purdue Pegboard suggests less speed or fine motor impairment and greater problems in gross motor strength. Poorer performance is defined by T-scores for one test being 10 points or more below the T-scores for the other test.

16. Lateralized deficits on the Purdue Pegboard that are greater than the lateralized deficit on Grip Strength indicate more speed or fine motor than strength problems in the affected hand. Similarly, greater lateralized deficits on Grip Strength than on Purdue Pegboard Tapping indicate greater problems with strength as opposed to basic speed or coordination.

17. A greater lateralized deficit can be calculated by computing the following ratio:

$$\frac{\text{PP (DOM)/PP (NON-DOM)}}{\text{GS (DOM)/GS (NON-DOM)}}$$

Purdue Pegboard (PP) is expressed as average taps per 10 seconds and Grip Strength (GS) is expressed as average strength.

18. In cases where DOM hand scores are higher than NON-DOM scores, a ratio of 1.2 or more indicates more lateralized Purdue Pegboard Performance while a ratio less than .83 indicates more lateralized Grip Strength Performance.

19. In cases where NON-DOM scores are higher than DOM scores for both tests, a ratio of 1.2 indicates more lateralized performance on Grip Strength while a ratio less than .83 indicates more lateralized performance on the Purdue Pegboard.

20. In general, deficits that are restricted to strength have little impact on most other neuropsychological tests. However, such clients may show faster rates of fatigue which can affect test scores. In such cases, shorter sessions or more frequent breaks may be necessary.

References for Grip Strength Test

Bornstein, R. A. (1983). Relationship of age and education to neuropsychological performance in patients with symptomatic carotid artery disease. *Journal of Clinical Psychology, 39*(4), 470–478.

Dee, H. L., & Van Allen, M. W. (1972). Psychomotor testing as an aid in the recognition of cerebral lesions. *Neurology, 22*, 845–848.

Dunwoody, L., Tittmar, H. G., & McClean, W. S. (1996). Grip strength and intertrial rest. *Perceptual and Motor Skills, 83*, 275–278.

Ernst, J. (1988). Language, grip strength, sensory-perceptual, and receptive skills in a normal elderly sample. *The Clinical Neuropsychologist, 2*(1), 30–40.

Haaland, K. Y., & Delaney, H. D. (1981). Motor deficits after left or right hemisphere damage due to stroke or tumor. *Neuropsychologia, 19*, 17–27.

Haaland, K. Y., Temkin, N., Randahl, G., & Dikmen, S. (1994). Recovery of simple motor skills after head injury. *Journal of Clinical and Experimental Neuropsychology, 16*(3), 448–456.

Lezak, M. D. (1995). *Neuropsychological Assessment* (2nd ed.). New York: Oxford University Press.

Montazer, M. A., & Thomas, J. G. (1991). Grip strength as a function of repetitive trials. *Perceptual and Motor Skills, 73*, 804–806.

O'Dennell, J. P. (1983). Lateralized sensorimotor asymmetries in normal learning-disabled and brain-damaged young adults. *Perceptual and Motor Skills, 57*, 227–232.

Reddon, J. R., Stefanyk, W. O., Gill, D. M., & Renney, C. (1985). Hand dynamometer: Effects of trials and sessions. *Perceptual and Motor Skills, 61*, 1195–1198.

Schwartz, F., Carr, A., Munich, R., Bartuch, E., Lesser, B., Rescigno, D., & Viegener, B. (1990). Voluntary motor performance in psychotic disorders: A replication study. *Psychological Reports, 66*, 1223–1234.

MOTOR FUNCTIONS SCALE (LNNB)

Motor Functions (Scale C1) is the longest scale in the Luria–Nebraska and one of the most useful. As the first scale, it includes initial items that are very easy and that most clients are capable of doing. At the same time, it gives the investigator the opportunity to explore the best methods of approaching the client and obtaining the client's highest level of functioning.

The scale consists of 51 tasks in which the client must perform motor behaviors in response to the given instruction. All of the items focus on the client's ability to perform motor tasks following the specific instruction. Along with verbal instructions, the motor behaviors are modeled for the client with the exception of seven items in the scale (items 19, 20, 25, 26, 27, 34, and 35). In this scale, the examiner is allowed to alter the verbal instructions as necessary to communicate to the client what is desired, as well as demonstrate the behaviors. With this flexibility, the examiner can quickly learn the best ways in which to communicate with the client for optimal test results. The examiner determines the degree to which there are disturbances in attention and concentration by closely observing the client.

When the scale is used independent of the full LNNB, the entire scale can be given (if T-scores are needed) or selected items can be given to screen for specific deficits or to confirm the presence of deficits suggested on other test instruments.

Interpretation

1. Overall impairment on the scale suggests problems in the broad area of motor execution using the hands. Detailed analysis by items is, however, necessary to make more specific diagnosis when the scale is administered alone. Impairment on this scale in the presence of normal performance on Finger Tapping and/or Purdue Pegboard suggests that

problems exist in more complex motor activities while basic motor speed and fine motor coordination are maintained. In such cases, items 1–4 are normal along with the bilateral coordination items (21–23), while other measures are relatively impaired on this scale. Impairment on Purdue Pegboard and/or Finger Tapping with a normal LNNB Motor scale score indicates overall problems in speed but that non-speeded fine and gross motor coordination is normal. In these cases, slowness will show on items 1–4 plus the bilateral speeded items (21–23) while other items will be relatively normal.

2. Deficits in items 1–4 reflect problems in motor speed. Results for each hand (left and right) should be identical, so raw score differences of more than 10% suggest impairment in the slower hand. Differences greater than 20% suggest moderate impairment and differences of over 30% suggest severe impairment.

3. Scaled scores of two on items 1–4 on any trial suggest severe impairment in motor speed or motor coordination. Good scores on items 3 and/or 4 with poor scores on items 1 and/or 2 indicate poor motor coordination while poor scores across the items suggest slowness.

4. Impairment on items 5–8 suggest impairment in kinesthetic feedback. Good scores on item 5 with a poor score on item 7 may suggest problems in cross-hemispheric transfer, as may a good score on item 6 and a poor score on item 8. Poor scores across items suggest poor sensory feedback from the muscles to the brain.

5. Deficits on items 9–18 reflect problems in the imitation of motor movements. In the absence of motor paralysis that prevents the task from being done at all, the most common errors are to repeatedly mirror image the examiner. In such cases, visual–spatial problems or confusion in general may be present. When the client persists on mirror imaged responses even when warned, this may indicate perseveration.

6. Items 19 and 20 measure the ability to interpret commands involving left and right. Failures on these items point to left right confusion or substantial problems in comprehension.

7. Item 24 may be missed as a result of visual–spatial problems in which case the figure is generally distorted or by perseveration in which case the item is repeated over the page, sometimes even running off the page. Perseveration should be inferred if simpler drawing items later in the scale are intact.

8. Items 21, 22, and 23 measure bilateral speed and coordination. When items 1–4 are normal, impairment in these items suggests difficulty in coordinating the two sides of the body. Deficits on item 21 alone point to a more complex motor organizational component, while normal performance on 21 but not 22 and 23 suggests difficulty in processing

motor-rhythmic patterns. Deficits on 22 but not 23 suggest mild impairment in the right-hand motor skills, while deficits on 23 but not 22 point to problems in left-hand motor skills.

9. Items 25 through 27 look at the ability to mimic an action from a verbal command without any concrete cues. Deficits on two or three of these items suggest ideational dyspraxia if motor coordination itself is normal on other measures.

10. Items 28 through 34 reflect oral motor skills. Deficits on more than three of these items indicate problems with motor oral skills which are often reflected in motor speech problems as well.

11. Items 36 through 47 reflect basic drawing skills. Because these items are so basic, scores of 2 indicating poor performance on time or accuracy of drawings point to construction dyspraxia. If motor abilities are generally intact, this may reflect a visual–spatial problem. Items 36–41 require drawing from verbal instructions and 42 through 47 require copying of the same figures. Deficits on only the verbal items suggest impairment in the following or initiating of commands, but not visual–motor deficits. Similarly, deficits on only 42–47 indicate the likelihood of visual problems but not visual–motor coordination.

12. Clients with visual–spatial deficits will have the most difficulties with item 47 (Green cross). Clients with moderate to severe visual–motor problems will generally show deficits in quality or speed across all the items.

13. Items 48–51 measure the ability of the client to inhibit simple and automatic motor movements. Deficits on 2 or more of these items indicate inhibitory problems, specifically related to the ability of internal speech to regulate motor output. Deficits in this area are generally associated with premotor or prefrontal deficits. These deficits may be characterized by perseverative behaviors as well. Perseverative behaviors will also be seen on executive tests such as Category or WCST.

References for Motor Functions Scale (LNNB)

Chelune, G. J. (1982). A reexamination of the relationship between the Luria–Nebraska and Halstead-Reitan batteries: Overlap with the WAIS. *Journal of Consulting and Clinical Psychology, 50,* 578–580.

Golden, C. J., Purisch, A. D., & Hammeke, T. A. (1985). *Luria–Nebraska Neuropsychological Battery: Forms I and II Manual.* Los Angeles: Western Psychological Services.

McKinney, R. K., Roecker, C. E., Puente, A. E., & Rogers, E. B. (1998). Performance of normal adults on the Luria–Nebraska Neuropsychological Battery, Form I. *Archives of Clinical Neuropsychology, 13*(4), 397–413.

Moses, J. A., & Pritchard, D. A. (1999). Performance scales for the Luria–Nebraska Neuropsychological Battery-Form I. *Archives of Clinical Neuropsychology, 14*(5), 285–302.

SENSORY–PERCEPTUAL EXAMINATION (HRNB)

This test consists of a series of sensory tests adapted from traditional neurological examinations. The client is given 20 trials on each hand of Finger Agnosia (identifying which finger is touched based on touch alone) and Finger Tip Number Writing (identifying numbers written on each finger tip). The exam also includes double simultaneous stimulation in which the client is touched in two places at the same time. This evaluates one's ability to feel only one, rather than both, of the touches. Extinction for double visual and auditory stimulation is also examined. For each of these procedures, the score is simply the number of errors on the right and left sides of the body. A final procedure asks the client to recognize simple shapes (circle, square, triangle, and cross) by touch (stereognosis). Each hand is scored for errors and for total time to do the individual tasks. Although this test cannot be directly compared to other procedures using T-scores, the presence of lateralization is significant for the presence of a central or peripheral disorder.

Interpretation

1. These subtests are very sensitive to disorders of concentration and attention; therefore these factors must be ruled out before interpreting deficits as due to specific sensory losses. This is best done by comparing the functions of the right and left sides of the body. In situations where there are bilateral deficits, interpretation should be cautious and considered in light of performance on tests of attention (TOVA) or working memory (Digit Span, Visual Span, Number–Sequencing).

2. On Finger Agnosia or Fingertip Number Writing, a deficit is indicated on the right hand if there are three more errors than on the left hand and left-hand errors do not exceed three. On Finger Agnosia or Fingertip Number Writing, a deficit is indicated on the left hand if there are three more errors than on the right hand and right-hand errors do not exceed three.

3. On Finger Agnosia or Fingertip Number Writing, a deficit is indicated at any time when right-hand errors exceed left-hand errors by six or more.

4. On Finger Agnosia or Fingertip Number Writing, a deficit is indicated at any time when left-hand errors exceed right-hand errors by six or more.

5. Suppression tests for all three modalities are based on the assumption that unilateral sensory stimulation (visual, auditory, or tactile) is intact. This is tested with four unilateral trials on each stimulus used in double simultaneous stimulation. If two or more errors are made on these tests, then the results of double simultaneous suppression are questionable.

6. If two or more errors are made during unilateral sensory stimulation in any modality, this may suggest injuries to the opposite hemisphere. Such losses may reflect cortical injuries, but injuries may also be in the

sensory organs themselves or in the sensory pathways. Such deficits must be interpreted cautiously based on the overall pattern of problems and an analysis of the sensory pathways that can create such a deficit.

7. When there are fewer than two unilateral sensory deficits in a given modality, two or more errors on one side when compared to the other during double simultaneous stimulation indicate the presence of a lesion. Double simultaneous stimulation errors in the left visual field point to right occipital lesions or left visual field pathways, while right visual field errors point to left occipital lesions or right visual field pathways.

8. Double simultaneous stimulation errors in the left ear point to right temporal lesions, while right ear errors point to left temporal lesions.

9. Double simultaneous stimulation errors in the left side of the body point to right parietal lesions, while right side errors point to left parietal lesions.

10. Stereognosis represents a more sensitive measure of tactile losses than the other tasks in the battery as it requires the integration and analysis of basic tactile information. Stereognostic losses are indicated when there are at least two more errors on one side than the other or when one side responds at least 20% slower than the other side (but this does not apply when both time scores across trials are less than 20 seconds on the shape recognition task and 30 seconds on object recognition). Although Stereognosis performance is affected by naming disorders, the focus on lateralization eliminates this as an interpretive issue. However, in cases where there are no errors on Stereognosis in either hand but errors exist on Boston Naming or other naming tests, visual problems rather than naming problems may be the cause of the naming disorder. However, rare cases exist in which visual naming is impaired while other forms of naming are intact.

11. Lateralized Stereognostic deficits reflect lesions in the opposite parietal lobe. However, if Finger Agnosia and Finger Number Writing are intact, these lesions may be more posterior toward the occipital–parietal areas or can reflect a serious spatial deficit arising from right parietal injuries. However, the latter deficit will be bilateral rather than unilateral.

12. Bilateral deficits may reflect attentional processes or a failure to understand the tasks. Performance on tasks of attention and receptive language should be employed to evaluate the impact of these factors. Naming disorders will also result in bilateral errors.

13. Consistent lateralized suppressions suggest destructive lesions to the appropriate area of the opposite hemisphere. Visual suppressions suggest injuries to the basic visual areas in the occipital lobe. Auditory suppressions suggest injuries to the core auditory areas in the temporal

lobe. Tactile suppressions suggest injuries to the anterior areas of the parietal lobe. Such injuries may be acute or in some cases can be the residual of serious destructive lesions.

14. Tactile sensory losses may impair motor tasks, especially those that are speeded or which cannot be compensated for by visual skills (Tactual Performance Test). Mile motor deficits may be related directly to tactile losses, while more severe losses are often a combination of motor and sensory loss. Motor and sensory deficits may be present at the same time, or may show relative independence depending on the exact location of the lesion.

15. Visual losses may have impact on all tests dependent on visual stimuli and construction skills, although many visual losses can be compensated for by simply turning the head (with the exception of cases of unilateral neglect). In such cases, impairment due to partial visual loss may be minor. In many cases, uncorrected peripheral visual disorders may result in significant problems seeing details or reading affecting any test requiring these skills (patients forgetting their glasses can be a major problem on many tests).

16. Auditory losses may also be compensated for if they are unilateral and if the lesions do not involve the cortex. In such cases, the client may favor one ear over the other. It is clearly essential that the examiner confirm that clients are perceiving instructions and information properly.

References for Sensory–Perceptual Examination (HRNB)

Henton, R. K., Grant, I., & Matthews, C. G. (1991). *Comprehensive norms for an expanded Halstead-Reitan battery: Demographic corrections, research findings, and clinical applications.* Odessa, FL: Psychological Assessment Resources.

Lezak, M. (1995). *Neuropsychological assessment* (3rd ed.). New York: Oxford University Press.

Reitan, R. M., & Wolfson, D. (1993). *The Halstead-Reitan neuropsychological test battery: Theory and clinical interpretation* (2nd ed.). S. Tucson, AZ: Neuropsychology Press.

Snyder, P. J., & Nussbaum, P. D. (1998). *Clinical neuropsychology: A pocket handbook for assessment.* Washington, D.C.: American Psychological Association.

Wood, D. G., & Bigler, E. D. (1995). Diencephalic changes in traumatic brain injury: Relationship to sensory perceptual function. *Brain Research Bulletin, 38*(6), 545–549.

Section VI: Achievement Tests

PEABODY INDIVIDUAL ACHIEVEMENT TEST (PIAT-R)

Based on the original version (PIAT; Dunn & Markward, 1970), the Peabody Individual Achievement Test-Revised (PIAT-R; Markwardt, 1989) is a wide-range screening device of overall academic achievement, as well as of functioning in six specific academic domains. Administration time is approximately 1 hour. It has been normed on a randomized national sample of children ranging in grade from kindergarten to 12th, as well as on age (5-0 to 18-11). Such normative practices have made this test useful in the assessment of all school-age children and teenagers, but it should be interpreted with caution in adults using the 18-11 norms.

Interpretation

1. In interpretation of findings on tests of achievement, it is always imperative to keep in mind the person's intellectual abilities, as intellectual ability has come to be seen as a measure of learning potential, whereas achievement tests are intended to measure what has been learned. Therefore, attempting to interpret achievement scores without a measure of intellectual ability offers the examiner much less information about the learning process. In general, standard scores for the PIAT-R should be within 15 points of the client's verbal IQ. When scores are below IQ by a greater amount, this indicates a failure to learn but does not specify the etiology.

2. In addition, standard scores for each scale should be within 15 points of the total test standard scores. Scores more than 15 points below this average suggest significant impairment in a given area, while scores more than 15 points above this level suggest strengths. Score ranges between the lowest and highest scores greater than 30 points are also a marker that there may be a deficit in one or more areas.

3. Situations where the PIAT-R scores are greater than the intelligence scores suggest the possibility of loss of intellectual skills (especially when aphasic symptoms are present). This may occur in strokes and more advanced cases of dementia as well as severe head trauma, but rarely in mild head injury. Generally, the Reading Recognition score is considered most indicative of premorbid functioning than are the other scores yielded by the test.

4. Spelling and Mathematics scores are very sensitive to brain injury in general in individuals whose skills were weak to begin with (IQs less than 100). However, weaknesses in these scores are frequently seen in normal individuals as well, so a correlation with history and school records is usually indicated before reaching a conclusion that there has been a decline.

5. Writing scores are also sensitive to brain injury. Disorders of written language may be associated with motor disorders in which the client knows that he or she wants to write but is unable to do so, or kinesthetic disorders of the dominant hemisphere in which letters that are written in a similar manner (o and a, or h and k, for example) are substituted for one another.

6. Parietal injuries of either hemisphere may result in disorders of grammar and sentence structure, with the more severe forms of loss associated with dominant hemisphere functions. These losses must be documented to represent a change from premorbid functioning.

7. Difficulty in using and understanding spatial words (above or below) or verbal relationships in writing or on the comprehension measure may indicate a nondominant lesion when there are no other signs of aphasia.

8. Disorders of primary reading skills in which they decline from a higher level of functioning is almost always related to posterior dominant hemisphere functioning. However, disorders that show up only in the reading of smaller print or dense pages may reflect a spatial or visual disorder which in turn may result from occipital–parietal lesions of either side.

9. Inability to read the left side of sentences or write on the left side of the page may indicate a neglect syndrome most characteristic of right posterior lesions.

10. Declines in arithmetic ability may result from anterior or posterior lesions. However, the loss of the meaning of numeric symbols is almost always associated with the posterior left hemisphere. Difficulties in understanding the spatial nature of numbers (such as the role of the tens place and hundreds place) may reflect lesions of either hemisphere in the parietal–occipital areas. Declines in only more complex arithmetic skills may reflect frontal lesions.

11. Losses in Reading Comprehension when all other achievement and intellectual areas are intact may reflect a dominant frontal lesion (which should also be visible on the more specific frontal tests). Given the visual nature of this subtest, specific problems will arise when there are any type of significant visual losses that can be seen on such tests as Picture Completion and the Visual Form Discrimination Test. Unilateral neglect will seriously affect RC scores. Reading Comprehension strengths in the presence of poor Recognition suggest strong adaptive (frontal) skills, which may be compensating for posterior losses.

12. The Total Test score is designed to give a composite index of wide-range achievement. It can be employed as a measure of an examinee's overall ability to learn, recall, and employ a number of skills acquired during his or her academic career. Low scores on this index are reflective of learning difficulties (either general or specific) and can be due to a learning disability or low cognitive abilities and may be interpreted only in the context of an intelligence score.

13. In cases where the Total Test score on the PIAT-R is low but remains consistent with the person's level of intellectual ability (within 15 points of FSIQ), the learning difficulties experienced are considered to be consistent with his or her cognitive ability.

14. Research with stroke victims (Heaton, Schmitz, Avitable, et al., 1987) has shown that clients with damage lateralized to the left hemisphere demonstrated significantly reduced scores on the Reading Comprehension and Spelling subtests in comparison to normal controls. This pattern was not significant for stroke patients suffering from damage to the right hemisphere. Further analysis demonstrated that performance on these subtests was particularly sensitive to damage of the left temporal and left occipital lobes.

15. The Reading Recognition subtest is more heavily rooted in the ability to discriminate and recognize phonemes. Although the Reading Comprehension subtest also relies on such fundamental skills, it further assesses higher level abilities such as the ability to obtain meaning from a word series, as well as the understanding of logical-grammatical structures and implied relationships. Therefore, a more drastically reduced score on Reading Comprehension, in comparison to Reading Recognition, is suggestive of difficulties in such higher level areas previously discussed, whereas a reduction in both reading subtests suggests difficulties in the more basic aspects of reading (i.e., phonemic processing).

16. Major deficits in expressive language will impair Reading Recognition and Information more than the other scores. In cases where language problems are present but the multiple-choice subtests are intact, these scores should likely be ignored as inaccurate.

17. The Information subtest is a good measure of incidental learning by the client during school but deficits are most often associated with a poor school learning history or an inability to access long-term or rarely used memories, most characteristic of frontal losses in the absence of aphasia. If aphasia is present, this score may reflect the language difficulties in either expressive or receptive language.

18. Higher scores on achievement tests that exceed intellectual scores by 15 points or more, especially on Reading Recognition and Spelling, may reflect a high level of organized practice on the tasks rather than a decline in IQ. In such cases, Reading Comprehension is typically closer to current IQ levels, although this may be seen in some brain injuries as well. Again, correlation with premorbid records and information is essential.

19. Comparison of similar tests on the PIAT and WRAT can be very useful in detecting specific deficits. The Reading Recognition scales of the two tests are essentially identical, so scores should be within 15 points of one another in most cases. When there are greater deviations, this may indicate motivational inconsistencies or fatigue.

20. The two spelling subtests differ considerably. On the WRAT, the client must spell each word by writing it. On the PIAT, the client picks from one of four choices.

21. If the PIAT Spelling Test is superior by 15 standard points or more, this indicates that the client is better at recognizing the right spelling than generating it. This suggests that the client is familiar with correct spelling but likely does not write much. Alternately, the client may have a writing disorder that impedes him or her from writing down the correct spelling. In such cases, clients may be able to dictate the correct spelling. If a writing disorder is not present, then this deficit likely reflects the client's educational, reading, and writing history rather than a brain injury.

22. If the WRAT Spelling test is superior by 15 standard points or more, this indicates that the client is likely confused by the multiple-choice format. This may indicate the presence of impulsivity or perseveration, which should show up across the subtests of the PIAT which use the multiple-choice format as well as such tests as Raven's Matrices and the Visual Form Discrimination Test. Alternately, if these signs are not present, the client's spelling may be more automatic and overlearned rather than "understood," causing the choice of items to confuse the client.

23. The PIAT and WRAT Arithmetic Scales differ more than any of the other similar subtests. The WRAT is a series of arithmetic problems that the client does on his or her own, writing down each problem. Many are problems that cannot be done in one's head. The PIAT consists of more verbally based items that can be solved in "one's head" and presents four alternate answers in a multiple-choice format. Items are given one by one by the examiner rather than all at once.

24. If the WRAT Arithmetic is performed better, then the client's strength is with purer mathematical problems. This may reflect a weakness with verbal mathematics problems. In such a case, Arithmetic on the WAIS-III will also be performed poorly. If this is not the case, this may indicate the presence of impulsivity or perseveration, which should show up across the subtests of the PIAT which use the multiple-choice format as well as such tests as Raven's Matrices and the Visual Form Discrimination Test. If neither hypothesis is supported, changes in motivation or fatigue should be considered.

25. If the PIAT Arithmetic is performed better, then the deficit may reflect problems with exact mathematical calculations often related to carelessness or to math anxiety, which is usually brought on more by the traditional test format of the WRAT. In some cases, however, the more complex problems of the WRAT may be impaired owing to the "spatial" aspects of arithmetic, primarily borrowing and carrying and aligning columns of numbers in multiplication, addition, and subtraction. Such errors can be identified by looking closely at the work of the client on the WRAT and can be verified through the LNNB Arithmetic Scale.

References for Peabody Individual Achievement Test (PIAT-R)

Cole, J. C., Muenz, T. A., Ouchi, B. Y., Kaufman, N. L., & Kaufman, A. S. (1997). The impact of pictorial stimulus on written expression output of adolescents and adults. *Psychology in the Schools, 34*(1), 1–9.

Dunn, L. M., & Markwardt, F. C. (1970). *Peabody Individual Achievement Test*. Circle Pines, MN: American Guidance Service.

Heaton, R. K., Schmitz, S. P., Avitable, N., & Lehman, R. A. (1987). Effects of lateralized cerebral lesions on oral reading, reading comprehension, and spelling. *Journal of Clinical & Experimental Neuropsychology, 9*(6), 711–722.

Mandes, E., & Gessner, T. (1989). The principle of additivity and it's relation to clinical decision making. *The Journal of Psychology, 123*(5), 485–490.

Markwardt, F. C. (1989). *Peabody Individual Achievement Test-Revised*. Circle Pines, MN: American Guidance Service.

Muenz, T. A., Ouchi, B. Y., & Cole, J. C. (1999). Item analysis of written expression scoring systems from the PIAT-R and WIAT. *Psychology in the Schools, 36*(1), 31–40.

Salvia, J., & Ysseldyke, J. E. (1988). *Assessment in special and remedial education* (4th ed.). Boston: Houghton Mifflin.

WIDE RANGE ACHIEVEMENT TEST (WRAT)

This is a quick and frequently used measure of achievement. Although it does not have the depth or detailed analysis seen in the PIAT, it offers a solid evaluation with minimal investment of time. It is therefore very useful in the quick assessment of adult subjects. Interpretive procedures are very similar to those used with the PIAT.

Interpretation

1. In interpretation of findings on tests of achievement, it is always imperative to keep in mind the person's intellectual abilities, as intellectual ability has come to be seen as a measure of learning potential, whereas achievement tests are intended to measure what has been learned. Therefore, attempting to interpret achievement scores without a measure of intellectual ability offers the examiner much less information about the learning process. In general, standard scores for the WRAT should be within 15 points of the client's verbal IQ. When scores are below IQ by a greater amount, this indicates a failure to learn but does not specify the etiology so that one cannot automatically diagnose a learning disability.

    In addition, standard scores for each scale should be within 15 points of the total test standard scores. Scores more than 15 points below this average suggest significantly impaired skills, while scores above this level suggest strengths. Score ranges greater than 30 points are also a marker that there may be a deficit in one or more areas.

2. Situations where the WRAT scores are greater than the intelligence scores suggest the possibility of loss of intellectual skills (especially when aphasic symptoms are present). This may occur in strokes and more advanced cases of dementia as well as severe head trauma, but rarely in mild to moderate head injury. Generally, the Reading Recognition score is considered most indicative of premorbid functioning than are the other scores yielded by the test.

3. Spelling and Mathematics scores are very sensitive to brain injury in general in individuals whose skills were weak to begin with (IQs less than 100). However, weaknesses in these scores are frequently seen in normal individuals as well, so a correlation with history and school records is usually indicated.

4. While writing it not formally evaluated, the spelling subtest yields a good sample of basic motor writing skills. Disorders of written language may be associated with motor disorders in which the client knows what he or she wants to write but is unable to do so, or kinesthetic disorders of the dominant hemisphere in which letters that are written in a similar manner (o and a, or h and k, for example) are substituted for one another. Spelling versus writing areas can be discriminated by asking the client to spell missed words out loud rather than writing them. Errors when writing but not speaking suggest a motor writing problem, while errors speaking but not writing suggest a motor speech problem or a disconnection syndrome between the receptive and expressive language areas.

5. Disorders of primary reading skills in which they decline from a higher level of functioning are almost always related to posterior dominant hemisphere functioning. However, disorders that show up only in the reading of smaller print or dense pages may reflect a spatial or visual disorder which in turn may result from occipital lesions of either side.

6. Ignoring the left side of words or ignoring the left side of the arithmetic pages may indicate a neglect syndrome most characteristic of right posterior lesions.

7. Declines in arithmetic ability may result from anterior or posterior lesions. However, the loss of the meaning of numeric symbols is almost always associated with the posterior left hemisphere. Difficulties in understanding the spatial nature of numbers (such as the role of the tens place and hundreds place) may reflect lesions of either hemisphere in the parietal–occipital areas. Declines in only more complex arithmetic skills may reflect frontal lesions.

8. Major deficits in expressive language will impair Reading Recognition more than the other scores.

9. Comparison of similar tests on the PIAT and WRAT can be very useful in detecting specific deficits. The Reading Recognition scales of the two tests are essentially identical, so scores should be within 15 points of one another in most cases. When there are greater deviations, this may indicate motivational inconsistencies or fatigue.

10. The two spelling subtests differ considerably. On the WRAT, the client must spell each word by writing it. On the PIAT, the client picks from one of four choices.

11. If the PIAT Spelling Test is superior by 15 standard points or more, this indicates that the client is better at recognizing the right spelling than generating it. This suggests that the client is familiar with correct spelling but likely does not write much. Alternately, the client may have a writing disorder that impedes him or her from writing down the correct spelling. In such cases, clients may be able to dictate the correct spelling. If a writing disorder is not present, then this deficit likely reflects the client's educational, reading, and writing history rather than a brian injury.

12. If the WRAT Spelling test is superior by 15 standard points or more, this indicates that the client is likely confused by the multiple-choice format. This may indicate the presence of impulsivity or perseveration, which should show up across the subtests of the PIAT which use the multiple-choice format as well as such tests as Raven's Matrices and the Visual Form Discrimination Test. Alternately, if these signs are not present, the client's spelling may be more automatic and overlearned rather than "understood," causing the choice of items to confuse the client.

13. The PIAT and WRAT Arithmetic Scales differ more than any of the other similar subtests. The WRAT is a series of arithmetic problems that the client does on his or her own, writing down each problem. Many are problems that cannot be done in one's head. The PIAT consists of more verbally based items that can be solved in "one's head" and presents four alternate answers in a multiple-choice format. Items are given one by one by the examiner rather than all at once.

14. If the WRAT Arithmetic is performed better, then the client's strength is with purer mathematical problems. This may reflect a weakness with verbal mathematics problems. In such a case, Arithmetic on the WAIS-III will also be performed poorly. If this is not the case, this may indicate the presence of impulsivity or perseveration, which should show up across the subtests of the PIAT which use the multiple-choice format as well as such tests as Raven's Matrices and

the Visual Form Discrimination Test. If neither hypothesis is supported, changes in motivation or fatigue should be considered.

15. If the PIAT Arithmetic is performed better, then the deficit may reflect problems with exact mathematical calculations often related to carelessness or to math anxiety which is usually brought on more by the traditional test format of the WRAT. In some cases, however, the more complex problems of the WRAT may be impaired due to the "spatial" aspects of arithmetic, primarily borrowing and carrying and aligning columns of numbers in multiplication, addition, and subtraction. Such errors can be identified by looking closely at the work of the client on the WRAT and can be verified through the LNNB Arithmetic Scale.

References to Wide Range Achievement Test (WRAT)

Groth-Marnet, G. (1997). *Handbook of psychological assessment* (3rd ed.). New York: John Wiley & Sons.

Sattler, J. M. (1992). *Assessment of children: Revised and updated third edition.* San Diego, CA: Jerome M. Sattler.

Snyder, P. J., & Nussbaum, P. D. (1998). *Clinical neuropsychology: A pocket handbook for assessment.* Washington, D.C.: American Psychological Association.

Wilkinson, G. S. (1993). *Wide Range Achievement Test (WRAT3): Administration manual.* Wilmington, DE: Wide Range.

READING SCALE (C8, LNNB)

The Reading Scale of the LNNB measures a client's ability to decode words. It differs from the other achievement tests in that it does not try to measure a grade level of achievement but rather the basic neurologically based skills necessary for reading and that may be impaired in injuries to the brain. It does not measure word-pronunciation skills but instead the ability to convert letters and letter combinations into sounds. It is primarily used to detect left hemisphere damage but can be used to identify other types of brain dysfunction as well. However, as reading is a "hold" skill this score may better represent premorbid levels of functioning. Deficits are seen most often in strokes or other focal destructive injuries of the brain located in the posterior temporal–parietal–occipital areas. It is best used within a general battery as a follow-up with clients who have reading problems in an attempt to identify specific underlying causes.

Interpretation

1. Items 188 and 189 generally measure the ability of the client to show integration of letters and auditory analysis from oral presentation of

material. In clients who cannot identify the visual presentation of letters, this allows for the testing of integrative skills important for reading without the visual component. Good performance on these items when the remainder of the scale is poor suggests that the reading problem is primarily visual rather than involving sound integration.

2. Difficulty on items 190 through 192 look at decoding basic phonemic sounds which may be impaired even when overlearned reading appears intact. Losses on these items suggest basic decoding problems and reflect (as do most of the items on this scale) lesions in the temporal–occipital area or in the temporal–parietal area of the left hemisphere. These deficits can exist even when the client is able to read words, usually because of overlearning. Such losses may not appear until the client needs to read words that are not overlearned (which will be related to premorbid levels and frequency of reading).

3. If the client is able to read simple words in items 193 through 196 but not sentences or paragraphs in items 197 through 199, possible injuries indicated are disorders of visual scanning that make it impossible for the client to grasp more than one word at a time. Such inability is usually a result of injuries in the secondary visual areas of the occipital lobe. These lesions are associated with visual–spatial problems on tests such as Trails A, Block Design, and the Rey Figure.

4. Items 193 through 196 look at the ability to read increasingly difficult words. In literate clients, the client will generally be able to do some items by simple recognition as a result of previous familiarity with the material and other words will require decoding. The dividing point will differ depending on premorbid achievement. Items that require decoding should be carefully evaluated not just for the presence of errors but for the nature of those errors. When errors suggest pronunciations that are not possible in English given the combination of letters, this is more serious and points to a lesion in the temporal–occipital areas of the left hemisphere. Errors that are possible in English are more benign and may simply reflect premorbid achievement levels.

5. When a client who could read prior to an injury has difficulty with this subtest, it is most often associated with a left hemisphere injury, usually posterior. However, some difficulty with complex words may appear in highly educated individuals with left frontal lesions. The exceptions to this are deficits that occur because of spatial disruption (inability to follow a line, which shows most clearly in the paragraph reading) or unilateral neglect. Both of these latter deficits suggest right hemisphere dysfunction.

6. Performance on this subtest must be carefully compared to premorbid levels of achievement. Deficits in many cases may reflect preexisting

deficits (such as a learning disability or a poor educational experience) rather than a current brain injury.

References for Reading Scale (C8, LNNB)

Chelune, G. J. (1982). A reexamination of the relationship between the Luria–Nebraska and Halstead–Reitan batteries: Overlap with the WAIS. *Journal of Consulting and Clinical Psychology, 50,* 578–580.

Golden, C. J., Purisch, A. D., & Hammeke, T. A. (1985). *Luria–Nebraska Neuropsychological Battery-Forms I and II Manual.* Los Angeles: Western Psychological Services.

Nagel, J. A., Harrell, E., & Gray, S. G. (1997). Prediction of achievement scores using the Luria–Nebraska Neuropsychological Battery Form II. *Psychology, 34*(1), 41–47.

WRITING SCALE (C7, LNNB)

The Writing Scale of the LNNB measures the client's spelling and motor writing skills. It assesses the ability to analyze words phonetically in English and then to do copying of increasing difficulty. Generally, this subtest detects left hemisphere dysfunction as writing disorders tend to localize around the temporal–parietal–occipital area, especially in and around the angular gyrus. This scale, however, can be used to identify other problematic areas. The goal of the scale is to identify specific problems that may relate to writing and spelling disorders. It is very useful as a follow-up to general achievement testing that reveals the possibility of a neurologically based deficit.

Interpretation

1. If the client is able to write from written material (items 177–179) but not from dictation (181–185), a specific lesion in the temporal lobe is indicated. If, on the other hand, the client can write from auditory material but not from written, a lesion in the occipital or occipital–parietal areas of the cerebral cortex may be present. These lesions are usually in the left hemisphere, but in some left-handed people they may be in the right hemisphere.

2. If the client is changing one letter to another and has difficulty forming letters even though he or she is able to write, there could be a kinesthetic feedback problem whereby the client mixes up letters that are formed by similar motor movements. An example would be substitution of an "h" for a "k" or an "o" for an "a."

3. If the client is unable to write as a result of paralysis, this is suggestive of a lesion to the motor strip of the posterior frontal lobe. In such cases

when a motor component is suspected, clients may be asked to orally spell words or point to letters on a page with the alphabet so that motor and cognitive components can be separated to some degree.

4. If the client writes at an angle to the page but has no other writing problems, this may suggest some spatial problems that may be associated with right hemisphere dysfunction. This should show up clearly in drawing and construction tasks as well.

5. The inability to write or read one's name is often indicative of general dementia. In some cases, it is indicative of a disorder of automatic writing that may occur with injuries to both hemispheres.

6. This scale can be split into spelling and writing subtests. Difficulty with spelling may be seen as an indication of either right or left hemisphere dysfunction. When the concept of spelling is completely lost (e.g., "CAT" is spelled "DBG"), it is most often associated with left hemisphere damage, especially in the parietal or temporal areas. Deficits in which the correct letters are retained but are placed in the wrong sequence have been seen in patients with a variety of injuries. Spelling deficits may also be the result of premorbid problems including poor educational experiences.

7. Motor writing errors are generally associated with the hemisphere opposite the client's writing hand, although one should be careful of the client who has switched writing hands as a result of an injury. In such cases, writing problems are reflective of ipsilateral dysfunction. Motor writing problems may simply be the result of problems in the motor area of the brain.

8. Motor writing impairments that are spatially disrupted (at large angles to the horizontal, or where words are written over one another) may be suggestive of right hemisphere dysfunction.

9. Writing problems in the absence of reading problems point to motor or kinesthetic lesions in the sensorimotor areas around the precentral gyrus.

10. Reading deficits without writing deficits indicate visual analysis problems most likely near the occipital–temporal areas.

References for Writing Scale (C7, LNNB)

Chelune, G. J. (1982). A reexamination of the relationship between the Luria–Nebraska and Halstead–Reitan batteries: Overlap with the WAIS. *Journal of Consulting and Clinical Psychology, 50,* 578–580.

Golden, C. J., Purisch, A. D., & Hammeke, T. A. (1985). *Luria–Nebraska Neuropsychological Battery: Forms I and II Manual.* Los Angeles: Western Psychological Services.

Nagel, J. A., Harrell, E., & Gray, S. G. (1997). Prediction of achievement scores using the Luria–Nebraska Neuropsychological Battery Form II. *Psychology, 34*(1), 41–47.

ARITHMETIC SCALE (C9, LNNB)

The Arithmetic Scale, of all the Luria–Nebraska Neuropsychological Battery (LNNB) scales, is the most sensitive of the LNNB scales to brain injury. However, it is also the most sensitive scale to educational deficits and strong fear reactions elicited by mathematical items in many normal individuals. As such, to ensure the client's best performance, the examiner must be aware of this issue and proceed slowly through the scale, while calming and/or gently pushing the client as needed. The scale as a unit does not allow for localization of brain dysfunction, although items can be analyzed individually for this purpose. Unlike the PIAT or WRAT, this scale does not try to identify grade level but rather tries to identify basic skill deficits that arise as the result of brain injury and that may impact the learning or execution of arithmetic skills. It serves as a good follow-up when more general achievement tests reveal the possibility of a problem.

Interpretation

1. Interpretations of the arithmetic scale must be made cautiously, as approximately 20% or more of the normal population in the normative sample exhibits deficits in this area often related to poor educational background or a negative attitude toward the subject. Having taken this into consideration, however, the scale appears to be very useful in detecting lesions in all parts of the brain.
2. Errors in arithmetic items may reflect deficits in disparate parts of the brain depending on the exact qualitative nature of the errors. Thus, it is very important to observe the client and determine how errors were made, including using testing-of-limits procedures if necessary.
3. On items 201 through 209, inability to read or write simple numbers suggests left hemisphere damage. This is especially true in those cases in which there is a failure to recognize individual numbers as numbers or symbols.
4. If clients can recognize individual numbers but fail to recognize the meaning of sequences of numbers, this may reflect lesions in the occipital–parietal areas of the dominant hemisphere.
5. Spatial dysfunctions, as manifested by a client's tendency to reverse the sequence of numbers, can also be seen on these same items. Individuals with severe spatial deficits often reverse even the most basic items. In contrast, clients with only subtle deficits are likely to reverse Roman numerals more often than they do Arabic numerals owing to their lack of familiarity with Roman numerals. Similarly, subtle spatial deficits also begin to show as the items progress in level of complexity. Deficits

in this area are indicative of right hemisphere or left occipital–parietal dysfunction.

6. On items 210 and 211, the client is asked to compare numbers to each other. Failure to perform this operation correctly suggests dysfunction of the left occipital–parietal area and a failure to again appreciate the importance of the sequence of digits in a number.

7. Items 212 through 214 involve the computation of simple arithmetic problems. Problems in this area are indicative of serious inability to understand what is being said and, thus, of severe left hemisphere dysfunction, mainly in the parietal lobe.

8. Items 215 through 220 involve complex mathematical manipulations, operations that are basic to the left parietal area. These types of problems are somewhat difficult and are often missed by clients with low educational attainment. As such, errors on these items are not considered as serious as deficits in other more basic sections of the scale. Clients with higher educational level, however, are expected to be able to complete these items. Consequently, a highly educated individual with a left parietal dysfunction will often not show deficits until this section.

9. Low scores on items 221 and 222 (serial 7s and serial 13s) are common among the normal population. Nevertheless, an extremely poor performance on these items is likely to be associated with brain dysfunction, especially when the rest of the scale is performed relatively well and the person seems to possess intact basic arithmetic skills. In the presence of normal mathematical skills, problems in this section are likely to be associated with attentional/concentration deficits and are indicative of left frontal lobe dysfunction.

10. The presence of arithmetic deficits without writing or reading deficits suggests either an occipital–parietal lesion of the left hemisphere, right hemisphere dysfunction, or simply weak premorbid learning of arithmetic skills.

11. An inability to understand what a basic number or a basic arithmetic sign is suggests a visual disorder that reflects dominant hemisphere function. This can exist independent of any other deficits or may reflect a more general pattern of deficits in the dominant parietal–occipital area.

12. For items involving the visual presentation of more than one number, failure to see the numbers on one side of the stimulus indicates unilateral neglect. These deficits reflect injuries to the posterior nondominant hemisphere and should be confirmed on other tests of writing and visual–spatial skills (such as the Benton).

13. Spatial arithmetic problems may be seen in several different circumstances. For example, an answer that shows the reversal of Arabic or

Roman numerals, as well as an answer that disregards the meaning of the ones, tens, or hundreds spaces. Inability to read multidigit numbers as a whole, single number as required on item 209 is also evidence of a spatial disorder. This can be seen if a client, on items 215 through 217, makes an error in carrying and lining up numbers when trying to solve mathematical problems. Such errors are associated with occipital-parietal lesions, most often in the dominant hemisphere, but can reflect nondominant hemisphere lesions as well, especially in an individual in whom arithmetic skills are not premorbidly overlearned.

References for Arithmetic Scale (C9, LNNB)

Chelune, G. J. (1982). A reexamination of the relationship between the Luria–Nebraska and Halstead-Reitan batteries: Overlap with the WAIS. *Journal of Consulting and Clinical Psychology, 50,* 578–580.

Golden, C. J., Purisch, A. D., & Hammeke, T. A. (1985). *Luria–Nebraska Neuropsychological Battery: Forms I and II Manual.* Los Angeles: Western Psychological Services.

Nagel, J. A., Harrell, E., & Gray, S. G. (1997). Prediction of achievement scores using the Luria–Nebraska Neuropsychological Battery Form II. *Psychology, 34*(1), 41–47.

SECTION VII: EXECUTIVE SKILLS

CONTROLLED ORAL WORD ASSOCIATION TEST (COWAT)

The purpose of the Controlled Oral Word Association Test (COWAT) is to evaluate the spontaneous production of words beginning with a given letter or belonging to a given category within a limited amount of time. In brief, the test is administered by instructing the individual to produce as many words in 1 minute as he or she can think of that begin with the given letter of the alphabet, excluding proper nouns and the same word with a different suffix. The most commonly used letters are FAS, although CFL and PRW are used as alternatives. Another alternative that is usually given in addition to letters, but that can be substituted for them, is the use of conceptual categories for which words must be generated. For example, the subject can be instructed to name as many fruits and vegetables or animals within a minute. However, the category alternative is considered to be somewhat different than the letter version because it allows the subject to draw on a conceptual category which may permit a form of fluency that is enhanced by cues inherent to the conceptual category. The basic idea here is that the conceptual category may activate verbal associations better and therefore allow for better access to appropriate responses.

Interpretation

1. Impairment in the understanding of language or the motor expression of language will have a profound effect on the completion of this test regardless of possible impairment in abstraction or flexibility. Interpretation is limited if there is any evidence of basic receptive or expressive speech problems (Aphasia Screen, LNNB Receptive Language, LNNB Expressive Language) or general verbal intellectual problems (WAIS-III).

2. Neuropsychological skills involved in the cognitive generation of responses at the preverbal output stage on the COWAT include production of internal speech, self-awareness, inhibition of inappropriate responses, and mental flexibility. Internal speech is involved to the degree that the examinee generates possible responses and contemplates their appropriateness. This involves an interface between processes involved in auditory comprehension and those involved in word retrieval. Normal scores on tests of receptive and expressive skills allow the COWAT to be analyzed from the perspective of frontal lobe skills of flexibility, inhibition, perseveration, and so on.

3. A major skill necessary for adequate performance is the ability to inhibit verbal output of responses that are not appropriate given the task at hand. Clients with deficits in this area will typically generate a number of responses that are not appropriate to the category selected or are perseverative. In such cases, similar disinhibited or perseverative responses will be expected on a variety of tests such as the WCST or Category tests which are more nonverbal in nature and Trails B which has a larger verbal content.

4. Mental flexibility deficits (and perseveration) will be reflected in the repetition of identical or very similar responses. In severe conditions, the same word or word form may be repeated many times.

5. Poverty of responses may reflect low IQ or poor language skills. However, if this poverty of responses is seen in the presence of normal intelligence and normal language skills, frontal lobe deficits regarding the inability to carry out a complex verbal task should be considered. If the deficits are limited to verbal tasks, this may not be associated with poor performance on similar nonverbal tasks (such as WCST or Category) but should be associated with poor performance on Trails B.

6. Responses should be examined for the presence of verbal disorders: paraphasias, neologisms, stuttering, awkward (disjointed) speech, and slurring. The speeded nature of this task and the intellectual demands will often make milder problems in these areas much more obvious.

Deficits in motor speech are generally associated with left anterior lesions, and paraphasias and neologisms with more posterior temporal–parietal injuries.

7. Because concept formation is often affected with lesions to the left temporal–parietal lobe, a examinee with such lesions may be unable to operate with complex systems of speech associations. Therefore, difficulties in classification may result in poor COWAT performance as manifest by inability to appropriately produce words guided by a particular classification (e.g., words beginning with "F" or "Animals").

8. An examinee with lesions to the left frontal lobe is likely to show a number of difficulties with COWAT performance. In receiving the instructions, the examinee may be unable to remain focused on the information given and irrelevant associations may easily emerge. This fact has implications not only for initial understanding of instructions and what is expected in terms of performance on the test, but also has implications for conflicting (or perhaps even tangential) signals that may arise in the examinee's internal speech. In the former, the examinee may experience a barrage of associations in response to one or a few elements of the instructions that draw him or her away from adequate comprehension of the instructions. For example, when asked to "produce as many words as you can …" the irrelevant association of vegetables (to the word produce) may arise, thereby distracting the examinee from the underlying meaning of the message. In the latter, the examinee may be distracted with irrelevant associations while attempting to produce alternatives. In this case the examinee may begin by producing words that begin with the letter S, but upon producing the word "suit" may be seized by the association "tie" and so on, rather than maintaining set.

9. Another possibility in frontal clients is that the examinee demonstrates perseveration on the task. In this scenario, once the examinee produces a word, the examinee may repeatedly offer the same word, unable to shift to other appropriate responses. This has a profound impact on verbal fluency, as a series of distinct responses does not flow naturally from the examinee. Overall, lesions to the left frontal lobe result in COWAT performance that is characterized by disinhibition of irrelevant responses, perseveration, and decreased verbal fluency.

10. Examinees with lesions to the deep subcortical region are likely to show lowered cortical activity. Performance on the COWAT is likely to be characterized by slowed performance wherein the number of words produced within the allotted time limit is very low. This impaired performance is perhaps best contrasted with the performance of one type of frontal lobe examinee whose speed is average or better, but

contains many perseverations. In cases of severe lesions of the deep subcortical region, the examinee may become disoriented, confabulatory, and often experience transient consciousness.

11. Good performance on the COWAT is inconsistent with low intelligence as well as problems in verbal fluency and flexibility (although nonverbal problems on other tests may exist). Good performance would be rare in any kind of significant brain injury involving the dominant hemisphere.

12. Profiles in which the WCST is impaired but Category, COWAT, Stroop, and Trails B are normal points to problems with the client figuring out the intent of the test. (See the WCST interpretation section for more detail.)

13. Profiles in which Category and TPT are impaired but WCST, COWAT, Trails B, and Stroop are normal suggest that the difficulties are with the visual–spatial nature of these tests. While there is a visual component to WCST, there is not a spatial component comparable to Category and TPT for most clients.

14. Profiles in which WCST, COWAT, Stroop, and Trails B are impaired but Category and TPT (frontal signs) are normal point to problems dealing with verbal executive skills, usually reflecting damage to the anterior left (dominant) hemisphere.

15. Profiles in which Category, WCST, and TPT (frontal signs) are impaired but COWAT, Stroop, and Trails B are intact suggest problems with visual executive skills, suggesting lesions in the anterior right (nondominant) hemisphere. In such cases, the client attempts to solve the WCST in a nonverbal manner.

16. Profiles in which the Stroop, COWAT, and Trails B are impaired but Category, WCST, and TPT are normal point to specific verbal analysis problems related to poor flexibility for verbal material.

References for Controlled Oral Word Association Test (COWAT)

Lezak, M. D. (1995). *Neuropsychological assessment* (2nd ed.). New York: Oxford University Press.
Luria, A. R. (1980). *Higher cortical functions in man* (2nd ed.). New York: Consultants Bureau.
Spreen, O., & Stauss, E. (1998). *A compendium of neuropsychological tests: Administration, norms, and commentary* (2nd ed.). New York: Oxford University Press.

WISCONSIN CARD SORTING TEST (WCST)

Executive functions, often referred to as problem-solving and abstraction, incorporate the ability to initiate appropriate sets of responses, maintain responses, and shift responses when required. Such functions are mediated mainly by the frontal lobe. One of the most common neuropsychological tools assessing such functions is the Wisconsin Card Sorting Test (WCST).

Interpretation

1. The complexity of the WCST makes interpretation for a specific cause or lesion difficult. Although the test has been reported to be a test of frontal lobe function, it has been recognized that many nonfrontal functions are involved including understanding of the instructions, verbal memory, visual analysis, visual memory, attention, concentration, and frustration analysis, in addition to the more frontal skills of sequencing, learning from experience, hypothesis formation, behavioral evaluation, planning, and conceptualization. An interpretation of frontal problems is stronger when the deficit occurs despite normal performance on tests of language comprehension (LNNB Receptive Language, Comprehension), Block Design, Digit Span, visual memory testing, and Picture Completion.

2. Difficulty sorting according to category is suggestive of impaired capacity for formulation of abstract concepts. This type of deficit is found to occur most frequently in subjects with frontal lobe dysfunction (particularly left frontal lobe damage). However, the examiner must make sure that the client understands what is to be done. In such cases, Category is often impaired as well as Trails B.

3. Frontal lobe clients achieve fewer sorting categories and make more perseverative errors than other brain-injured clients. The presence of excessive perseverative responses is the strongest indicator both of brain damage and the involvement of the frontal areas. Perseverative response score cutoffs greater than 19 are indicative of impairment.

4. Individuals with Alzheimer's disease, Pick's disease, and Parkinson's disease also show significantly more deficits on the WCST.

5. Perseveration on the WCST and erratic error patterns illustrated by disruptions and impersistence characterize the performance of long-term alcoholics. The client may form categories easily and shift sets readily several times, but end up losing track of the present category and become totally confused.

6. Individuals with focal frontal lesions show significantly more perseveration on the WCST than those with focal nonfrontal lesions. Clients with focal nonfrontal lesions may be misclassified as normal when using just the perseveration measure.

7. Older clients appear to show more perseverations regardless of neurological status. Increasing the perseverative response cutoff to around 35 may be appropriate for clients age 60 and above. The norms of Heaton,

Grant, and Matthews (1991) are useful in classifying these responses in older individuals.

8. Clients with diffuse cerebral lesions may perform similar to frontal patients.

9. Failure to maintain set was conceived as a measure of frontal dysfunction but appears to load independently of other measures in factor studies. The presence of more than two failures suggests either a memory problem or easy distractibility, but the absence of such findings appears to have no meaning.

10. Interpretation must be very cautious in any client with aphasia (especially relating to language comprehension) or significant visual spatial deficits. In each case, frontal-like behavior may be seen which reflects a more posterior rather than anterior focus. Interpretation can be made much more confidently in the absence of these deficits.

11. In some cases of dementia and others involving memory problems, the client's errors will be due to forgetting the instructions or what he or she has been doing. In such cases, the client should be asked to explain what he is doing to see if he has forgotten what is happening.

12. Some intelligent clients may do poorly because they make the task more difficult. In such cases, they may figure that a combination of color and form or form and number is being used. When faced with error, they adopt more difficult schemata which further disrupts their performance. This is rarely indicative of brain injury and can be detected only by asking the client to explain his or her performance.

13. After the test is completed poorly, the examiner can directly explain how the test works and ask the client to do it again. Clients with significant frontal injuries will find the task impossible even under such conditions.

14. Scores are affected by anxiety, depression, and low frustration tolerance. When these are present, scores should be interpreted cautiously.

15. Profiles in which the WCST is impaired but Category, COWAT, Stroop, and Trails B are normal point to problems with the client figuring out the intent of the test. On all of the other tests the fact that demands across the test change is stated explicitly in the instructions, while on WCST the client must infer this when he or she begins to make errors after completing the first Category. Clients with milder frontal problems may be able to handle the other tests but react badly to the sudden change in feedback on the WCST and be further confused by the fact that they accidentally get some right by following the old category when an item matches on more than one category.

16. Profiles in which Category and TPT are impaired but WCST, COWAT, Trails B, and Stroop are normal suggest that the difficulties are with the

visual–spatial nature of these tests. While there is a visual component to WCST, there is not a spatial component comparable to Category and TPT for most clients.

17. Profiles in which WCST, COWAT, Stroop, and Trails B are impaired but Category and TPT (frontal signs) are normal point to problems dealing with verbal executive skills, usually reflecting damage to the anterior left (dominant) hemisphere.

18. Profiles in which Category, WCST, and TPT (frontal signs) are impaired but COWAT, Stroop, and Trails B are intact may indicate problems with visual executive skills, suggesting lesions in the anterior right (nondominant) hemisphere. In such cases, the client attempts to solve the WCST in a nonverbal manner.

19. Profiles in which the Stroop, COWAT, and Trails B are impaired but Category, WCST, and TPT are normal point to specific verbal analysis problems related to poor flexibility for verbal material.

20. Good performance on the WCST can occur with low verbal intelligence.

21. Because of the length of the WCST, it generally demands more sustained attention than do other memory tests. Thus, problems in sustained attention as reflected in poor IVA or TOVA performance (particularly on visual portions) may correlate with poor performance. In such cases, impairment will also be seen on Faces, TPT, Category, and the Rey Figure, which also require sustained attention for good performance. Similar tests that require less sustained attention (e.g., BVRT, Stroop, COWAT, Trails B, Working Memory) will generally be normal if this is the primary problem except in the more severe deficits which can potentially affect any test.

References for Wisconsin Card Sorting Test (WCST)

Elliot, R., McKenna, P. J., Robbins, T. W., & Sahakian, B. J. (1995). Neuropsychological evidence for frontostriatal dysfunction in schizophrenia. *Psychological Medicine, 25*, 619–630.

Gansler, D. A., Covall, S., McGratil, N., & Oscar-Berman, M. (1996). Measures of prefrontal dysfunction after closed head injury. *Brain and Cognition, 30*, 194–204.

Greve, K. W., Ingram, F., & Bianchini, K. J. (1998). Latent structure of the Wisconsin Card Sorting Test in a clinical sample. *Archives of Clinical Neuropsychology, 1*(7), 597–609.

Heaton, R. K., Grant, I., & Matthews, C. G. (1991). *Comprehensive norms for an expanded Halstead–Reitan battery: Demographic corrections, research findings, and clinical applications.* Odessa, FL: Psychological Assessment Resources.

Merello, M., Sabe, L., Teson, A., Migliorelli, R., Petracchi, M., Leiguarda, R., & Starkstein, S. (1994). Extrapyramidalism in Alzheimer's disease: Prevalence, psychiatric, and neuropsychological correlates. *Journal of Neurology, Neurosurgery, and Psychiatry, 57*, 1503–1509.

Seidenberg, M., Hermann, B., Noe, A., & Wyler, A. R. (1995). Depression in temporal lobe epilepsy: Interaction between laterality of lesion and Wisconsin Card Sort performance. *Neuropsychiatry, Neuropsychology, and Behavioral Neurology, 8*(2), 81–87.

Wiegner, S., & Donders, J. (1999). Performance on the Wisconsin Card Sorting Test after traumatic brain injury. *Assessment*, 6(2), 179–187.

HALSTEAD CATEGORY TEST

The Halstead Category Test, which measures higher order cognitive functions of a nonverbal nature and the ability to determine general principles from sets of specific stimulus items, is a complex visual abstraction concept-formation assessment tool requiring the utilization of abstract concept formation, cognitive flexibility, and aspects of visual–spatial functioning and memory. It is considered to be an excellent discriminator between brain-damaged and neurologically intact groups.

The adult version of the test is divided into seven subtests grouped by abstract principles, and consists of 208 stimulus figures varying in number, shape, size, color, intensity, and location. The test can be administered manually with the booklet version, or by an automated version. The first six subtests involve a single principle. The seventh subtest is without one single unifying principle and requires the subject to remember the correct responses for stimulus items previously presented. The client must generate hypotheses and utilize examiner feedback to modulate response patterns. There is no time limit and administration averages 40–60 minutes. After completion of the test, incorrect responses are totaled. The Category Test is strongly influenced by age and education. To address issues of age, education, and gender effects on subtests of the Halstead–Reitan battery, Heaton, Grant, and Matthews (1991) developed age, education, and gender corrections norms. The test was originally introduced as a measure of frontal lobe functioning. Although such functions are clearly tapped by the test, it also clearly measures other skills as well, making it a measure sensitive to many forms of brain injury.

Interpretation

1. The Category Test alone has been found to be as effective as 90% in discriminating brain injury from intact individuals and is considered the single most sensitive test of brain damage in the Halstead–Reitan Battery. Reitan's cutoff was originally over 50 errors, but the recent normative data (Heaton et al., 1993) have supplied age and education-corrected norms. Because the Category Test identifies clients with so many different lesions, it cannot be considered a test of just frontal lobe function in isolation.
2. Interpretation of the test as showing frontal disorders can be done only after all other possible causes have been ruled out, including visual

identification (Picture Completion, Boston Naming, PPVT), visual–spatial skills (Block Design, Matrices, BVRT), fatigue, frustration tolerance, comprehension of instructions (Aphasia Screen, LNNB Receptive Language), depression, and anxiety. Good performance on Block Design, Digit Span, Trails Making-Part A, language comprehension tests, and Raven's Matrices enhances the interpretation of poor Category Test performance as indicating frontal deficits.

3. For clients with IQs in the average or above range, a low Category Test score may be indicative of a functional decrease in the integrity of higher order functioning. The number of errors on the Category Test is negatively correlated with IQ. The Category Test has been indicated as having significant correlation with Performance IQ measures on the WAIS and WAIS-R in both brain-injured and normal populations, but as inconsistent with regard to correlation with Verbal IQ.

4. Increasing age will lower Category Test performance in normals, often to levels suggestive of brain injury.

5. The pattern of errors within the Category Test is of important consideration. Patterns of error may be different within the first six subtests. Unless severely impaired, most individuals commit very few errors on the first two subtests. Those with moderate impairment usually begin to commit errors on subtests three and four. When a majority of a client's errors appear on Subtest three, the profile may not be indicative of brain injury, as this subtest is very difficult for a large number of normal individuals.

6. Incorrect responses at the beginning of each subtest are common as the client attempts to learn the criterion principle via trial and error. A large error percentage within a subtest may be indicative of deficient learning abilities, ineffective strategy use in problem solving, perseverative style, or inability to shift set. An inconsistent error pattern may suggest attentional difficulties or the inability to maintain set. A prevalence of perseverative responses or inability to shift set (which may result in different answers made on the wrong principle) is suggestive of frontal patterns.

7. Inferences about memory can be made if errors are lower on the first six subtests and higher on the memory subtest by at least 15%.

8. Debriefing clients to understand their reasoning is useful in comprehending the nature of the client's deficits.

9. After the test is over, one may "test the limits" by explaining the principle to the client on the subtest in which he or she did the worse. While frontal clients will continue to do poorly due to shifts in the type of items within each subtest, anxious normals or those with mild injuries will show normal performance.

10. Although the test has been presented as "culture free" there is some accumulating evidence that this is not the case. As with other tests in this book, it is strongly suggested that the test not be used for cultural or ethnic groups that differ significantly from the normal sample.

11. The acuteness or chronicity of brain damage does not appear to have a role in the outcome of the test score.

12. There is some indication that the Category Test has the capability to distinguish between cortical and subcortical dementia. Individuals with cortical dementia have been found to score in the severely impaired range. Those with subcortical dementia typically score in the mildly impaired range.

13. The Category Test is very sensitive to chronic excessive alcohol consumption. A poor Category Test score is usually obtained despite intact scores on intellectual measures. The deterioration has been noted to resemble that of early aging. Deficits are revealed in an inability to maintain set, rather than in learning the principle or in difficulty shifting sets.

14. Schizophrenics have been shown to score so poorly on the Category Test that it is difficult to distinguish them from clients with organic injury. It has been argued that this is because many schizophrenics have a brain injury, which led to chronic schizophrenia. The test should not be administered during acute exacerbations of schizophrenia, as the results are questionable.

15. A poor score obtained with a very fast test taking time (less than 30 minutes) is usually indicative of impulsivity and lack of motivation.

16. The Category Test subtests differ on the reasoning skills necessary to complete each subtest, so an analysis can be made from the distribution of errors. Subtests one and two, symbol recognition and counting, are limited in their relation to other subtests and serve mainly to introduce the client to the measure. A spatial reasoning factor is identified with subtest three, which requires recognition of the row of location. Subtest four involves linear and quadrant positioning but provides training for the individual in the initial items. Some normal individuals make errors on this subtest because they reverse the location of quadrants III and IV, preferring to go left to right on each row rather than in a clockwise direction around the square. Subtests five and six are indicated as proportional reasoning factors which involve the determination of percentages based on quartiles. Subtest seven is the memory subtest.

17. Profiles in which the WCST is impaired but Category, COWAT, Stroop, and Trails B are normal point to problems with the client figuring out the intent of the test. (See the WCST interpretation section for more detail.)

18. Profiles in which Category and TPT are impaired but WCST, COWAT, Trails B, and Stroop are normal suggest that the difficulties are with the visual–spatial nature of these tests. While there is a visual component to WCST, there is not a spatial component comparable to Category and TPT for most clients.

19. Profiles in which WCST, COWAT, Stroop, and Trails B are impaired but Category and TPT (frontal signs) are normal point to problems dealing with verbal executive skills, usually reflecting damage to the anterior left (dominant) hemisphere.

20. Profiles in which Category, WCST, and TPT (frontal signs) are impaired but COWAT, Stroop, and Trails B are intact suggest problems with visual executive skills, suggesting lesions in the anterior right (nondominant) hemisphere. In such cases, the client attempts to solve the WCST in a nonverbal manner.

21. Profiles in which the Stroop, COWAT, and Trails B are impaired but Category, WCST, and TPT are normal point to specific verbal analysis problems related to poor flexibility for verbal material.

22. Category performance is very sensitive to age. At ages above 60, it becomes difficult to discriminate between impairment due to normal aging and that due to known pathological processes.

23. Because of the length of Categories, it generally demands more sustained attention than do other memory tests. Thus, problems in sustained attention as reflected in poor IVA or TOVA performance (particularly on visual portions) may correlate with poor performance. In such cases, impairment will also be seen on the WCST, TPT, Faces, and the Rey Figure, which also require sustained attention for good performance. Similar tests that require less sustained attention (e.g., BVRT, Stroop, COWAT, Trails B, Working Memory) will generally be normal if this is the primary problem except in the more severe deficits which can potentially affect any test.

References for Halstead Category Test

Berger, S. G., Chibnall, J. T., & Gfeller, J. D. (1997). Construct validity of the computerized version of the category test. *Journal of Clinical Psychology, 53*(7), 723–726.

Choca, J. P., Laatsch, L., Wetzel, L., & Agresti, A. (1997). The Halstead category test: A fifty year perspective. *Neuropsychology Review, 7*(2), 61–75.

Golden, C. J., Zillmer, E., & Spiers, M. (1992). *Neuropsychological assessment and intervention.* Springfield, IL: Charles C Thomas.

Heaton, R. K., Grant, I., & Matthews, C. G. (1991). *Comprehensive norms for an expanded Halstead–Reitan battery: Demographic corrections, research findings, and clinical applications.* Odessa, FL: Psychological Assessment Resources.

Johnstone, B., Holland, D., & Hewett, J. E. (1997). The construct validity of the category test: Is it a measure of reasoning or intelligence? *Psychological Assessment, 9*(1), 28–33.

Mercer, W. N., Harrell, E. H., Miller, D. C., Childs, H. W., & Rockers, D. M. (1997). Performance of brain-injured versus healthy adults on three versions of the category test. *The Clinical Neuropsychologist, 11*(2), 174–179.

Wiegner, S., & Donders, J. (1999). Performance on the Wisconsin Card Sorting Test after traumatic brain injury. *Assessment, 6*(2), 179–187.

TRAIL MAKING TEST (TMT)

The Trail Making Test (TMT) is easily administered and has been utilized as a test of visual conceptual abilities, cognitive flexibility, set shifting, sequencing ability, visual–motor tracking, and visual–spatial functioning. It involves a large attentional component and has proven to be highly sensitive to the effects of brain injury in general, but not useful in lateralizing the damage. It consists of two parts, Trails A and Trails B. Trails B is considered one of the best general indicators of cerebral dysfunction.

Interpretation

1. Normal performance on Trails A should be 40 seconds or less, and for Trails B, 91 seconds or less. The combined time to complete both parts should be less than 110 seconds. These norms will overdiagnose problems in older people, and age-adjusted norms should be used in such groups.
2. The ratio of the Trails B time to the Trails A time (Trails B/Trails A) is a useful index of the comparative performance of the two subtests.
3. A ratio less than 2 suggests good performance on Trails B.
4. A ratio of less than 1.5 suggests impairment in the performance of Trails A. This is most often due to motor impairment or slow visual scanning. However, if Trails A is less than 30 seconds, then the ratio may be interpreted as excellent performance on Trails B.
5. If the ratio is greater than 3, this suggests impaired performance on Trails B. This is almost always due either to the verbal content of Trails B (in clients who do not know the alphabet well) or to the switching between numbers and letters.
6. Deficits on Trails B due to poor learning of the alphabet often suggest longstanding problems (which can be documented by history) that may be related to the function of the dominant hemisphere.
7. Good performance on Trails A in terms of the absolute norms, combined with overlearned alphabetic skills, suggests that B/A ratios of 3.0 or more are due to the alternating (task switching) demands of Trails A. Such problems point to dysfunction of the anterior frontal areas of the brain, particularly in the dominant hemisphere.

8. Poor performance on Trails A, which is indicated by a time over the cutoff and a ratio of less than 1.5, is generally due to motor speed problems. This can be confirmed by the comparison to Finger Tapping or other basic tests of motor speed. If motor speed is intact, visual scanning is likely defective. Such scanning may reflect right posterior spatial deficits or limited analysis of the visual fields as seen in some frontal disorders.

9. In cases of poor number awareness or simple counting, scores on both Trails A and B will be substantially elevated or the test will not be completed. This can be the result of injuries to the posterior dominant hemisphere in clients in whom the disorder is more recent, or can reflect long-term cognitive impairment such as moderate to severe mental retardation.

10. Performance more than two standard deviations away from the mean on both Trails A and B (Heaton et al., 1993) may indicate poor number awareness, generalized cognitive problems, severe motor problems, visual scanning deficits, memory problems, or a failure to understand the task. Although the test is accurate in such cases as identifying the presence of a problem, it offers few clues to cause except through qualitative observations.

11. Large A/B ratios when Trails A has an absolute time of less than 20 seconds may be deceptive. In very bright clients, the ratio may indicate subtle frontal problems, which are not clearly evident on other tests because of the client's intelligence. In clients with IQs under 100, the ratio may indicate relatively weaker verbal as opposed to visual skills, but will not reliably indicate the presence of a brain disorder.

12. The Trail Making Test is an excellent screen for brain injury. Good performance, especially on the more complex Trails B, is inconsistent with substantial brain injuries although more subtle disorders (especially in intelligent people) may be missed.

13. Clients with mild head injury are slower than those of non-brain-injured populations, slowing increases on the Trail Making Test with severity of damage.

14. Both Parts A and B are sensitive to progressive cognitive decline in dementia. Part A alone has been shown to differentiate demented clients from control subjects.

15. Error types made during completion of the Trail Making Test provide useful information. Impulsive errors (e.g., most typical is a jump from 12 to 13 on Trails B, omitting "L" in an otherwise correct performance) and perseveration (difficulty shifting from number to letter) on Trails B are common among head trauma patients.

16. Emotionally disturbed clients tend to perform more poorly than nor-

mals. Depression has a slowing effect on Trails B. This can interact with the slowing of aging, causing elderly depressed clients to require a disproportionately greater amount of time to complete Trails B than emotionally stable elderly clients or depressed younger subjects. However, Trails B is generally a more sensitive screening instrument in the elderly than traditional mental status examinations.

17. The Trail Making Test's diagnostic effectiveness in differentiating brain-injured from psychiatric patients (not identified as such) has been inconsistent. In such cases, conclusions should not be reached on the basis of the Trail Making Test alone, although good performances in psychiatric clients may rule out significant brain injury in most cases.

18. Profiles in which the WCST is impaired but Category, COWAT, Stroop, and Trails B are normal point to problems with the client figuring out the intent of the test. (See the WCST interpretation section for more detail.)

19. Profiles in which Category and TPT are impaired but WCST, COWAT, Trails B, and Stroop are normal suggest that the difficulties are with the visual–spatial nature of these tests. While there is a visual component to WCST, there is not a spatial component comparable to Category and TPT for most clients.

20. Profiles in which WCST, COWAT, Stroop, and Trails B are impaired but Category and TPT (frontal signs) are normal point to problems dealing with verbal executive skills, usually reflecting damage to the anterior left (dominant) hemisphere.

21. Profiles in which Category, WCST, and TPT (frontal signs) are impaired but COWAT, Stroop, and Trails B are intact suggest problems with visual executive skills, suggesting lesions in the anterior right (nondominant) hemisphere. In such cases, the client attempts to solve the WCST in a nonverbal manner.

22. Profiles in which the Stroop, COWAT, and Trails B are impaired but Category, WCST, and TPT are normal point to specific verbal analysis problems related to poor flexibility for verbal material.

References for Trail Making Test (TMT)

Arnold, B. R., Montgomery, G. T., Castaneda, I., & Longoria, R. (1994). Acculturation and performance of Hispanics on selected Halstead–Reitan neuropsychological tests. *Assessment, 1*(3), 239–248.

Bornstein, R. A. (1983). Relationship of age and education to neuropsychological performance in patients with symptomatic carotid artery disease. *Journal of Clinical Psychology, 39*(4), 470–478.

Bornstein, R. A. (1985). Normative data on selected neuropsychological measures from a nonclinical sample. *Journal of Clinical Psychology, 41*(5), 651–659.

Bornstein, R. A. (1986). Classification rates obtained with "standard" cut-off scores on selected neuropsychological measures. *Journal of Clinical and Experimental Neuropsychology, 8*(4), 413–420.

Choca, J. P., Laatsch, L., Wetzel, L., & Agresti, A. (1997). The Halstead category test: A fifty year perspective. *Neuropsychology Review, 7*(2), 61–75.

Cicerone, K. D. (1997). Clinical sensitivity of four measures of attention to mild traumatic brain injury. *Clinical Neuropsychologist, 11*(3), 266–272.

Ernst, J. (1987). Neuropsychological problem-solving skills in the elderly. *Psychology and Aging, 2*(4), 363–365.

Golden, C. J., Zillmer, E., & Spiers, M. (1992). *Neuropsychological assessment and intervention.* Springfield, IL: Charles C Thomas.

Hays, J. R. (1995). Trail making test norms for psychiatric patients. *Perceptual and Motor Skills, 80,* 187–194.

Heaton, R. K., Grant, I., & Matthews, C. G. (1991). Comprehensive norms for an expanded Halstead–Reitan battery: Demographic corrections, research findings, and clinical applications. Odessa, FL: Psychological Assessment Resources.

Heilbronner, R. L., Henry, G. K., Buck, P., & Adams, R. L. (1991). Lateralized brain damage and performance on trail making A and B, digit span forward and backward, and TPT memory and location. *Archives of Clinical Neuropsychology, 6*(4), 251–258.

Keyser, D. J., & Sweetland, R. C. (1984). The Halstead–Reitan Neuropsychological Battery and Allied Procedures. In *Test Critiques,* Vol. I. Kansas City, MO: Test Corporation of America.

Leon, J., Pearlman, O., Doonan, R., & Simpson, G. M. (1996). A study of bedside screening procedures for cognitive deficits in chronic psychiatric inpatients. *Comprehensive Psychiatry, 37*(5), 328–335.

Prigatono, G. P., & Parsons, O. A. (1976). Relationship of age and education to Halstead test performance in different patient populations. *Journal of Consulting and Clinical Psychology, 44*(4), 527–533.

Reitan, R. M., & Wolfson, D. (1993). *The Halstead-Reitan neuropsychological test battery: Theory and clinical interpretation* (2nd ed.). S. Tucson, AZ: Neuropsychology Press.

Russell, E. W., Neuringer, C., & Goldstein, G. (1971). *Assessment of brain damage: A neuropsychological key approach.* New York: Wiley-Interscience.

Searight, H. R., Dunn, E. J., Grisso, T., & Margolis, R. B. (1992). The relation of the Halstead–Reitan neuropsychological battery to ratings of everyday functioning in a geriatric sample: Clarification. *Neuropsychology, 6*(4), 394.

Snyder, P. J., & Nussbaum, P. D. (1998). *Clinical neuropsychology: A pocket handbook for assessment.* Washington, D.C.: American Psychological Association.

Stringer, A. Y., & Green, R. C. (1996). Stimulus Imperception. In *A guide to adult neuropsychological diagnosis.* Philadelphia, PA: F. A. Davis.

Thompson, L. L., & Heaton, R. K. (1991). Pattern of performance on the tactual performance test. *Clinical Neuropsychologist, 5*(4), 322–328.

Welch, L. W., Cunningham, A. T., Eckardt, M. J., & Martin, P. R. (1997). Fine motor speed deficits in alcoholic Korsakoff's syndrome. *Alcoholism: Clinical & Experimental Research, 21*(1), 134–139.

STROOP COLOR AND WORD TEST

The Stroop Color and Word Test is a simple, 5-minute test used both for screening of brain damage as well as part of a more detailed neuropsychological battery. It has been used most frequently as a test of frontal lobe damage, but can be used to detect other types of damage as well. Although it can be used as a screening test by itself, the test is best used in combination with other tests as part of a more comprehensive battery. Its extremely short administration time makes it an ideal addition to any test battery.

Interpretation

1. The Word score reflects basic reading speed and reaches near adult levels before age 10. Low scores in this measure may reflect a motor speech problem (in which case the clinician might try having the client read the items to himself rather than out loud). In such cases, the client's words are generally halting, slurred, mispronounced, or stiff not only in the testing situation but in all speech. Low scores may also reflect poorly developed reading skills. In such cases, the speech itself is fluent but the decoding of the words is slow and remains slow throughout the test. Such cases may suggest a developmental learning disorder or simply the lack of an opportunity to learn to read. This is also consistent with relatively poor dominance for reading skills as may be seen in a Learning Disability or when testing someone in his or her second language. Word reading disorders are consistent with posterior left hemisphere dysfunction in acquired brain injuries.

2. Slow scores on Color in the presence of normal Word scores can suggest an inability to identify color names (in which the client can point out the similar colors but cannot name them) or color blindness. Occasionally, low Color scores are seen in psychiatric clients in whom the colors may arouse emotional rather than cognitive reactions. Low Color scores combined with low Word scores are consistent with speech impairment or low intelligence. In cases of individuals with normal intelligence, low scores on both may be related to malingering or lack of effort. Low Color scores by themselves (in the absence of color blindness) may indicate disorders of the dominant temporal–occipital areas or the posterior right hemisphere.

3. Slow scores on Color–Word in the presence of normal scores on Color and Word are indicative of interference. Such scores indicate the possible presence of either prefrontal pathology (in which case the dominant word naming cannot be inhibited) or emotional turmoil (in clients who are hysterical or acutely agitated). T-scores on Color–Word that are significantly better than T-scores on Color or Word, combined with raw Color–Word scores that are at least 20% below raw Color scores and 30% below raw Word scores, suggest good ability to inhibit conflicting responses.

4. Protocols in which Color and Word are normal (T-scores above 40) but that show raw Color–Word scores of more than 80% of the raw Color

score may reflect a client who has discovered a way to "cheat" by covering all but the first letter of the words with his finger or squinting his eyes so that the words cannot be clearly seen. Such clients should be retested.

5. Score patterns in which Color is normal, Word is low, and the raw Color–Word score is more than 80% of the raw Color score suggests either acquired or developmental dyslexia. This pattern is very common in reading disabilities and in brain injuries to the left parietal–temporal areas of the brain. When these disorders occur in early childhood, however, this may indicate a simple delay rather than an injury.

6. Score patterns in which Word is low, Color is normal, and Color–Word is low may suggest malingering or lack of motivation on the Word or Color–Word task. Such profiles show significant interference which should not occur when Word is low.

7. Score patterns in which Word and Color are low, and the raw Color–Word score is at least 80% of the raw Color score, may indicate a generalized disorder in adults (which can be associated with low intelligence) or the presence of a nondominant or diffuse disorder in children.

8. Score patterns in which the Color–Word raw score is higher than the Color raw score are invalid and the test should be repeated.

9. Low Interference scores (negative scores, especially below -7) in the presence of normal Color and Word scores suggest the presence of prefrontal disorders.

10. Normal Interference scores in the presence of normal Color and Word scores suggest good flexibility and ability to respond to task demands. In some cases, this may reflect poor dominance of the word naming system over the color naming system in an individual who reads but in whom reading is not automatic. This is commonly seen developmentally in many first through third grade students, for example, as well as older children with learning disabilities whose reading skills may be improving but in whom the verbal system is impaired. This is an especially likely interpretation when interference scores are above average.

11. Interference scores are generally meaningless when Color or Word are below average by more than one standard deviation, with the exception of substantial Interference in the presence of low Word and normal Color scores (see no. 6).

12. When used as a screening test, performance more than one standard deviation below average of any of the three basic scores or the Interference score suggests the need for further investigation. Reduction on more than one score strengthens the likelihood of a cognitive disorder.

13. Profiles in which the WCST is impaired but Category, COWAT, Stroop, and Trails B are normal points to problems with the client figuring out

the intent of the test. (See the WCST interpretation section for more detail.)

14. Profiles in which Category and TPT are impaired but WCST, COWAT, Trails B, and Stroop are normal suggest that the difficulties are with the visual–spatial nature of these tests. While there is a visual component to WCST, there is not a spatial component comparable to Category and TPT for most clients.

15. Profiles in which WCST, COWAT, Stroop, and Trails B are impaired but Category and TPT (frontal signs) are normal point to problems dealing with verbal executive skills, usually reflecting damage to the anterior left (dominant) hemisphere.

16. Profiles in which Category, WCST, and TPT (frontal signs) are impaired but COWAT, Stroop, and Trails B are intact suggest problems with visual executive skills, suggesting lesions in the anterior right (nondominant) hemisphere. In such cases, the client attempts to solve the WCST in a nonverbal manner.

17. Profiles in which the Stroop, COWAT, and Trails B are impaired but Category, WCST, and TPT are normal point to specific verbal analysis problems related to poor flexibility for verbal material.

References for Stroop Color and Word Test

Corbett, B., & Stanczak, D. E. (1999). Neuropsychological performance of adults evidencing attention-deficit hyperactivity disorder. *Archives of Clinical Neuropsychology, 14*(4), 373–387.

Degl'Innocenti, A., Agren, H., & Bäckman, L. (1998). Executive deficits in major depression. *Acta Psychiatrica Scandinavica, 97*(3), 182–188.

Golden, C. J. (1978). *Stroop Color and Word Test.* Chicago, IL: Stoelting.

Klein, M., Ponds, R W. H., Houx, P. J., & Jolles, J. (1997). Effect of test duration on age-related differences in stroop interference. *Journal of Clinical and Experimental Neuropsychology, 19*(1), 77–82.

Lannoo, E., & Vingerhoets, G. (1997). Flemish normative data on common neuropsychological tests. Influence of age, education, and gender. *Psychologica Belgica, 37*(3), 141–155.

Leahy, B. J., & Lam, C. S. (1998). Neuropsychological testing and functional outcome for individuals with traumatic brain injury. *Brain Injury, 12*(12), 1025–1035.

Lezak, M. D. (1995). *Neuropsychological assessment* (3rd ed.). New York: Oxford University Press.

Snyder, P. J., & Nussbaum, P. D. (1998). *Clinical neuropsychology: A pocket handbook for assessment.* Washington, D.C.: American Psychological Association.

SECTION VIII: MEMORY TESTS

WECHSLER MEMORY SCALE-III

Because of the popularity of the Wechsler Intelligence Tests and its close tie-in with the WAIS-III, the WMS-III has quickly become one of the most popular memory test batteries in the field. Although it is not without its detractors, the test's psychometric and clinical characteristics are clearly superior to the earlier versions of the test (WMS and WMS-R). This section focuses on the interpretation of the basic indexes generated by the test, while individual sections on the major and most useful subtests focus on the interpretation of those individual scores.

Interpretation

1. The WMS-III generates eight major scores. Working Memory is calcu-
    lated by combining Letter–Number Sequencing and Visual Spatial
    Span. (While the WAIS-III has a Working Memory Index as well, it is
    made up of Arithmetic, Digit Span, and Letter–Number Sequencing.)
    Auditory Immediate Memory is determined by combining the immedi-
    ate recall trials of Logical Memory and Verbal Paired Associates.
    Visual Immediate Memory is determined by combining the immediate
    recall trials of Faces and Family Pictures. Immediate Memory is deter-
    mined by combining both of these indices.

    Delayed Verbal Memory is calculated by combining the 30-
    minute delayed version of the same tests in the Immediate Verbal
    Index, Logical Memory, and Visual Paired Associates. Similarly, De-
    layed Visual Memory is calculated by combining the delayed versions
    of the same tests in the Visual Immediate Index, Faces, and Family
    Pictures. In addition, there is an Auditory Delayed Recognition Index,
    which is based on a single score combining the delayed recognition
    versions of the tests in the Immediate Verbal Index, Logical Memory,
    and Verbal Paired Associates. Finally, General Memory is a combina-
    tion of the scores in the Visual Delayed Index, Verbal Delayed Index,
    and the Auditory Delayed Index.

2. While the General Memory Index on the WMS-R encompassed both
    immediate and delayed memory, this score reflects only delayed perfor-
    mance. Delayed Memory has been found to be much more sensitive to
    brain injury than Immediate or Working Memory. Low scores on
    General Memory compared to Immediate Memory by 15 or more points
    may point to problems in the retention of learned material. This can be
    related to the effects of a wide range of brain injuries including mild
    head injuries. Direct comparison of the scores is hampered by the
    addition of the delayed recognition score to the General Memory Index
    when there is not a similar test score in the Immediate Memory Index.
    In cases where the Auditory Recognition score differs from the Verbal
    Delayed and Visual Delayed scores by 20 Standard Scores or more
    (higher or lower), any differences may be due solely to this score.

3. If the General Memory Index is significantly better than the Immediate

Memory Index and the Auditory Recognition Delayed Index is more than 20 points above both Visual Delayed and Verbal Delayed, then the client is likely showing consistent recall scores but has relatively superior recognition skills. This suggests that the client is retaining more information than evident on recall which can be elicited through recognition trials. This may reflect less of a memory problem but rather a problem in organizing the information, responding to open-ended questions, or in communicating his or her knowledge. Such deficits may reflect problems in language or executive areas of the brain.

4. If the General Memory Index is worse than the Immediate Memory Index and the Auditory Recognition Delayed Index is more than 20 points below both Visual Delayed and Verbal Delayed scores, then the client is likely again showing consistent recall scores but failing to show the expected improvement in Recognition skills. This suggests that the client clearly has not learned the information at any level, which can be due to attentional processes (the information was never processed at all), characterized by inattention or focusing only on initial or final information to the exclusion of the other material. Such deficits reflect executive problems that may coexist with other memory problems. In other cases, such a pattern may suggest a lack of cooperation or even malingering.

5. A more direct comparison of the General and Immediate Indices can be achieved by eliminating the effects of the Delayed Score. This requires recomputing the General Memory index by adding up the scale scores of the four delayed recall subtests (Logical Memory II, Visual Paired Associates II, Faces II, and Family Pictures II). This total is multiplied by 1.25 to yield a sum of scaled scores for General Memory which can be converted to a standard score using the General Memory Table in the test manual.

6. In cases where eliminating the effect of recognition wipes out any difference between the scores, the above interpretations should be considered. In cases where this procedure creates a difference in favor of Immediate Memory, this indicates that there is a deficit in delayed recall.

7. In cases where eliminating the effect of recognition creates a difference in favor of General Memory, this suggests either executive problems or much better than average retention of what is initially learned. By looking at the raw scores, one can determine if the client has recalled more in delayed phase on each test or simply just a very high percentage (usually 90% or more) of the initial performance. In cases where the retention is more, there is likely an executive problem or in some cases a disorder of motivation. In cases where rentention is less or equal

to the initial score, then this is evidence of excellent retention skills. Such a finding is inconsistent with a primary memory deficit except in cases where the scores are very low (under 70 SS) to begin with.

8. Direct comparisons may also be made between Immediate Verbal and Delayed Verbal Memory. As these use the same tests, the comparison is uncomplicated. A higher Immediate than Delayed Memory by 15 SS points or more is consistent with an impairment in delayed memory and the most frequent finding after brain injury. Such individuals can function in simple everyday conversation but cannot retain information over extended periods of time or when there is excessive interference.

9. A more rare finding is when Delayed Verbal Memory is better than Immediate Verbal Memory by 15 points or more. This is an inconsistent finding, as the performance on delayed memory is dependent on what was remembered in the initial phase. In some cases, this occurs because of excellent retention, in which the client retains 100% of the material. In the case of Logical Memory, the Delayed raw score should be compared to the sum of the raw score on the first story and the raw score on the second reading of the second story. In the case of Paired Associates, the delayed raw score should be compared against the best raw score on any single trial in the immediate repetition. If these comparisons yield delayed raw scores that are 100% or less, that performance reflects excellent retention. This finding suggests that there is not a memory problem, but rather a problem in concentration or in organizing the immediate task.

10. In cases where retention is greater than 100%, this also suggests an absence of memory problems but points to confusion, possible malingering, or lack of initial cooperation.

11. Direct comparisons may also be made between Immediate Visual and Delayed Visual Memory. Since these use the same tests, the comparison is uncomplicated. A higher Immediate than Delayed Memory by 15 SS points or more is consistent with an impairment in delayed memory and is the most frequent finding after brain injury. Such individuals can function in simple everyday conversation but cannot retain information over extended periods of time or when there is excessive interference.

12. A more rare finding is when Delayed Verbal Memory is better than Immediate Verbal memory by 15 points or more. This is an inconsistent finding, as the performance on delayed memory is dependent on what was remembered in the initial phase. In some cases, this occurs because of excellent retention, where the client retains 100% of the material. This finding suggests that there is not a memory problem, but rather a problem in concentration or in organizing the immediate task.

13. In cases where retention is greater than 100%, this also suggests an

absence of memory problems but points to confusion, possible malingering, or lack of initial cooperation.

14. Comparisons can also be made between Immediate Verbal Memory and Immediate Visual Memory. Profiles in which Immediate Visual Memory is more than 20 SS points above Immediate Verbal Memory suggest a strength in visual memory, while the opposite finding suggests a strength in verbal memory. However, no conclusions should be reached until one also compares Delayed Visual and Verbal Memory looking for a 20-point difference as well. A conclusion that Verbal or Visual Memory is a relative strength must be based on findings from both comparisons rather than only one.

15. In cases where there are inconsistent findings regarding the superiority of verbal or visual memory, interpretation must be cautious. In some cases, there is a clear tendency for both sets of scores to favor one modality but the scores do not reach the 20-point cutoff. If one reaches 20 and the other is at least 15 points above, this can be interpreted as a clear superiority. If this criterion is not reached, one can interpret a tendency toward stronger skills in one modality.

16. In cases where the delayed and immediate comparisons yield opposite results, this is likely related to issues in concentration, attention, cooperation, test conditions, or other nonmemory conditions.

17. Interpretation of the visual tests requires the assumption that visual skills are adequate. Normal scores on any of these establishes visual competency: Picture Completion, Visual Form Discrimination, Picture Arrangement, Boston Naming, or Benton. One exception to this is facial memory, where an individual may have a specific focal loss in identifying faces called prosopagnosia. In such cases, however, the scores will be at random levels in both trials of Faces.

18. Interpretation of the verbal tests requires the assumption that verbal skills are adequate. Normal scores on any of the following establishes basic verbal competency: Comprehension, Vocabulary, or LNNB Receptive Language.

19. Working Memory appears as a measure of attention and immediate working memory processes. This score should be within 15 points of General Memory. In situations involving head injury and most brain disorders, this score will generally stay within the expected range when compared to other memory scores. A low working memory score, when compared to other indices, often suggests an emotional or motivational process rather than a brain injury, as this score should be less affected by a brain injury than would the other scores.

20. Working Memory on the WAIS-III may be compared with Working Memory on the WMS-III. The two indexes overlap, with the WAIS-III

index based on Arithmetic, Digit Span, and Letter–Number Sequencing. On the WMS-III, the index is based on Spatial Span and Letter–Number Sequencing. As a result, lower scores on the WAIS-III measure generally suggest problems working with numbers while lower scores on the WMS-III measure point to problems with short-term visual–spatial retention.

21. Working Memory is very different from the same measures on the WAIS-R and WMS-R owing to the inclusion of Letter–Number Sequencing. This task is akin to Digits Backwards in the demands it places on the client and is very difficult for clients with a wide range of problems. As a result, we would expect the new Working Memory measure to be frequently lower than the old measure by as much as one standard deviation in clients without there being any sign of clinically reliable deterioration from an earlier testing with the WAIS-R or WMS-R. As a consequence, differences of more than two standard deviations (which are quite unlikely) would be necessary before deterioration could be confirmed.

22. It has often been suggested that visual memory deficits are related to right hemisphere lesions while verbal memory deficits are related to left hemisphere lesions. While this holds when there are other clear signs of lateralized involvement to support such a statement, this has not been the case when only memory problems exist or the memory problems are the major deficit. Attempts at localization from memory findings alone should be tentative and cautious at best given our current state of knowledge.

References for Wechsler Memory Scale-III

Bernard, L. C., Houston, W., & Natoli, L. (1993). Malingering on neuropsychological memory tests: Potential objective indicators. *Journal of Clinical Psychology, 49*(1), 45–53.

Brooker, A. E. (1995). Performance on the Wechsler Memory Scale-Revised for patients with mild traumatic injury and mild dementia. *Perceptual and Motor Skills, 84*(1), 131–138.

Chelune, G. J., & Bornstein, R. A. (1988). WMS-R patterns among patients with unilateral brain lesions. *Clinical Neuropsychologist, 2*(2), 121–132.

Guilmette, T. J., & Rasile, D. (1995). Sensitivity, specificity, and diagnostic accuracy of three verbal memory measures in the assessment of mild brain injury. *Neuropsychology, 9*(3), 338–344.

Hawkins, K. A. (1998). Indicators of brain dysfunction derived from graphic representations of the WAIS-III/WMS-III Technical Manual clinical samples data: A preliminary approach to clinical utility. *Clinical Neuropsychologist, 12*(4), 535–555.

Larrabee, G. J., & Crook, T. H. (1989). Dimensions of everyday memory in age-associated memory impairment. *Psychological Assessment: A Journal of Consulting and Clinical Psychology, 1*(2), 92–97.

Lezak, M. D. (1995). *Neuropsychological assessment* (3rd ed.). New York: Oxford University Press.

Luria, A. R. (1962). *Higher cortical functions in man.* New York: Consultants Bureau.

Luria, A. R. (1980). *Higher cortical functions in man* (2nd ed.). New York: Consultants Bureau.

Mutchnick, M. G., Ross, L. K., & Long, C. J. (1991). Decision strategies for cerebral dysfunction IV: Determination of cerebral dysfunction. *Archives of Clinical Neuropsychology, 6,* 259–270.

Ryan, J. J., & Ward, L. C. (1999). Validity, reliability, and standard error of measurement for seven-subtest short forms on the Wechsler Adult Intelligence Scale-III. *Psychological Assessment, 11*(2), 207–211.

Vangel, S. J., Lichtenberg, P. A., & Ross, T. P. (1995). Clinical utility of the logical memory subtests and the relationship of demographic factors to test performance. *Journal of Clinical Geropsychology, 1*(1), 67–77.

Webster, J. S., Godlewski, M. C., Hanley, G. L., & Sowa, M. V. (1992). A scoring method for logical memory that is sensitive to right-hemisphere dysfunction. *Journal of Clinical & Experimental Neuropsychology, 14*(2), 222–238.

Wechsler, D. (1945). *Wechsler Memory Scale.* New York: Psychological Corporation.

Wechsler, D. (1955). *Manual for the Wechsler Adult Intelligence Scale.* New York: Psychological Corporation.

Wechsler, D. (1987). *Wechsler Memory Scale-Revised manual.* San Antonio, TX: The Psychological Corporation.

Wechsler, D. (1997). *Wechsler Memory Scale-Third Edition.* San Antonio, TX: The Psychological Corporation.

DIGIT SPAN (WAIS-III)

Digit Span has been a subtest of Wechsler's batteries for intellectual and memory assessment since the inception of the Wechsler–Bellevue Intelligence Scales (Wechsler, 1939). Although the format has remained unaltered, the randomized strings of numbers vary across versions of the Wechsler Adult Intelligence Scales (Wechsler; WAIS-R, 1981; WAIS-III, 1997). While initially the scale was considered a measure of attention and concentration as well as verbal memory, the WAIS-III conceives of the test as a measure of working memory.

Interpretation

1. The overall performance on the Digit Span subtest is sensitive to a wide variety of influences. Performance can be reduced by disruptions of working memory, attention, emotional disorders, anxiety, and math/ number phobias. Thus, performance must be compared against measures or observations of current stress and anxiety levels before making a neuropsychological interpretation. In addition, cases in which problems show up only on numeric problems should be viewed very cautiously.

2. Cases of left frontal/temporal/parietal injuries that result in aphasia may have drastic effects on Digit Span scores. Right hemisphere lesions to the same areas will have much more minor effects. Lesions that do not result in aphasia may also affect Digit Span, but generally to a lesser degree.

3. Head-injured patients generally show better performance on measures of working memory (such as Digit Span) than on more complex and delayed measures of memory. As a result, if Digit Span is substantially reduced after mild to moderate head injury (with the exception of those cases with focal injuries of the left hemisphere) the individual may be malingering or showing signs of anxiety. It must be emphasized that this does not apply to cases of left hemisphere stroke or head injuries, which are accompanied by intracranial bleeding.

4. Comparison of Digit Span Forward and Backwards is a valuable way of gaining additional information. The maximum number of digits learned backwards on any trial is subtracted from the maximum number of digits learned forward on any trial. A difference greater than plus 3 (Digit Forwards > Digits Backwards) may be suggestive of problems in holding the digits in memory and resequencing them and can be associated with a problem in the right anterior areas of the brain.

5. A difference between forward and backwards that is zero or negative (Digits Backwards > Digits Forward) suggests inappropriate motivation of even malingering, as Digits Backwards should never be better than Digits Forward in terms of absolute number of digits learned.

6. A poor absolute score on Digits Forward (less than a sequence of 5) suggests poor attentional processes or poor memory.

7. If Digits Backwards is less than 4 in terms of absolute length of best sequence while Digit Forward is normal, this may indicate sequencing problems or poor retention of verbal material beyond a few seconds.

8. Good performance on Digit Span is not inconsistent with most forms of brain injury including dementia, although in dementia cases a larger than expected difference may exist between Digits Forwards and Digit Backwards.

9. Digit Span and other measures of working memory may be used as a baseline in nonaphasic cases to compare changes in other forms of immediate and delayed memory.

10. Digit Span can be compared to Visual Span of the WMS-III. Comparisons are best made on the basis of the size of the largest sequence correct for forward and backwards rather than the raw or scaled scores for the test.

11. If Digits Forward is more than 2 greater than Visual Span Forward, this suggests an advantage for verbal working memory if this is confirmed by a similar advantage on Digits Backwards versus Visual Span Backwards. An advantage for visual working memory can be determined using the same criteria in reverse. Such an advantage, however, is meaningful only if confirmed by more general comparisons of verbal and visual memory (see section on WAIS-III). In many cases, an

advantage may reflect basic visual or verbal processing problems rather than a memory advantage per se.

References for Digit Span (WAIS-III)

Boone, D. E. (1998). Specificity of the WAIS-R subtests with psychiatric inpatients. *Assessment, 5,* 123–126.

Campbell, J. M., & McCord, D. M. (1996). The WAIS-R comprehension and picture arrangement subtests as measures of social intelligence: Testing traditional interpretations. *Journal of Psychoeducational Assessment, 14,* 240–249.

Golden, C. J., Zillmer, E., & Spiers, M. (1992). *Neuropsychological assessment and intervention.* Springfield, IL: Charles C Thomas.

Kramer, J. H. (1990). Guidelines for interpreting the WAIS-R subtest scores. *Psychological Assessment, 2,* 202–205.

Matarazzo, J. D. (1972). *Wechsler's measurement and appraisal of adult intelligence* (5th ed.). New York: Oxford University Press.

Sprandel, H. Z. (1995). *The psychoeducational use and interpretation of the Wechsler Adult Intelligence Scale-Revised* (2nd ed.). Springfield, IL: Charles C Thomas.

Wechsler, D. (1981). *WAIS-R manual.* New York: The Psychological Corporation.

Wechsler, D. (1986). *WAIS-R administration and scoring manual.* San Antonio, TX: The Psychological Corporation.

Wechsler, D. (1997). *WAIS-III administration and scoring manual.* San Antonio, TX: The Psychological Corporation.

SPATIAL SPAN (WMS-III)

Spatial Span has been recently added as a subtest as a nonverbal version of Digit Span. Like Digit Span, the WMS-III conceives of the test as a measure of working memory.

Interpretation

1. The overall performance on the Spatial Span subtest is sensitive to a wide variety of influences. Performance can be reduced by disruptions of working memory, attention, emotional disorders, and anxiety. In general, however, it is better received than Digit Span, in which the presence of numbers upsets many clients.

2. Cases of right frontal/temporal/parietal injuries that result in aphasia may have drastic effects on Digit Span scores. In general, such lesions will affect Spatial Span Backwards more than Forwards. A deficit is inferred when the longest Spatial Backwards performance is at least 3 below the longest Spatial Forward sequence.

3. Head-injured patients generally show better performance on measures of working memory than on more complex and delayed measures of mem-

ory. As a result, if Spatial Span is substantially reduced after mild to moderate head injury (with the exception of those cases with focal injuries of the left hemisphere) may be malingering or showing signs of anxiety. It must be emphasized that this does not apply to cases of left hemisphere stroke or head injuries, which are accompanied by intracranial bleeding.

4. A difference between forward and backwards that is zero or negative (Spatial Backwards > Digits Forward) suggests inappropriate motivation or even malingering, as Digits Backwards should never be better than Digits Forward in terms of absolute number of digits learned.

5. A poor absolute score on Spatial Forward (less than a sequence of 5) suggests poor attentional processes or impaired visual–spatial skills.

6. Good performance on Spatial Span is not inconsistent with most forms of brain injury including dementia, although in dementia cases a larger than expected difference may exist between Forwards and Backwards.

7. Spatial Span and other measures of working memory may be used as a baseline in nonaphasic clients to compare changes in other forms of immediate and delayed memory.

8. Digit Span can be compared to Spatial Span. Comparisons are best made on the basis of the size of the largest sequence correct for Forward and Backwards rather than the raw or scaled scores for the test.

9. If Digits Forward is more than 2 greater than Spatial Span Forward, this suggests an advantage for verbal working memory if this is confirmed by a similar advantage on Digits Backwards versus Spatial Span Backwards. An advantage for visual working memory can be determined using the same criteria in reverse. Such an advantage, however, is meaningful only if confirmed by more general comparisons of verbal and visual memory (see section on WAIS-III). In many cases, an advantage may reflect basic visual or verbal processing problems rather than a memory advantage per se.

References for Spatial Span (WMS-III)

Bernard, L. C., Houston, W., & Natoli, L. (1993). Malingering on neuropsychological memory tests: Potential objective indicators. *Journal of Clinical Psychology, 49*(1), 45–53.

Brooker, A. E. (1995). Performance on the Wechsler Memory Scale-Revised for patients with mild traumatic injury and mild dementia. *Perceptual and Motor Skills, 84*(1), 131–138.

Chelune, G. J., & Bornstein, R. A. (1988). WMS-R patterns among patients with unilateral brain lesions. *Clinical Neuropsychologist, 2*(2), 121–132.

Guilmette, T. J., & Rasile, D. (1995). Sensitivity, specificity, and diagnostic accuracy of three verbal memory measures in the assessment of mild brain injury. *Neuropsychology, 9*(3), 338–344.

Larrabee, G. J., & Crook, T. H. (1989). Dimensions of everyday memory in age-associated memory impairment. *Psychological Assessment: A Journal of Consulting and Clinical Psychology, 1*(2), 92–97.

Lezak, M. D. (1995). *Neuropsychological assessment* (3rd ed.). New York: Oxford University Press.

Luria, A. R. (1962). *Higher cortical functions in man.* New York: Consultants Bureau.

Luria, A. R. (1980). *Higher cortical functions in man* (2nd ed.). New York: Consultants Bureau.

Mutchnick, M. G., Ross, L. K., & Long, C. J. (1991). Decision strategies for cerebral dysfunction IV: Determination of cerebral dysfunction. *Archives of Clinical Neuropsychology, 6,* 259–270.

Vangel, S. J., Lichtenberg, P. A., & Ross, T. P. (1995). Clinical utility of the logical memory subtests and the relationship of demographic factors to test performance. *Journal of Clinical Geropsychology, 1*(1), 67–77.

Webster, J. S., Godlewski, M. C., Hanley, G. L., & Sowa, M. V. (1992). A scoring method for logical memory that is sensitive to right-hemisphere dysfunction. *Journal of Clinical & Experimental Neuropsychology, 14*(2), 222–238.

Wechsler, D. (1945). *Wechsler Memory Scale.* New York: Psychological Corporation.

Wechsler, D. (1955). *Manual for the Wechsler Adult Intelligence Scale.* New York: Psychological Corporation.

Wechsler, D. (1987). *Wechsler Memory Scale-Revised manual.* San Antonio, TX: The Psychological Corporation.

Wechsler, D. (1997). *Wechsler Memory Scale-Third Edition.* San Antonio, TX: The Psychological Corporation.

REY–OSTERRIETH COMPLEX FIGURE TEST (CFT)

The Rey–Osterrieth Complex Figure Test (CFT) was developed by Rey (1942) and was later normed on a population of 60 adults by Osterrieth (1944). Additional normative data sets including the young and elderly have been recently offered (i.e., Spreen & Strauss, 1991). This test has been commonly seen as a useful screening tool for constructional ability, perceptual–organizational ability, and visual–perceptual memory (Tupler, Welsh, Asare-Aboagye, & Dawson, 1995). However, it has also been found to be valuable in discriminating malingered memory impairments (Bernard, Houston, & Natoli, 1993), as well as localizing hemispheric involvement in cases of temporal lobe epilepsy (Loring, Lee, & Meador, 1988). Another factor which makes this test a valuable part of a neuropsychological assessment is that performance on this measure has been found to be insensitive to the effects of extraneous factors such as gender, education, personality variables, and psychosis (Boone, Lesser, Hill-Gutierrez, Berman, & D'Elia, 1993; Cornell, Roberts, & Oram, 1997; Sautter, McDermott, Cornwell, Borges, Johnson, Vasterling, & Marcontell, 1997).

Interpretation

1. According to the Spreen & Strauss (1991) normative data set average adult performance on the Copy Phase ranges from 35.53 ± .8 (ages 50–59) to 32.9 ± 2.7 (over 70).
2. It is important to ensure that the client is able to understand what is required of him or her. If basic receptive speech abilities are intact, the

client should have little difficulty comprehending what is to be done on this task. However, if the client has a disruption of receptive language ability, the examiner must ensure that the client has full comprehension of the task before proceeding. If such deficits interfere with a client's ability to understand what is required, then the client's subsequent errors are a vivid reflection of a receptive language deficit, and nothing more. In cases where the copy is incomplete because details have been left out, it is useful to inquire why this occurred and allow for completion of the copy task.

3. As the copy phase of this examination is designed as a screening tool for constructional difficulties, it is not designed (with use of the 18-point scoring system) to pinpoint which of the many possible deficits are causing the appearance of constructional apraxia. To best differentiate whether the underlying deficits are rooted in visual–perceptual difficulties or visual–motor coordination problems, a more thorough investigation of these specific abilities should be employed by comparison with more basic measures of drawing (such as the Bender or BVRT), with spatial measures that require no motor component (Raven's Matrices), and pure motor measures (such as Finger Tapping and Purdue Pegboard).

4. Qualitative observations regarding the quality of lines drawn, the difficulty with which the motor task is carried out, the presence of tremors, and the presence of partial or complete paralysis all indicate the presence of motor problems independent of any spatial problems.

5. All copied figures can be classified into one of several groups for purposes of identifying possible lesions. Figures that are complete and look like the original in the absence of motor problems are classified as normal and suggest intact visual–motor and visual–spatial skills.

6. Figures that preserve the general outline and shape of the figure but lack detail even with prompting suggest possible left hemisphere dysfunction.

7. Figures that are badly distorted and cannot be recognized as the general figure suggest right posterior deficits.

8. Figures with the left half of the figure missing or drawn only on the left side of the page suggest unilateral neglect, typically seen in right posterior lesions.

9. Clients who finish the figure without drawing problems but who are impulsive in their drawing, show perseveration and repetition of specific parts of the figure, or who must be prompted repeatedly to include detail and finish the figure may be showing anterior frontal dysfunction.

10. The Immediate and Delayed Recall sections of this test were designed to give the examiner an assessment of the client's visual–perceptual

memory across both immediate and short-term memory. The key to this assessment is how well the client does compared to his or her initial performance. Scores typically decline about one third from the copying to memory phase. Losses greater than 50% suggest impairment in memory skills.

11. Profiles in which the client loses less than 33% of his or her score from copying to memory suggest that visual memory skills are relatively intact. However, when the client achieves a very poor score on the copying phase (less than a score of 24), the interpretation of this change must be cautious.

12. Normal performance on the Copy and Recall phases with reduced performance on the delayed section suggests problems in longer term consolidation of memory as well as susceptibility to interference. In some frontal lobe clients, there will be more evidence of perseveration on the delayed phase.

13. In many diffuse injuries such as mild to moderate head trauma, delayed performance will be the worst overall compared to both the copy and recall stages, which may be relatively normal.

14. Normal performance on copying and delayed memory with poor performance on recall suggests motivational problems or inconsistent effort, or may indicate malingering.

15. Occasionally, some clients will improve from copying to recall phases. This may indicate poor initial motivation, impulsivity in the copy phase, or slow information processing which should be evident on other tests as well.

16. Clients with mild frontal injuries may show no problems on this test. Others may perform the task in a haphazard manner with no regard to the organizational aspects of the stimuli. Interestingly, however, such clients may manage to finish the figure correctly but will have no sense of the overall gestalt of the figure which will interfere with recall. In other cases, the lack of organization will result in a loss of details, which the client cannot identify when asked to compare his or her drawing and the initial figure.

17. The Rey is sensitive to the presence of dementia and may be a good nonverbal screening test in a suspected client.

18. Performance on the copy phase below 30 after a mild head injury or in the absence of a clear neurological disorder may suggest malingering. While such performances may indeed indicate substantial pathology, such significant conditions can usually be verified on MRI or SPECT scans.

19. Some cases of frontal disorders will result in defective scanning of the visual field, leading to omission of significant details or even whole

sections of the figure. Such clients, however, can reproduce these details when they are pointed out to them.

20. Because of the complexity of the Rey Figure, it generally demands more sustained attention than do other memory tests. Thus, problems in sustained attention as reflected in poor IVA or TOVA performance (particularly on visual portions) may correlate with poor Rey performance. In such cases, impairment will also be seen on the WCST, TPT, Category, and Faces, which also require sustained attention for good performance. Similar tests that require less sustained attention (e.g., BVRT, Stroop, COWAT, Trails B, Working Memory) will generally be normal if this is the primary problem except in the more severe deficits which can potentially affect any test.

21. Block Design can be performed at an average level using verbal mediation strategies, unlike the Rey Figure. This pattern of using verbal mediation generally includes good block design performance, good Matrices Performance, and good reproduction of simple drawings put poor reproduction of complex drawings (such as the Rey) and poor performance on measures of facial memory and other tasks that are not easily encodable. This is also accompanied by strong performance on verbal tests in general.

22. While the Rey is presented in this section as a memory test, it is clearly also a test of complex visual–spatial performance. Normal performance on the copy phase rules out visual–motor as well as visual–spatial problems.

23. Impaired performance on the Rey when other memory tests and visual–spatial tasks are intact may point to significant impairment in organizational skills related to frontal injuries. In such cases, impaired performance will also be seen on WCST or Category.

24. Good performance on the Rey while other visual–spatial tests are abnormal suggests inconsistent motivation that may be related to fatigue, a lack of cooperation, malingering, or other noncognitive factors.

25. Memory for complex designs as measured by the Rey may be independent of other forms of visual memory tapped by Faces or Family Pictures. Across the board impairment suggests impairment of general visual memory skills, while specific patterns of losses points to more specific injuries to nonmeaningful design memory (Rey), facial memory (Faces), or meaningful picture memory (Family Pictures).

References for Rey–Osterrieth Complex Figure Test (CFT)

Bernard, L. C., Houston, W., & Natoli, L. (1993). Malingering on neuropsychological memory tests: Potential objective indicators. *Journal of Clinical Psychology, 49,* 52–58.

Bigler, E. D. (1988). Frontal damage and neuropsychological assessment. *Archives of Clinical Neuropsychology, 3*, 279–297.

Binder, L. M. (1982). Constructional strategies on complex figure drawings after unilateral brain damage. *Journal of Clinical Neuropsychology, 4*, 51–58.

Boone, K. B., Lesser, I. M., Hill-Gutierrez, E. H., Berman, N. G., & D'Elia, L. F. (1993). Rey–Osterrieth complex figure performance in healthy, older adults: Relationship to age, education, sex, and IQ. *The Clinical Neuropsychologist, 7*(1), 22–28.

Cherrier, M. M., Mendez, M. F., Dave, M., & Perryman, K. M. (1999). Performance on the Rey–Osterrieth Complex Figure test in Alzheimer's disease and vascular dementia. *Neuropsychiatry, Neuropsychology, and Behavioral Neurology, 12*(2), 95–101.

Cornell, D. G., Roberts, M., & Oram, G. (1997). The Rey–Osterrieth complex figure test as a neuropsychological measure in criminal offenders. *Archives of Clinical Neuropsychology, 12*(1), 47–56.

Delaney, R. C., Prevey, M. L., Cramer, J., Mattson, R. H., & V. A. Epilepsy Cooperative Study #264 Research Group (1992). Test–retest comparability and control subject data for the Rey–auditory verbal learning test and the Rey–Osterrieth/Taylor complex figures. *Archives of Clinical Neuropsychology, 7*, 523–528.

Denman, S. (1984). *Denman Neuropsychology Memory Scale.* Charleston, S. C.: S. B. Denman.

Hamby, S. L., Wilkins, J. W., & Barry, N. S. (1993). Organizational quality on the Rey–Osterrieth and Taylor complex figures tests: A new scoring system. *Psychological Assessment, 5*(1), 27–33.

Hartman, M., & Potter, G. (1998). Sources of age differences on the Rey–Osterrieth Complex Figure Test. *Clinical Neuropsychologist, 12*(4), 513–552.

Kaplan, E. (1993). Neuropsychological Assessment. In T. Boll & B. K. Bryant (Eds.). *Clinical neuropsychology and brain function: Research, measurement, and practice.* Washington, D. C.: American Psychological Association.

Kuehn, S. M., & Snow, W. G. (1992). Are the Rey and Taylor figures equivalent? *Archives of Clinical Neuropsychology, 7*, 445–448.

Lezak, M. D. (1995). *Neuropsychological assessment* (2nd ed.). New York: Oxford University Press.

Loring, D. W., Lee, G. P., & Meador, K. J. (1998). Revising the Rey–Osterrieth: Rating right hemisphere recall. *Archives of Clinical Neuropsychology, 3*, 239–247.

Meyers, J. E., & Meyers, K. R. (1995). Rey complex figure test under four different administration procedures. *The Clinical Neuropsychologist, 9*(1), 63–67.

Milberg, W. P., Hebben, N., & Kaplan, E. (1986). The Boston process approach to neuropsychological assessment. In I. Grant & K. M. Adams (Eds.). *Neuropsychological assessment of neuropsychiatric disorders.* New york: Oxford University Press.

Osterrieth, P. A. (1944). Le test du copie d'une figure complexe. *Archives de Psychologie, 28*, 206–356.

Rapport, L. J., Farchione, T. J., Dutra, R. L., Webster, J. S., & Charter, R. A. (1996). Measures of hemiinattention on the Rey-figure copy for the Lezak-Osterrieth scoring method. *The Clinical Neuropsychologist, 10*(4), 450–454.

Rey, A. (1942). L'examen psychologique dans le cas d'encephalopathie traumatique. *Archives de Psychologie, 28*, 286–340.

Sautter, F. J., McDermott, B. E., Cornwell, J. M., Borges, A., Johnson, J., Vasterling, J. J., Marcontell, D. K. (1997). A comparison of neuropsychological deficits in familial schizophrenics, nonfamilial schizophrenics, and normal controls. *Journal of Nervous and Mental Disorders, 185*(10), 641–644.

Spreen, O., & Strauss, E. (1991). *A compendium of neuropsychological tests: Administration, norms, and commentary.* New York: Oxford University Press.

Stern, R. A., Singer, E. A., Duke, L. M., Singer, N. G., Morey, C. E., Daughtery, E. W., & Kaplan, E. (1994). The Boston qualitative scoring system for the Rey–Osterrieth complex figure: Description and interrater reliability. *The Clinical Neuropsychologist, 8*(3), 309–322.

Strauss, E., & Spreen, O. (1991). A comparison of the Rey and Taylor figures. *Archives of Clinical Neuropsychology, 7*, 449–456.

Taylor, L. B. (1969). Localization of cerebral lesions by psychological testing. *Clinical Neurosurgery*, *16*, 269–287.

Tombaugh, T. M., & Hubley, A. M. (1991). Four studies comparing the Rey–Osterrieth and Taylor complex figures. *Journal of Clinical and Experimental Neuropsychology*, *13*, 587–599.

Tupler, L. A., Welsh, K. A., Asare-Aboagye, Y., & Dawson, D. V. (1995). Reliability of the Rey–Osterrieth Complex Figure in use with memory-impaired patients. *Journal of Clinical & Experimental Neuropsychology*, *17*(4), 566–579.

Visser, R. S. H. (1973). *Manual of the complex figure test*. Amsterdam: Swets & Zietlinger.

REY AUDITORY VERBAL LEARNING TEST (RAVLT)

The Rey Auditory Verbal Learning Test (RAVLT) is an easily administered measure of verbal learning and memory. Designed to gauge indices such as immediate memory span, learning and learning strategies, retroactive and proactive interference, and comparisons of types of errors (e.g., intrusions, perseverations) (Lezak, 1983), the RAVLT provides qualitative measures of learning and memory that are not easily discernible from other tests that approach memory as a unitary entity. The RAVLT is similar to the California Verbal Learning Test in its administration and scoring. However, the two tests differ with regards to stimuli. The RAVLT consists of a semantically unrelated word list (List A) and a similar interference list (List B). As such, many clinicians and researchers regard the RAVLT as a more pure measure of verbal memory functioning.

Interpretation

1. A low score on immediate free recall of List B words as compared to Trial 1 immediate free recall of List A words may be related to a high degree of proactive interference. Such deficits are often related to retrieval problems and associated with anterior lesions. However, in some cases this may reflect cognitive fatigue, as the repeated trials are very demanding on arousal and attention skills.

2. A low score on Trial 6 for List A words relative to Trial 5 may be indicative of either high degrees of forgetting during the short delay or retroactive interference or a combination of these problems. These may reflect subcortical lesions in cases where information cannot be stored over time. A recognition test is useful to see if this is a true inability to retain new memories or reflects a retrieval problem as well.

3. A low score on the 30-minute delay recall trial, which reflects the examinee's ability to retain verbal information over time, indicates a problem in retaining the material over time. This again may indicate a subcortical storage problem. However, if there are many intrusion

errors, this would indicate a retrieval problem, as material has clearly been stored.

4. Poor recall of primacy-region words relative to recency-region words may signify that the examinee has a passive learning style characteristic of clients with frontal disorders. Brain-injured clients generally do better with recent words rather than with those presented first when they actively try to learn a list. Clients with difficulty forming new memories will more likely remember the most recent words, while the passive frontal clients focus on the initial words and ignore or fail to process the additional words even across trials.

5. Low recall consistency (i.e., the percentage of target words recalled on one of the first four trials that are also recalled on the very next trial) reflects a disorganized learning style and may denote that the examinee has difficulty formulating or maintaining a learning plan. This also may reflect anterior injuries although frontal patients may also show consistent but low levels of learning across trials.

6. Repetition of the same word in recall shortly after it is said initially suggests disinhibition, which is associated with anterior lesions. Perseverations on the RAVLT can be subdivided into two types. Repetition of the same word much farther along in the recall process may indicate attentional problems, memory problems, and some disorganization seen most often in subcortical disorders.

7. Intrusions by words not in either list and unrelated to the words in the list indicate that the client has difficulty in making the distinction between information coming from the outside and his or her own associations. This may suggest a breakdown in frontal self-evaluation skills. Such clients are generally unaware that their performance is unrelated to the task they are supposed to do.

8. Clients with retrieval deficits will do better on a recognition trial, while clients with storage deficits will do poorly on recognition and recall trials. In cases where recall is better than recognition, the client may be showing impulsivity in reacting to the nonlist words or perseverating on saying yes or no to the question of recognition.

9. In mild head injury, recognition should be much better than recall. An absence of this effect may suggest low effort of malingering. Mild head-injured clients should also do better in short-term recall (immediate list learning) and worse on delayed trials. A reversed pattern also may indicate fluctuating effort. In more severe head injuries, both may be lower but delayed memory will be poorer than immediate memory.

10. Learning over trials indicate that some memory traces are being retained and are often a more sensitive indicator of low-level memory

scores. However, long list tests such as this may overwhelm the client, leading to poorer performance than if a seven-word list has been used, for example. Thus the client may remember only 3 of 15 words after five trials, but manage 5 of 7 words after five trials. Thus, these tests should not be interpreted as showing a maximum level of learning across situations.

11. Deficits in memory are an early sign of Alzheimer's disease.

12. In a study by Powell, Cripe, and Dodrill (1991), scores for Trials 1–7 and the total score (i.e., the sum of Trials 1–5) successfully differentiated non-neurological from mixed neurologically impaired study participants, with Trial 5 showing the best performance. In contrast, the derived indices (i.e., words learned after Trial 1, words forgotten over the interference trial, and percentage of words forgotten) were not effective in differentiating these groups.

13. Scores on the RAVLT and CVLT should be similar. Major discrepancies of more than one standard deviation (15 SS points) indicate inconsistency in performance due to varying levels of cooperation, fatigue, malingering, or other noncognitive factors.

14. List memory is a distinctly independent task from Story memory (Logical Memory) or paired associate learning (Paired Associates). Each of the latter tasks provides the client with more organization as well as meaning. Impairment on only list learning suggests that the client is overwhelmed by the organizational tasks required by long list learning rather than verbal memory per se. (Such clients may do better on short list learning, as can be partially determined by looking at their performance on Digit Span.) Deficits on only story memory suggest that rote memory is intact but that the client cannot take advantage of the story's meaning to show normal improvement in performance over base rote learning. Deficits on only Paired Associates type tasks indicate that the client cannot sequence the order of the material together. (This can be evaluated as well by looking at the sequence in which they perform the other verbal memory tasks.)

15. Deficits on Paired Associates and List Learning but not Logical Memory indicate the client has trouble with rote memory but can use the meaning in the story as an effective cue in aiding memory.

16. Deficits on Paired Associates and Logical Memory but not on List Learning tasks indicate strong rote memory but poor skills at taking advantage and responding to organizational and meaning cues in the impaired tasks.

17. Meaningful picture memory is analogous to meaningful verbal memory as seen in Logical Memory and can be separated theoretically from those tasks that represent rote memory (such as List Learning, Verbal

Paired Associates, Faces). In theory, strong performance on Logical Memory and Family Pictures compared to impaired performance on Faces, Verbal Paired Associates, and List Learning task suggests that the client is using high cognitive skills to augment weak memory skills across the board. This comparison, however, is not perfect in that Faces is a recognition rather than a recall task and Verbal Paired Associates requires a specific organization of the material which may make it easier or harder to a specific client. However, the general comparison is still useful in clear-cut cases.

18. Similarly, weak performance on Logical Memory and Family Pictures compared to strong performance on Faces, Verbal Paired Associates, and List Learning task suggests that the client is not using higher cognitive skills to augment memory skills and is generally relying on rote memory skills alone.

References for Rey Auditory Verbal Learning Test (RAVLT)

Kin J. H., Gfeller, J. D., & Davis, H. P. (1998). Detecting simulated memory impairment with the Rey Auditory Verbal Learning Test: Implications of base rates and study generalizability. *Journal of Clinical and Experimental Neuropsychology, 20*(5), 603–612.

Lezak, M. D. (1983). *Neuropsychological Assessment* (2nd ed.). New York: Oxford University Press.

Miranda, J. P., & Valencia, R. R. (1997). English and Spanish versions of a memory test: Word-length effects versus spoken-duration effects. *Hispanic Journal of Behavioral Sciences, 1*(2), 171–181.

Powell, J. B., Cripe, L. I., & Dodrill, C. B. (1991). Assessment of brain impairment with the Rey Auditory Verbal Learning Test: A comparison with other neuropsychological measures. *Archives of Clinical Neuropsychology, 6*(4), 241–249.

Rey, A. (1964). *L'examen clinique en psychologie*. Paris: Presses Universitaries de France.

Savage, R. M., & Gouvier, W. D. (1992). Rey Auditory-Verbal Learning Test: The effects of age and gender, and norms for delayed recall and story recognition trials. *Archives of Clinical Neuropsychology, 7*(5), 407–414.

CALIFORNIA VERBAL LEARNING TEST (CVLT)

The California Verbal Learning Test (CVLT) is a measure of verbal learning and memory. Derived from principles of cognitive neuroscience, the CVLT was created to provide qualitative indices of learning and memory such as learning strategies (e.g., semantic versus serial clustering), comparisons of types of errors (e.g., intrusions and perseverations), and the effects of interference on recall. This sets the CVLT apart from other measures of cognitive dysfunction that are scored for global achievement only and, as such, do not easily lend themselves to the gauging of these qualitative aspects of learning and memory. The CVLT has been useful in characterizing the memory deficits associated with a number of neurological and psychiatric conditions, including head injury (Crosson, Novack,

Trenerry, & Craig, 1988), Alzheimer's disease, Huntington's disease, and alcoholic Korsakoff's syndrome (Delis, Massman, Butters, Salmon, Cermak, & Kramer, 1991), multiple sclerosis and Parkinson's disease (Delis, Freeland, Kramer, & Kaplan, 1988), and adult attention-deficit/hyperactivity disorder (ADHD) (Downey, Stelson, Pomerleau, & Giordani, 1997).

Factor-analytic studies of the CVLT generally indicate either a five- or six-factor solution. In a sample of 286 normal participants, Delis, Freeland, Kramer, and Kaplan (1988) found a six-factor solution: (1) General Verbal Learning; (2) Response Discrimination; (3) Learning Strategy; (4) Proactive Effect; (5) Serial Position Effect; and (6) Acquisition Rate. When the scores of 113 participants with neurological disorders were analyzed, these same authors found a five-factor solution:. (1) General Verbal Learning; (2) Response Discrimination; (3) Serial Position Effect; (4) Learning Strategy; and (5) Retroactive/Short Delay Effect. These findings are in contrast to past factor-analytic studies of other clinical memory tests which commonly produce a single verbal learning factor.

Interpretation

1. The CVLT's recall measures lend themselves to the following interpretations. A low score on immediate free recall of List B as compared to Trial 1 of immediate free recall of List A may be associated with a high degree of proactive interference.
2. A low score on short-delay free recall of List A relative to Trial 5 of immediate free recall of List A may be indicative of either high degrees of forgetting during the delay interval or retroactive interference or a combination thereof. Poor free-recall performance relative to cued-recall performance may indicate that the client has problems in retrieval that may be contributing to her or his memory deficits. If, however, free and cued recall are both impaired, then problems in encoding may account for the client's memory deficits. With regards to long-delay testing (i.e., free and cued recall), a low score indicates "impaired 20-minute retention."
3. Interpretation of low scores on Trials 1–5 of immediate free recall for List A requires an evaluation of the following learning characteristics. Low semantic clustering scores may indicate that the client is using less effective learning strategies such as serial clustering. Semantic clustering involves the reorganization of target words into categorical groups and is considered a highly effective learning strategy. Low semantic clustering scores correlate with poor performance on many other CVLT indices.
4. High serial clustering scores correlate with poor performance on other CVLT indices. Serial clustering scores indicate the degree to which the

client recalls words in the same order as they are presented. As mentioned, this is considered a less effective learning strategy and may reflect a "stimulus-bound" response style.

5. Primacy and recency effects and recall consistency should be examined. Poor recall of words presented first (primacy) relative to words presented last in the list (recency) may signify that the client has a passive learning style. Low recall consistency (remembering a word on the next trial after initially learning it) reflects a disorganized learning style and may denote that the client has difficulty formulating or maintaining a learning plan.

6. Perseverations can be subdivided into two types. A proximal perseveration is indicated when a word is repeated shortly after the original response. This type of perseveration may reflect a problem in response inhibition and is often observed in clients with frontal lobe pathology. In contrast, a distal perseveration is indicated when the client repeats a response a considerable time after it was initially reported. Such perseverations are commonly found in clients with attention or memory deficits.

7. Problems in discriminating relevant from irrelevant responses are indicated by a high number of intrusions. These may occur in either the recall of List B trial or the delay trials of List A. When the intrusion score is elevated, this indicates a high degree of proactive and/or retroactive interference.

8. The last trial on the CVLT is the long-delay recognition trial. Accurate recognition (i.e., recognition hits) denotes that the target items were encoded. Difficulties in discriminating target items from distractor items or a "Yes" response bias may be indicated by a high number of false-positives.

9. On delayed recall, the most impaired performance is indicated by a high number of "Neither List-Unrelated" false-positives and the least impaired performance is denoted by only a few "List B-Shared" false-positives.

10. The best indicator of recognition performance is the "Discriminability" index. A low score on this index may indicate problems in differentiating target items from distractor items, suggesting that encoding difficulties contribute to the client's memory impairment.

11. Alzheimer's disease (AD) and alcoholic Korsakoff's syndrome (AK) patients share similar CVLT profiles. The two groups exhibited impaired immediate recall, flat learning rates across trials, inconsistent recall across trials, low scores on semantic clustering, a tendency to recall words passively from the recency region of the list, poor retention over delay intervals, high intrusion rates, poor recognition discrim-

inability, high false-positive rates, a "Yes" response bias, and no improvement on recognition relative to free recall.

12. Huntington's disease (HD) patients exhibited low levels of free- and cued-recall, flat learning rates, inconsistent recall, a large recency effect, and low scores on semantic clustering. In contrast to AD and AK patients, HD patients displayed better retention on delayed recall, lower intrusion rates on free- and cued-recall trials, less vulnerability to interference, lower false-positive rates, higher recognition discriminability, and greater improvement on recognition relative to free recall. Contrasts between AD and HD CVLT profiles may reflect differences in memory functioning between subcortical (i.e., HD) and cortical (i.e., AD) dementias.

13. Head-injured persons demonstrate low scores across learning trials, high levels of intrusions, and low scores on semantic clustering, indicating that they are unable to take advantage of more efficient learning strategies (i.e., semantic clustering). Their performance improved on cued recall trials.

14. Scores on the RAVLT and CVLT should be similar. Major discrepancies of more than one standard deviation (15 SS points) indicate inconsistency in performance due to varying levels of cooperation, fatigue, malingering, or other noncognitive factors.

15. List memory is a distinctly independent task from story memory (Logical Memory) or paired associate learning (Paired Associates). Each of the latter tasks provides the clients with more organization as well as meaning. Impairment on only List Learning suggests that the client is overwhelmed by the organizational tasks required by long list learning rather than verbal memory per se. (Such clients may do better on short list learning, as can be partially determined by looking at their performance on Digit Span.) Deficits on only story memory suggest that rote memory is intact but that the client cannot take advantage of the story's meaning to show normal improvement in performance over base rote learning. Deficits on only Paired Associates type tasks indicate that the client cannot sequence the order of the material together (This can be evaluated as well by looking at the sequence in which he or she performs the other verbal memory tasks.)

16. Deficits on Paired Associates and List Learning but not Logical Memory indicate the client has trouble with rote memory but can use the meaning in the story as an effective cue in aiding memory.

17. Deficits on Paired Associates and Logical memory but not on List Learning tasks indicate strong rote memory but poor skills at taking advantage of and responding to organizational and meaning cues in the impaired tasks.

18. Meaningful picture memory is analogous to meaningful verbal memory

as seen in Logical Memory and can be separated theoretically from those tasks that represent rote memory (such as List Learning, Verbal Paired Associates, Faces). In theory, strong performance on Logical Memory and Family Pictures compared to impaired performance on Faces, Verbal Paired Associates, and list learning task suggests that the client is using higher cognitive skills to augment weak memory skills across the board. This comparison, however, is not perfect in the Faces is a recognition rather than a recall task and Verbal Paired Associates requires a specific organization of the material which may make it easier or harder to a specific client. However, the general comparison is still useful in clear-cut cases.

19. Similarly, weak performance on Logical Memory and Family Pictures compared to strong performance on Faces, Verbal Paired Associates, and list learning task suggests that the client is not using higher cognitive skills to augment memory skills and is generally relying on rote memory skills alone.

References for California Verbal Learning Test (CVLT)

Benton, A. L., Hamsher, K. de S., Varney, N. R., & Spreen, O. (1983). *Contributions to neuropsychological assessment.* New York: Oxford University Press.

Crosson, B., Novack, T. A., Trenerry, M. R., & Craig, P. L. (1988). California Verbal Learning Test (CVLT) performance in severely head-injured and neurologically normal adult males. *Journal of Clinical and Experimental Neuropsychology, 10*(6), 754–768.

Delis, D. C., Freeland, J., Kramer, J. H., & Kaplan, E. (1988). Integrating clinical assessment with cognitive neuroscience: Construct validity of the California Verbal Learning Test. *Journal of Consulting and Clinical Psychology, 56*(1), 123–130.

Delis, D. C., Massman, P. L., Butters, N., Salmon, D. P., Cermak, L. S., & Kramer, J. H. (1991). Profiles of demented and amnesic patients on the California Verbal Learning Test: Implications for the assessment of memory disorders. *Psychological Assessment, 3*(1), 19–26.

Downey, K. K., Stelson, F. W., Pomerleau, O. F., & Giordani, B. (1997). Adult attention deficit hyperactivity disorder: Psychological test profiles in a clinical population. *Journal of Nervous and Mental Disease, 185*(1), 32–38.

Eslinger, P. J., & Benton, A. L. (1983). Visuoperceptual performances in aging and dementia: Clinical and theoretical implications. *Journal of Clinical Neuropsychology, 5*, 213–220.

Golski, S., Zonderman, A. B., Malamut, B. L., & Resnick, S. M. (1998). Verbal and figural recognition memory: Task development and age associations. *Experimental Aging Research, 24*, 359–385.

Kibby, M. Y., Schmitter-Edgecomb, M., & Long, C. J. (1998). Ecological validity of neuropsychological tests: Focus on the California Verbal Learning Test and the Wisconsin Card Sorting Test. *Archives of Clinical Neuropsychology, 1*(6), 523–534.

Mittenberg, W., Seidenberg, M., O'Leary, D. S., & DiGiulio, D. V. (1989). Changes in cerebral functioning associated with normal aging. *Journal of Clinical and Experimental Neuropsychology, 11*, 918–932.

Rapport, L. J., Axelrod, B. N., Theisen, M. E., Brines, D. B., Kalechstein, A. D., & Rick, J. H. (1997). Relationship of IQ to verbal learning and memory: Test and retest. *Journal of Clinical and Experimental Neuropsychology, 19*(5), 655–666.

WMS-III LOGICAL MEMORY SUBTEST

Logical Memory has been a subtest of the Wechsler Memory Scales (WMS; Wechsler, 1955, 1987, 1997) since their inception. It has provided each battery with a method of assessing memory for verbally presented conceptual material. The basic premise and design of this subtest have remained relatively consistent, although some changes were noted with the WMS-III, which are discussed in Chapter 2.

Interpretation

1. Performance on the Logical Memory subtest is dependent on several factors other than memory: the subject's ability to hear and process speech sounds, the ability to understand logical–grammatical structures, and concentration. As the stores must be orally reproduced, expressive language problems, in general, and word-finding problems will influence scores.

2. Disruption of the receptive speech processes would impair performance on this task. Poor performance on this task resulting from sensory or receptive language deficits would occur concurrently with deficits on tasks of speech comprehension, and in cases of severe deficits, and with a difficulty understanding directions which may be evidenced through multiple requests to repeat questions and instructions. A comparison should be made with tests of aphasia or basic language comprehension.

3. Deficits in speech production would likewise disrupt performance as the subject may be able to hear, comprehend, and retain the material, but may not be able to effectively communicate this knowledge verbally. This process could be disrupted in a number of areas in the process of producing speech ranging from lesions of the peripheral motor/sensory system related to the vocal apparatus, lesions of the motor homunculus involved in movement of the vocal apparatus, or lesions of the left temporal lobe that cause productive impairments seen in various forms of aphasias. Patients would also show impaired speech production which is universal to all tasks that require the production of speech, and not specific to this task.

4. Word-finding difficulties have been found subsequent to left-temporal or left-frontal–temporal disruption (Carlson, Khoo, Yaure, & Schneider, 1990). On Story A the subject is required to give a specific key word to obtain credit on 9 of the 25 "story units." For Story B the use of specific key words is required for the client to receive credit on 5 of the 25 recall elements. Under these scoring criteria, persons with word-

finding difficulties may demonstrate reduced performance on the recall portion of this task, as they may have difficulty producing some of the key words and would lose credit for this deficit, even under circumstances where they were able to convey the general idea.

5. Qualitatively, an individual with word-finding difficulties (in the absence of gross verbal memory deficits) would often be able to demonstrate memory of specific key words through talking around the missing word. This disturbance of performance on recall and delayed recall items with stringent scoring criteria would tend to be seen in the absence of difficulty on items with more general and relaxed scoring guidelines. Therefore, there would likely be little to no disruption of performance on the Thematic total score when compared to the normative sample.

6. Education has been found to be significantly correlated with performance on the Logical Memory subtest. As an interpretive guideline it is important to ensure that the client's level of education is consistent with that of the normative sample. If the client's level of education is found to be significantly lower than that of the normative sample, attributing impaired performance on this subtest to anything other than a low educational level would be of questionable validity.

7. Lesions to the left hemisphere have been found to reduce performance on LM I and LM II in comparison to clients with right hemispheric lesions and normals (Chelune & Bornstein, 1988). The performance reduction on the LM subtests in cases of left hemisphere lesions has been found to occur in the midst of corresponding reductions on other verbally mediated memory subtests (i.e., Verbal Paired Associates I & II). While performance on visually mediated memory subtests (most predominantly Visual Reproduction I & II) was relatively intact and significantly better than that seen in patients with right hemispheric lesions.

8. Patients with neurodegenerative conditions affecting the memory process (i.e., Alzheimer's dementia, Parkinson's disease, Huntington's disease) have been found to perform quite poorly on Logical Memory I & II, as well as Verbal Paired Associates I & II. The pattern of scores reported by Wechsler (1997) indicates that Working Memory (a measure of attention) was far less affected than Logical Memory. A difference between Logical Memory and Working Memory of 20 or more standard score points should raise substantial concerns.

9. Logical Memory requires more active processing of information than do the Working Memory measures, Paired Associate Learning, and List Learning. While those tasks may successfully be approached using a rote memory approach, Logical Memory stories are too long to simply memorize. They must be understood and categorized so that informa-

tion may be stored more economically. A specific deficit on Logical Memory compared to those tests (by 20 or more SS points) suggests that this higher level organizing process is incomplete, pointing to anterior lesions of the dominant hemisphere.

10. Patients with left hemisphere lesions tend to demonstrate errors in producing elements essential to the plot of the stories, whereas patients with right hemisphere lesions show a tendency to omit nonessential elements and also tend to add elements that were not part of the original story. This sensitivity to some right hemisphere lesions reduces the effectiveness of the test as a measure of laterality of lesions.

11. More than a 3 scale point difference in favor of Immediate versus Delayed recall of this subtest suggests difficulty in consolidating and retaining memories. This is commonly seen in the subtests that have immediate and delayed components.

12. More than a 3-point difference in favor of Delayed versus Immediate recall of this subtest suggests difficulty in organizing and repeating information rather than memory. This may reflect frontal lobe problems, psychiatric disorders, or motivational issues.

13. Logical Memory requires more sustained and active concentration than the other subtests of the WMS-III. Specific problems here but not on other memory tests suggest that sustained concentration is impaired, a problem in attending to details by perseverating on what is presented first or last, or an inability to comprehend the meaning of the story.

14. Sustained concentration may be ruled out by investigation with the tests of attention and concentration such as the IVA or the TOVA.

15. Profiles in which Logical Memory is better than all of the other subtests, including working memory measures, suggest that the client is using intellectual skills to organize and retain information despite memory impairment. Such a procedure reflects a compensation that is usually seen in higher IQ clients, for deficits in memory that are relatively specific. Such individuals will do better on thematic scores and those items that require the gist of the information rather than specific detail, similar to the profile seen in clients with expressive language problems but in the absence of deficits in fluency. Lesions in these cases are usually subcortical.

16. List memory is a distinctly independent task from story memory (Logical Memory) or paired associate learning (Paired Associates). Each of the latter tasks provide the client with more organization as well as meaning. Impairment on only List Learning suggests that the client is overwhelmed by the organizational tasks required by long list learning rather than verbal memory per se. Such clients may do better on short list learning, as can be partially determined by looking at their perfor-

mance on Digit Span. Deficits on only story memory suggest that rote memory is intact but that the client cannot take advantage of the story's meaning to show normal improvement in performance over base rote learning. Deficits on only Paired Associates type tasks indicate that the client cannot sequence the order of the material together. (This can be evaluated as well by looking at the sequence in which they perform the other verbal memory tasks.)

17. Deficits on Paired Associates and List Learning but not Logical Memory indicate the client has trouble with rote memory but can use the meaning in the story as an effective cue in aiding memory.

18. Deficits on Paired Associates and Logical Memory but not on List Learning tasks indicate strong rote memory but poor skills at taking advantage and responding to organizational and meaning cues in the impaired tasks.

19. Meaningful picture memory is analogous to meaningful verbal memory as seen in Logical Memory and can be separated theoretically from those tasks that represent rote memory (such as List Learning, Verbal Paired Associates, Faces). In theory, strong performance on Logical Memory and Family Pictures compared to impaired performance on Faces, Verbal Paired Associates, and List Learning task suggests that the client is using higher cognitive skills to augment weak memory skills across the board. This comparison, however, is not perfect in that Faces is a recognition rather than a recall task and Verbal Paired Associates requires a specific organization of the material which may make it easier or harder to a specific client. However, the general comparison is still useful in clear-cut cases.

20. Similarly, weak performance on Logical Memory and Family Pictures compared to strong performance on Faces, Verbal Paired Associates, and List Learning task suggests that the client is not using higher cognitive skills to augment memory skills and is generally relying on rote memory skills alone.

References for WMS-III Logical Memory Subtest

Bernard, L. C., Houston, W., & Natoli, L. (1993). Malingering on neuropsychological memory tests: Potential objective indicators. *Journal of Clinical Psychology*, *49*(1), 45–53.

Brooker, A. E. (1995). Performance on the Wechsler Memory Scale-Revised for patients with mild traumatic injury and mild dementia. *Perceptual and Motor Skills*, *84*(1), 131–138.

Carlson, R. A., Khoo, B. H., Yaure, R. G., & Schneider, W. (1990). Acquisition of problem-solving skill: Levels of organization and use of working memory. *Journal of Experimental Psychology: General*, *119*(2), 193–214.

Chelune, G. J., & Bornstein, R. A. (1988). WMS-R patterns among patients with unilateral brain lesions. *Clinical Neuropsychologist*, *2*(2), 121–132.

Guilmette, T. J., & Rasile, D. (1995). Sensitivity, specificity, and diagnostic accuracy of three verbal memory measures in the assessment of mild brain injury. *Neuropsychology, 9*(3), 338–344.

Larrabee, G. J., & Crook, T. H. (1989). Dimensions of everyday memory in age-associated memory impairment. *Psychological Assessment: A Journal of Consulting and Clinical Psychology, 1*(2), 92–97.

Lezak, M. D. (1995). *Neuropsychological assessment* (3rd ed.). New York: Oxford University Press.

Luria, A. R. (1962). *Higher cortical functions in man.* New York: Consultants Bureau.

Luria, A. R. (1980). *Higher cortical functions in man* (2nd ed.). New York: Consultants Bureau.

Mutchnick, M. G., Ross, L. K., & Long, C. J. (1991). Decision strategies for cerebral dysfunction IV: Determination of cerebral dysfunction. *Archives of Clinical Neuropsychology, 6,* 259–270.

Vangel, S. J., Lichtenberg, P. A., & Ross, T. P. (1995). Clinical utility of the logical memory subtests and the relationship of demographic factors to test performance. *Journal of Clinical Gerospychology, 1*(1), 67–77.

Webster, J. S., Godlewski, M. C., Hanley, G. L., & Sowa, M. V. (1992). A scoring method for logical memory that is sensitive to right-hemisphere dysfunction. *Journal of Clinical & Experimental Neuropsychology, 14*(1), 222–238.

Wechsler, D. (1945). *Wechsler Memory Scale.* New York: Psychological Corporation.

Wechsler, D. (1955). *Manual for the Wechsler Adult Intelligence Scale.* New York: Psychological Corporation.

Wechsler, D. (1987). *Wechsler Memory Scale-Revised manual.* San Antonio, TX: The Psychological Corporation.

Wechsler, D. (1997). *Wechsler Memory Scale-Third Edition.* San Antonio, TX: The Psychological Corporation.

WMS-III VERBAL PAIRED ASSOCIATES SUBTEST (VPA)

The Verbal Paired Associates Subtest (VPA) is a task of verbal cued recall and learning (Wechsler, 1997). This subtest is included in the all editions of the Wechsler Memory Scales (WMS, WMS-R, & WMS-III; Wechsler, 1945, 1987, 1997). The format of this subtest has remained consistent. In the first section of this subtest (VPA I) subjects are administered several word pairs in succession. Then, the examiner cues the subject with the first word of each pair, and the subject is to respond with the associated word. This procedure is then repeated over several trials. The initial trial is intended to assess recall for verbally cued material, and the subsequent repeated trials are designed to examine cued learning of verbally presented material. A delayed readministration of a single trial (VPA II) is then administered approximately 30 minutes following the administration of the last learning trial to assess delayed recall and retention of verbally learned material. In all trials, the same word-pairs are used, but the order is randomized to ensure learning of the word-pairs.

In reviewing the information provided, in this new version of the VPA there appear to be well rationalized alterations and improved internal consistency and stability. Although very little research has been done on the latest version of this subtest it will likely prove to be a valuable screening instrument for verbal memory and learning processes, as well as a valuable component to the assessment of general memory ability.

Interpretation

1. As items are all verbally administered to the subject there is a heavy reliance on the ability to process spoken language, as well as the ability to produce speech. However, unlike its other verbal memory counterpart (Logical Memory), this subtest requires these capacities at a more basic and fundamental level, as the language heard needs only to be repeated, whereas Logical Memory further relies on the ability to comprehend more complex logical–grammatical structures.

2. The lack of a demand by the test for an understanding of more complex grammatical structures allows users to employ the test with clients whose language is not as strong as required by Logical Memory. However, although such clients may take the test, the standard norms cannot be applied. In such clients the symbolic value of the words is lost, making the task much more difficult, approaching the difficulty of nonsense word type tasks. Losses in such individuals—whether the language problem is due to brain injury or cultural background—may be indicative not of memory disorders but of language processing issues.

3. With these abilities intact, the ability to recall verbal material is best depicted by the first Recall Score of Trial A (VPA I). This score is a new addition to the WMS-III and lends the examiner insight into the subject's immediate storage and retrieval capacities for verbally presented material. As the raw score can be compared to the normative data yielding a scaled score, the examiner can easily compute the subject's level of functioning in this area. Reduced performance on this score (in a subject with intact prerequisite skills) is suggestive of deficient immediate cued recall for verbally presented material.

4. This immediate first trial score may be compared to other tests of List Learning first trial performance (such as on the CVLT) or to the first trial of Logical Memory. This task differs from Word List Learning in that the words are cued but must be given in a specific order. On Word Lists there is no cueing but there is also no need to keep words together.

5. Better performance on Word List first trials suggest an impairment in associating words together. Such clients often respond with words on the association list but mix up which word is associated with the other. This performance suggests that rote memory is more intact and points to higher level deficits in many cases.

6. Better performance on Paired Associates suggests that memories are

being stored but need to be cued for retrieval. Such clients will typically do better on recognition than recall tasks as well.

7. Both Logical Memory and Paired Associates involve a form of cuing. In Paired Associates the clues are concrete and externally generated; in Logical Memory, they are internally generated. Better performance on PA suggests the need for external organization. In such cases, PA will be better than both LM and tests involving the memory of simple words.

8. Better performance on LM when compared to PA suggests the use of higher cognitive structures rather than word memory to complete the tasks. Such clients will typically do poorly on word lists as well while scoring well on intelligence and achievement measures.

9. The total score for the VPA I subtest is comprised of the total number of correct responses obtained across the initial trial and the three repeated learning trials. Improvement from first trial performance to last trial suggests an active and effective learning strategy even when memory itself is poor. This pattern suggests subcortical disorders.

10. Worse performance after four trials compared to the first trial suggests poor learning strategy, which points to an organizational and planning component, an indication of possible frontal disorders.

11. Performance on VPA I recall is reduced by lesions to either hemisphere, with more severe performance deficits being seen in left hemisphere lesions. Performance is mildly to moderately reduced in cases of right hemisphere lesions while more severely impaired in left hemisphere lesions.

12. Dementia clients generally have substantial difficulty with this subtest, especially the new more difficult version.

13. The VPA II Recall Score is designed to assess the short-term retention of verbally learned material. Findings on this score demonstrate that it is more sensitive to left versus right hemisphere lesions, most likely due to the fact that this task requires memory for verbal rather than nonverbal material (Chelune & Bornstein, 1988). As this subtest is performed after a 30-minute delay, it provides a better assessment of the subject's ability to encode, store, and retrieve information that is reflected by the recall score. Impairment in VP II compared to VP I is most likely associated with memory.

14. The recent retention is a score that gives the examiner information regarding the amount of verbal information retained at a half hour after the last recall trial of VPA I. A retention composite can be computed using this score in combination with percent retention score from the Logical Memory II subtest. This composite provides the examiner with information concerning the retention of material under cued and free

recall conditions. We generally expect this score in normal individuals to be around 70% or better. Scores below 50% suggest impairment in delayed memory.

15. Better performance on VPI compared to verbal IQ (by 15 or more SS points) suggests a reliance on rote memory processes in day-to-day activities, especially if LM is also at least 15 points below VPI.

16. List memory is a distinctly independent task from story memory (Logical Memory) or paired associate learning (Paired Associates). Each of the latter tasks provides the client with more organization as well as meaning. Impairment on only List Learning suggests that the client is overwhelmed by the organizational tasks required by long list learning rather than verbal memory per se. (Such clients may do better on short list learning, as can be partially determined by looking at their performance on Digit Span.) Deficits on only story memory suggest that rote memory is intact but that the client cannot take advantage of the story's meaning to show normal improvement in performance over base rote learning. Deficits on only Paired Associates type tasks indicate that the client cannot sequence the order of the material together. (This can be evaluated as well by looking at the sequence in which they perform the other verbal memory tasks.)

17. Deficits on Paired Associates and List Learning but not Logical Memory indicate the client has trouble with rote memory but can use the meaning in the story as an effective cue in aiding memory.

18. Deficits on Paired Associates and Logical Memory but not on List Learning tasks indicate strong rote memory but poor skills at taking advantage and responding to organizational and meaning cues in the impaired tasks.

19. Meaningful picture memory is analogous to meaningful verbal memory as seen in Logical Memory and can be separated theoretically from those tasks that represent rote memory (such as List Learning, Verbal Paired Associates, Faces). In theory, strong performance on Logical Memory and Family Pictures compared to impaired performance on Faces, Verbal Paired Associates, and List Learning task suggests that the client is using higher cognitive skills to augment weak memory skills across the board. This comparison, however, is not perfect in that Faces is a recognition rather than a recall task and Verbal Paired Associates requires a specific organization of the material which may make it easier or harder to a specific client. However, the general comparison is still useful in clear-cut cases.

20. Similarly, weak performance on Logical Memory and Family Pictures compared to strong performance on Faces, Verbal Paired Associates, and List Learning task suggests that the client is not using higher

cognitive skills to augment memory skills and is generally relying on rote memory skills alone.

References for WMS-III Verbal Paired Associates Subtest (VPA)

Bernard, L. C., Houston, W., & Natoli, L. (1993). Malingering on neuropsychological memory tests: Potential objective indicators. *Journal of Clinical Psychology, 49*(1), 45–53.

Brooker, A. E. (1995). Performance on the Wechsler Memory Scale-Revised for patients with mild traumatic injury and mild dementia. *Perceptual and Motor Skills, 84*(1), 131–138.

Chelune, G. J., & Bornstein, R. A. (1988). WMS-R patterns among patients with unilateral brain lesions. *Clinical Neuropsychologist, 2*(2), 121–132.

Guilmette, T. J., & Rasile, D. (1995). Sensitivity, specificity, and diagnostic accuracy of three verbal memory measures in the assessment of mild brain injury. *Neuropsychology, 9*(3), 338–344.

Larrabee, G. J., & Crook, T. H. (1989). Dimensions of everyday memory in age-associated memory impairment. *Psychological Assessment: A Journal of Consulting and Clinical Psychology, 1*(2), 92–97.

Lezak, M. D. (1995). *Neuropsychological assessment* (3rd ed.). New York: Oxford University Press.

Luria, A. R. (1962). *Higher cortical functions in man.* New York: Consultants Bureau.

Luria, A. R. (1980). *Higher cortical functions in man* (2nd ed.). New York: Consultants Bureau.

Mutchnick, M. G., Ross, L. K., & Long, C. J. (1991). Decision strategies for cerebral dysfunction IV: Determination of cerebral dysfunction. *Archives of Clinical Neuropsychology, 6,* 259–270.

Vangel, S. J., Lichtenberg, P. A., & Ross, T. P. (1995). Clinical utility of the logical memory subtests and the relationship of demographic factors to test performance. *Journal of Clinical Geropsychology, 1*(1), 67–77.

Webster, J. S., Godlewski, M. C., Hanley, G. L., & Sowa, M. W. (1992). A scoring method for logical memory that is sensitive to right-hemisphere dysfunction. *Journal of Clinical & Experimental Neuropsychology, 14*(2), 222–238.

Wechsler, D. (1945). *Wechsler Memory Scale.* New York: Psychological Corporation.

Wechsler, D. (1955). *Manual for the Wechsler Adult Intelligence Scale.* New York: Psychological Corporation.

Wechsler, D. (1987). *Wechsler Memory Scale-Revised manual.* San Antonio, TX: The Psychological Corporation.

Wechsler, D. (1997). *Wechsler Memory Scale-Third Edition.* San Antonio, TX: The Psychological Corporation.

WMS-III FACES I AND FACES II SUBTESTS

The most recent revision of the Wechsler Memory Scale occurred in 1997 and included the introduction of two new subtests, Faces I and Faces II. Both subtests are described as being tasks of visual memory that incorporate the use of forced choice recognition paradigms. The purpose of the Faces I Subtest is to assess immediate memory for visual stimuli, whereas the purpose of the Faces II Subtest is to assess visual delayed memory. Although these subtests are new to the Wechsler Memory Scale, the attempt to assess how brain-injured patients differ in their ability to recognize unfamiliar faces is not. Overall, each subtest is easy to administer, takes approximately 5–10 minutes to complete, and is quick to score.

A number of neuropsychological skills are involved in the successful performance of the Faces I and II Subtests. At the most basic level, the patient must be conscious and able to visually perceive the test stimuli. Therefore, individuals who are legally blind are not appropriate for this test. In addition, this test should not be administered if an individual who requires corrective lenses to see at the specified testing distance does not bring them to the testing session. The ability to sustain attention is also required to successfully complete this task, as the patient is required to visually focus on a series of 72 items (pictures of faces) during Faces I and 48 items during Faces II. The patient must also be able to understand the directions to the subtests. This requires that the peripheral auditory system be intact or that another mode of communication is used, such as sign language. The Faces subtests do not heavily incorporate motor abilities. However, eye movement is required for the eyes to scan the stimuli.

Interpretation

1. Memory for faces is reported to be sensitive to right hemisphere deficits. Therefore, a patient who performs poorly on this subtest may have a deficit in one of several areas, including the right temporal lobe, right hippocampal region, or right parietal lobe. Patients with right hemisphere lesions may have difficulty executing the task. For example, they may have difficulty processing the stimuli, especially when they are only allowed 2 seconds to view each of the pictures in the first portion of Faces I (24 items). Anosognosia (also known as Anton's syndrome), in which there is neglect of one side (i.e., body or visual field), can result from massive lesions of the posterior zones of the right hemisphere. If such neglect was present, the patient would likely ignore the left side of his or her visual field. This would make it difficult for the patient to memorize the material, as the visual information was not being adequately input and processed.

2. Lesions involving the left hemisphere affect an individual's ability to quickly recognize and process frequently occurring and overlearned patterns. It is unlikely that performance on the Faces I and II Subtests would be significantly changed with lesions in the left hemisphere, as the stimuli are novel (unfamiliar) and are not presented enough to become overlearned.

3. Vision is one of the primary neuropsychological skills needed to complete these two WMS-III subtests. Aleksandr Romanovick Luria indicated that visual perception of an object is a complex and active reflex process that requires sensory and motor skills. This process begins with the identification of individual parts of the object (such as a picture of a face), which also incorporates the use of eye movements (i.e., scan-

ning). The next step that is required is the ability to integrate these parts into groups, followed by the ability to select or differentiate the stimuli from a series of alternative stimuli (Is it familiar, unfamiliar, are there specific characteristics that are recognizable?) Given this complex process, lesions to the occipital lobes are likely to cause noticeable changes in test performance. For example, lesions to the right and left primary areas of the visual cortex (area 17) can result in cortical blindness. Lesions of the optic chiasm, optic tract, and optic radiations can lead to a variety of visual field defects. For example, lesions of the optic chiasm can cause bitemporal hemianopsia. Pituitary gland tumors (which press from below on the chiasm) and aneurysms in the anterior cerebral or anterior communicating artery are the major causes of this deficit. Lesions of the right optic tract can lead to left homonymous hemianopsia. In addition, lesions of the right side of the visual radiation fibers in Meyer's loop pathway can cause left superior homonymous quadrantanopia. Temporal lobe lesions, enlargement of the lateral ventricles, and tumors are the likely causes of such deficits. A lesion of the right side of the visual radiation fibers running through the parietal lobe can cause left inferior homonymous quandrantanopia. Overall, individuals are typically able to compensate for these visual deficits (except cortical blindness) by repositioning their heads or producing compensatory eye movements so that visual integration can occur.

Lesions that extend beyond the primary visual cortical fields are quite different than those that occur predominantly in the visual cortex. Such lesions can cause one side of the visual field to be lost, as indicated earlier. However, the ability of the individual to compensate for this deficit is blocked and therefore the hemianopsia becomes permanent. This is often referred to as unilateral spatial agnosia, which is defined as a disturbance of visual attention or a unilateral disintegration of the visual process.

Perceptual impairment can arise from lesions that do not extend beyond areas 18 and 19, yet involve the right and left hemispheres (or their connections). Such lesions cause the processes of visual perception of the object and mental representation to be grossly impaired. This can also be referred to as optic agnosia. Overall, this deficit causes the structure of the visual act to be incomplete, perhaps owing to the inability to integrate all of the parts of the stimulus into a recognizable and understandable whole.

4. Lesions involving the primary sensorimotor regions do not typically affect visual perception or visual spatial abilities. However, lesions of the oculomotor area (area 8) may decrease the patient's ability to focus

on and scan the visual stimuli (i.e., faces). If the patient is not able to focus on the stimuli, then the ability to memorize the stimuli is also decreased.

5. Performance on the Faces I subtest is not likely to be equally affected by lesions to the right and left temporal lobes. Right temporal lobe lesions generally affect the ability to discriminate pitch and performance on rhythmic patterns. Although the test instructions are presented verbally, they are short and straightforward and therefore are unlikely to be misunderstood. Left temporal lobe lesions can disturb phonetic hearing, articulation of speech, and retention and/or retrieval of words. However, performance on the Faces II subtest has been found to be sensitive to right temporal lobe damage owing to the delayed memory component (nonverbal information). Lesions to the medial zones of the temporal region, especially the hippocampal, are thought to affect memory for faces as this region is involved with the regulation of the state of activity of the cerebral cortex as a whole. Memory for faces has also been reported to increase cerebral blood flow in the right temporal lobe. A patient who has a massive lesion of the medial temporal zones and adjacent formations will likely show an impairment in imprinting.

Researchers have attempted to identify material-specific memory deficits, such as memory for faces, in patients with right versus left temporal lobe epilepsy. However, the findings have been mixed. Beardsworth and Zaidel (as cited in WMS-III technical manual, 1997) found that right temporal lobe epilepsy was associated with impaired memory for faces. Similarly, Smith and Milner (as cited in WMS-III technical manual, 1997) found that right temporal lobe epilepsy was associated with impaired spatial memory. It appears that the right temporal lobe deals more with visual material, whereas the left temporal lobe deals with auditory material.

6. Lesions to the left parietal lobe outside the sensorimotor area would not necessarily affect performance on the Faces I and II subtests as this area is concerned predominantly with the ability to synthesize individual words. Complex verbal production is not required to complete this task, even though the patient must provide a response of either yes or no. If the patient has difficulty verbalizing his or her answer to the test questions, then alternative responses, such as eye blinking or head nodding, can be used.

7. The ability to see faces is mediated by the right parietal lobe. An individual who has a lesion to the right parietal lobe outside the sensorimotor area may have difficulty with spatial relationships. This

could negatively affect performance on memory for faces. Memory for faces has also been reported to be associated with increased metabolism in the right parietal area.

8. The Faces subtests are not likely to be affected by lesions to the right or left sensorimotor regions, as these areas are concerned predominantly with receptive and expressive speech. However, if receptive speech is compromised, the ability to understand the verbal instructions is limited.

9. The frontal lobes are involved with the preliminary integration of new or incoming stimuli. Lesions to the premotor area may cause disturbances in planned voluntary movement. For example, an individual who must compensate for a visual deficit by repositioning the head may not be able to do so if there is damage to this region of the brain. Frontal lobe lesions can also cause the patient to show a decrease in activity due to inattention and loss of interest in the task. Ultimately, if the patient is unable to attend to the pictures of the faces, memory for the stimuli is impossible.

10. Effects of lesions to the deep subcortical region can result in disorientation and inability to focus on the test. Such lesions are found to lower cortical activity which affects performance, despite the higher cortical processes (such as speech, thinking, praxis, and agnosia) being intact. A patient who has massive deep lesions to this region may find it difficult to complete the Faces subtests, especially subtest I, due to being allowed to view the stimuli for only 2 seconds. The ability to store the new information may also be compromised.

11. Memory for Faces can also be used to assess for malingering since you are able to compare immediate recognition versus delayed recognition scores.

12. Because of the length of Faces, it generally demands more sustained attention than do other memory tests. Thus, problems in sustained attention as reflected in poor IVA or TOVA performance (particularly on visual portions) may correlate with poor performance. In such cases, impairment will also be seen on the WCST, TPT, Category, and the Rey Figure, which also require sustained attention for good performance. Similar tests that require less sustained attention (e.g., BVRT, Stroop, COWAT, Trails B, Working Memory) will generally be normal if this is the primary problem except in the more severe deficits which can potentially affect any test.

13. Memory for Faces can be independent of memory for complex designs as measured by the Rey as well as other forms of visual memory tapped by Faces or Family Pictures. Across the board impairment suggests impairment of general visual memory skills, while specific patterns of

losses point to more specific injuries to nonmeaningful design memory (Rey), facial memory (Faces), or meaningful picture memory (Family Pictures).

14. Meaningful picture memory is analogous to meaningful verbal memory as seen in Logical Memory and can be separated theoretically from those tasks that represent rote memory (such as List Learning, Verbal Paired Associates, Faces). In theory, strong performance on Logical Memory and Family Pictures compared to impaired performance on Faces, Verbal Paired Associates, and List Learning task suggests that the client is using higher cognitive skills to augment weak memory skills across the board. This comparison, however, is not perfect in that Faces is a recognition rather than a recall task and Verbal Paired Associates requires a specific organization of the material which may make it easier or harder to a specific client. However, the general comparison is still useful in clear-cut cases.

15. Similarly, weak performance on Logical Memory and Family Pictures compared to strong performance on Faces, Verbal Paired Associates, and List Learning task suggests that the client is not using higher cognitive skills to augment memory skills and is generally relying on rote memory skills alone.

References for WMS-III Faces I and Faces II Subtests

Bernard, L. C., Houston, W., & Natoli, L. (1993). Malingering on neuropsychological memory tests: Potential objective indicators. *Journal of Clinical Psychology, 49*(1), 45–53.

Brooker, A. E. (1995). Performance on the Wechsler Memory Scale-Revised for patients with mild traumatic injury and mild dementia. *Perceptual and Motor Skills, 84*(1), 131–138.

Chelune, G. J., & Bornstein, R. A. (1988). WMS-R patterns among patients with unilateral brain lesions. *Clinical Neuropsychologist, 2*(2), 121–132.

Guilmette, T. J., & Rasile, D. (1995). Sensitivity, specificity, and diagnostic accuracy of three verbal memory measures in the assessment of mild brain injury. *Neuropsychology, 9*(3), 338–344.

Larrabee, G. J., & Crook, T. H. (1989). Dimensions of everyday memory in age-associated memory impairment. *Psychological Assessment: A Journal of Consulting and Clinical Psychology, 1*(2), 92–97.

Lezak, M. D. (1995). *Neuropsychological assessment* (3rd ed.). New York: Oxford University Press.

Luria, A. R. (1962). *Higher cortical functions in man*. New York: Consultants Bureau.

Luria, A. R. (1980). *Higher cortical functions in man* (2nd ed.). New York: Consultants Bureau.

Mutchnik, M. G., Ross, L. K., & Long, C. J. (1991). Decision strategies for cerebral dysfunction IV: Determination of cerebral dysfunction. *Archives of Clinical Neuropsychology, 6*, 259–270.

Vangel, S. J., Lichtenberg, P. A., & Ross, T. P. (1995). Clinical utility of the logical memory subtests and the relationship of demographic factors to test performance. *Journal of Clinical Geropsychology, 1*(1), 67–77.

Webster, J. S., Godlewski, M. C., Hanley, G. L., & Sowa, M. V. (1992). A scoring method for logical memory that is sensitive to right-hemisphere dysfunction. *Journal of Clinical & Experimental Neuropsychology, 14*(2), 222–238.

Wechsler, D. (1945). *Wechsler Memory Scale*. New York: Psychological Corporation.

Wechsler, D. (1955). *Manual for the Wechsler Adult Intelligence Scale*. New York: Psychological Corporation.

Wechsler, D. (1987). *Wechsler Memory Scale-Revised manual*. San Antonio, TX: The Psychological Corporation.

Wechsler, D. (1997). *Wechsler Memory Scale-Third Edition*. San Antonio, TX: The Psychological Corporation.

FAMILY PICTURES (WMS-III)

This is also a new subtest of the WAIS-III. As a result, there is a paucity of research on the neuropsychological implications of this test. In theory, the test measures the ability to remember a meaningful picture that cannot be easily verbally encoded in the 10 seconds given to study the picture.

Interpretation

1. Higher verbal IQ clients who listen closely to the instructions may get clues on what to look for which may aid verbal encoding of the stimulus.

2. Basic visual skills and visual memory are necessary for this task. Intact performance on simple visual memory tests (Spatial Scan, BVRT) is necessary to interpret the test fully.

3. The test requires intact spatial memory as well as visual memory. Intact basic spatial skills should be demonstrated on Block Design or a similar task.

4. Memory for complex designs as measured by the Rey may be independent of other forms of visual memory tapped by Faces or Family Pictures. Across the board impairment suggests impairment of general visual memory skills, while specific patterns of losses points to more specific injuries to nonmeaningful design memory (Rey), facial memory (Faces), or meaningful picture memory (Family Pictures).

5. Meaningful picture memory is analogous to meaningful verbal memory as seen in Logical Memory and can be separated theoretically from those tasks that represent rote memory (such as List Learning, Verbal Paired Associates, Faces). In theory, strong performance on Logical Memory and Family Pictures compared to impaired performance on Faces, Verbal Paired Associates, and List Learning task suggests that the client is using higher cognitive skills to augment weak memory skills across the board. This comparison, however, is not perfect in that Faces is a recognition rather than a recall task and Verbal Paired Associates requires a specific organization of the material which may make it easier or harder to a specific client. However, the general comparison is still useful in clear-cut cases.

6. Similarly, weak performance on Logical Memory and Family Pictures compared to strong performance on Faces, Verbal Paired Associates, and List Learning task suggests that the client is not using higher cognitive skills to augment memory skills and is generally relying on rote memory skills alone.

References for Family Pictures (WMS-III)

Bernard, L. C., Houston, W., & Natoli, L. (1993). Malingering on neuropsychological memory tests: Potential objective indicators. *Journal of Clinical Psychology*, *49*(1), 45–53.

Brooker, A. E. (1995). Performance on the Wechsler Memory Scale-Revised for patients with mild traumatic injury and mild dementia. *Perceptual and Motor Skills*, *84*(1), 131–138.

Chelune, G. J., & Bornstein, R. A. (1988). WMS-R patterns among patients with unilateral brain lesions. *Clinical Neuropsychologist*, *2*(2), 121–132.

Guilmette, T. J., & Rasile, D. (1995). Sensitivity, specificity, and diagnostic accuracy of three verbal memory measures in the assessment of mild brain injury. *Neuropsychology*, *9*(3), 338–344.

Larrabee, G. J., & Crook, T. H. (1989). Dimensions of everyday memory in age-associated memory impairment. *Psychological Assessment: A Journal of Consulting and Clinical Psychology*, *1*(2), 92–97.

Lezak, M. D. (1995). *Neuropsychological assessment* (3rd ed.). New York: Oxford University Press.

Luria, A. R. (1962). *Higher cortical functions in man*. New York: Consultants Bureau.

Luria, A. R. (1980). *Higher cortical functions in man* (2nd ed.). New York: Consultants Bureau.

Mutchnick, M. G., Ross, L. K., & Long, C. J. (1991). Decision strategies for cerebral dysfunction IV: Determination of cerebral dysfunction. *Archives of Clinical Neuropsychology*, *6*, 259–270.

Vangel, S. J., Lichtenberg, P. A., & Ross, T. P. (1995). Clinical utility of the logical memory subtests and the relationship of demographic factors to test performance. *Journal of Clinical Geropsychology*, *1*(1), 67–77.

Webster, J. S., Godlewski, M. C., Hanley, G. L., & Sowa, M. V. (1992). A scoring method for logical memory that is sensitive to right-hemisphere dysfunction. *Journal of Clinical & Experimental Neuropsychology*, *14*(2), 222–238.

Wechsler, D. (1945). *Wechsler Memory Scale*. New York: Psychological Corporation.

Wechsler, D. (1955). *Manual for the Wechsler Adult Intelligence Scale*. New York: Psychological Corporation.

Wechsler, D. (1987). *Wechsler Memory Scale-Revised manual*. San Antonio, TX: The Psychological Corporation.

Wechsler, D. (1997). *Wechsler Memory Scale-Third Edition*. San Antonio, TX: The Psychological Corporation.

INTERMEDIATE MEMORY SCALE (C12, LNNB)

The Intermediate Memory Scale (C12) on the LNNB is available only on Form II of the battery. It measures delayed, intermediate memory, and the delays elapse over the course of the battery administration time itself. For instance, during this final scale of the battery, a client might be asked to replicate from memory a figure that was originally the object of a drawing task from the beginning of the battery. Items on the Intermediate Memory Scale involve both recall and recognition tasks and both verbal and nonverbal tasks. Ideally, C12 follows a consecutive administration of C1–C11. However, as noted in the administration section, the test may be given independent of the remainder of the LNNB.

Ten items comprise C12. The first five items (270–275) plus 277 and 279 test recall, and 276 and 278 are designed in a recognition format. Items 272 through 275, 277, and 279 specifically target verbal memory, whereas items 270, 271, 276, and 278 rely on nonverbal memory. The remaining items require specific recall from the client.

Interpretation

1. Should qualitative analysis show a pattern of deficits only in a single sensory modality, it is critical to distinguish between a sensory problem and an actual memory deficit.
2. Analysis of performance on recall and recognition items can help differentiate a storage problem from a retrieval problem. If a client cannot recall adequately but exhibits improved performance during recognition trials, his may be a retrieval problem. Any such suspicion calls for additional examination of memory and of the client's real-life behavior.
3. C12 is highly sensitive to psychiatric disturbances, and the score may improve as the disturbances are treated. If, however, the score does not show concomitant improvement, it may be indicative of an organic, rather than psychiatric, disorder.
4. Impaired C12 performance may be one of the first signals of a degenerative disease (e.g., Alzheimer's disease). This is especially true when a client manifests deficits on executive function tasks as well.
5. Below average performance on C12 is probable in the case of head injury. Good scores on the scale argue against a substantial memory problem.
6. This acts as a good short screening test for delayed memory problems when given separately from the remainder of the LNNB. Deficits in specific visual or verbal areas should be followed up with more detailed testing.

References for Intermediate Memory Scale (C12, LNNB)

Chelune, G. J. (1982). A reexmaination of the relationship between the Luria–Nebraska and Halstead–Reitan batteries: Overlap with the WAIS. *Journal of Consulting and Clinical Psychology, 50,* 578–580.

Golden, C. J., Purish, A. C., & Hammeke, T. A. (1985). *Luria–Nebraska Neuropsychological Battery: Forms I and II Manual.* Los Angeles: Western Psychological Services.

Makatura, T. J., Lam, C. S., Leahy, B. J., Castillo, M. T., & Kalpakjian, C. Z. (1999). Standardized memory tests and the appraisal of everyday memory. *Brain Injury, 13*(5), 355–367.

Mayes, A. R. (1995). The assessment of memory disorders. In A. D. Baddeley, B. A. Wilson, et al. (Eds.), *Handbook of memory disorders* (pp. 367–391). Chichester, England: John Wiley & Sons.

MEMORY SCALE (C10-LNNB)

The LNMS, or the C10 scale on the LNNB, is designed to measure short-term memory. It accomplishes this by using items both with and without interference and in both auditory and visual modalities. Items included in the C10 scale tap verbal as well as nonverbal memory abilities, so the C10 score is comprehensive in this regard. Having only 13 items, the LNMS takes only about 15 minutes to administer. Its duration coupled with the feasibility of individual item analysis makes the LNMS useful as a quick screen for areas of memory that need further examination (Mayes, 1995).

The first three items challenge the client to remember and repeat an orally presented list of seven words; also, prior to each trial, the client must predict how many words he will be able to recall (e.g., metamemory). The next four tasks involve nonverbal memory: (1) matching shapes and colors from one card to another, (2) redrawing the image of a shape, (3) reproducing a rhythm, and (4) repeating finger positions. The final six items test the client's verbal memory, utilizing different combinations of interference and modality.

Given that a client's performance on the LNMS is dependent on his attention, and especially because no stimulus repetitions are permitted, it is crucial that the examiner take measures to encourage the client to attend fully to each item. Standard instructions are provided for each item, but to enhance communication, the clinician may paraphrase and give illustrative examples when deemed necessary. Within administration of each item, however, the modality must remain consistent, such that oral examples are given for auditory items and visual examples for visual items.

The goal of the scale is to look for areas of significant deficit that may suggest a focal injury to a specific form of memory. Unlike the other more complex memory tests described in this book, it is less susceptible to issues of attention and concentration, and the influence of other cognitive skills.

Interpretation

1. Large discrepancies between the number of words a client predicts he will recall on items 223–225 and the true number he recalls may suggest frontal lobe impairment. The prediction task measures metamemory, for which insight and judgement are necessary. Therefore, if a client predicts he will remember seven words for each trial and really reproduces no

more than four words in any trial, he may be exhibiting frontal lobe dysfunction.

2. Inability to learn seven words across five trials points to a clear memory deficit, although this performance may be normal in some older groups. Such deficits strongly indicate problems in either storing or retrieval of information.

3. Items 226 through 230 tap sensorimotor aspects of memory, such as visual memory, rhythmic memory, and tactile visual memory. Impaired performance on these items may suggest left hemisphere dysfunction, but more likely suggests right hemisphere deficits. The right hemisphere is an especially likely hypothesis when the client performs within normal limits on verbal tasks but not on items 226 through 230.

4. Poor performance on items 231 through 234 may indicate generalized short-term memory problems. When a client experiences difficulty on items following their interference portions, it is possible that insult to subcortical areas involved in long-term memory encoding is at fault.

5. Item 235 challenges the client to associate an auditory, verbal stimulus with a visual, nonverbal stimulus. Either left or right hemisphere disturbance would affect performance on this task of higher order memory functions. Because of the cueing involved in this task, it is generally easier than the other memory tasks. Thus, significant deficits suggest at least moderate memory problems. If this item is impaired but the remainder of the scale shows no problem, the client may be overwhelmed by the length of the task, pointing to either frontal or anxiety-based problems.

6. Total memory scale elevations that are very high (e.g., 80T) generally are attributed to problems with verbal memory and therefore left hemisphere or bilateral impairment. Even a score of 60T may be indicative of nonverbal dysfunction, in which case the right hemisphere may be involved. It is advisable, however, to analyze the pattern of items missed before speculating if and what lateralization is present. If there is widespread impairment on this scale, subcortical dysfunction, specifically of the temporal lobes, may be suggested.

7. General impairment on the C10 scale would not be unusual from clinically depressed test-takers.

8. As with all memory tests, poor performance on the LNMS would support suspicion of dementia.

References for Memory Scale (Scale C10-LNNB)

Chelune, G. J. (1982). A reexamination of the relationship between the Luria–Nebraska and Halstead–Reitan batteries: Overlap with the WAIS. *Journal of Consulting and Clinical Psychology, 50,* 578–580.

Golden, C. J., Purisch, A. D., & Hammeke, T. A. (1985). *Luria–Nebraska Neuropsychological Battery: Forms I and II Manual.* Los Angeles: Western Psychological Services.

Makatura, T. J., Lam, C. S., Leahy, B. J., Castillo, M. T., & Kalpakjian, C. Z. (1999). Standardized memory tests and the appraisal of everyday memory. *Brain Injury, 13*(5), 355–367.

Mayes, A. R. (1995). The assessment of memory disorders. In A. D. Baddeley, B. A. Wilson, et al. (Eds.), *Handbook of memory disorders* (pp. 367–391). Chichester, England: John Wiley & Sons.

SECTION IX: SUSTAINED ATTENTIONAL TESTS

TEST OF VARIABLES OF ATTENTION (TOVA)

Test of Variables of Attention (TOVA) (Greenberg, 1985) is a continuous performance test using non-language-based stimuli. The tests measure a cognitive element of Attention (Corman & Greenberg, 1996). There are two stimulus versions available for the test, visual (the TOVA) and auditory (TOVA-A).

Each test (TOVA and TOVA-A) has independent norms. The TOVA has norms developed for years 4 through adulthood. For years 4 through 19, norms are stratified by year and by gender. Over age 19, norms are stratified by decade (i.e., 20–29, etc.) and by gender. Subjects aged 4 and 5 receive a shortened format Of the test (11.3 minutes). The TOVA-A was developed for years 6 through 19 with norms stratified by year and gender. The TOVA-A is currently in the process of norm development for ages over 19 years.

In addition to the basic scales, their are two supplemental scales—the ADHD Score and d' prime. Each of these is empirically derived from the subject's performance on the test. The ADHD Score consists of the scores that best predicted placement between the normal control group and the ADHD clinical group (Leark, 1996). To determine this, a receiver-operated character discriminant analysis was conducted to determine the test's ability to accurately predict group placement (Greenberg, 1996). This analysis yielded an overall 80% sensitivity and 80% specificity.

Interpretation

1. Measures of individual test profile validation consist of the multiple-response and anticipatory response scores.
2. Multiple response (MR) is defined as pressing the microswitch button more than once per stimulus interval. Normals rarely perform this way, so such responses may indicate invalidity of the test profile.
3. An Anticipatory Response (AR) is defined as the subject pressing the microswitch button any time within a time frame window from 200 microseconds prior to stimulus onset to 200 microseconds after stim-

ulus onset. This 400-microsecond window is the AR. Normals rarely perform in this fashion, so these responses suggest invalidity.

4. The Omission and Commission scores are affected by AR. Increased AR can artificially alter the Omission and Commission score. Both MR and AR errors were unusual in the standardization sample. Further analysis of these two scores is given below.

5. Scores are presented by standard scores based upon a mean of 100 and a standard deviation of 15. Thus, normalized scores are those from 85 to 115. Further, norms were developed on normal IQ range subjects. In using the TOVA for subjects whose IQ scores may fall out of that range, caution is urged.

6. Standardization data were obtained up until 1:00 p.m. (1300 hours); caution is warranted for tests administered after that time frame.

7. The test consists of two conditions: target infrequent (Quarters 1 and 2) and target frequent (Quarters 3 and 4). Differences between Quarters 1 and 2, and between Quarters 3 and 4, should be minimal. Standard errors of measurement (SEM) to assess these differences are provided in the manual (Leark, 1996). Quarters 1 and 2 are of the target infrequent condition. There are only 26 targets presented during each quarter. Omission scores less than 85 are clinically significant.

8. If the subject has a poorer omission performance in Quarter 1 but a normal or an improved Quarter 2, then the subject does display an ability to learn tasks. ADHD clients generally fail to demonstrate this learning.

9. Subjects who show poor omission scores on Quarter 1 typically are those individuals who are slow to warm up to a task. They can be described as being easily distracted early in a task. If this is the case, the subject will usually show definite improvement on the second quarter.

10. Continued poor performance on Quarter 2 is indicative of a subject who not only shows poor sustained attention to task at task onset, but also of one who fails continuously. During Quarters 1 and 2, the subject waits and waits for a target before experiencing one; then, boom it is gone, only to wait again. For many subjects, this represents their experience in the classroom—it is far too boring.

11. Poor performance on omission errors on Quarter 2, but intact performance on Quarter 1, represents subjects who begin tasks well in the classroom or work setting, but without adequate structure begin to fail. Quarter 2 poor subjects may well present like normals in some circumstances, but in a brief time this aura of normality declines. They are not able to be vigilant to task.

12. Omission error differences between Quarters 3 and 4 can be of significance. Non-normals demonstrated a failure to either maintain perfor-

mance or improve performance when comparing Quarter 4 to Quarter 3. This represents a failure to learn over time. Poor performance in omissions during Quarter 3 (less than 85) suggests an inability to shift in response to a more intense demand load. Stimulus appear much more frequently, so the task is not boring. Rather, the task represents a heightened need for vigilance. When Quarter 3 is the only low score, this demonstrates an inability to shift attention, especially if Quarter 4 is higher than Quarter 3.

13. Increased Omission errors in Quarter 4 reflect a poor ability to sustain attention and vigilance over time and task demand. This is the opposite of a poor Quarter 1 only score. Hear the subject displays an ability to sustain focus to task, but declines over time. These subjects may actually perform adequately on other continuous performance tests that are abbreviated in length. But, when given a task of sufficient time, clinical loss of function can be highlighted. This may be seen in higher functioning ADHD clients. Although it may be intuitive to interpret poor Omission scores as indicating the DSM IV ADHD Inattentive Type, no research yet supports this conclusion.

14. Too high of a dose of stimulant medication often causes a poorer performance on Omissions. Thus, this can be watched to monitor ideal stimulant dosage.

15. The Omission Total Score is the summation of performance over both conditions. The clinician must take into account the performance over the Half 1 and Half 2 when interpreting the Total score. Differences in task demand can become obvious. Omission Total Scores below 85 are clinically significant. It is also important to review the raw data for this score. Sometimes, though rarely, it is technically possible for a raw score of only a few errors (e.g., 2 or 3) to have a standard below 85 because normals made few errors of Omission on the visual stimuli.

16. The Commission scores are measures of sustained impulse control. Quarter 1 poor Commission scores reflect poor impulse control. The subject waits and waits for a target, only to misidentify the nontarget.

17. If Quarter 2 Commission performance is normalized following a poor Quarter 1 performance, then the subject is able to demonstrate task learning. ADHD subjects do not show this pattern of task learning; rather, they show continued or further decline in performance.

18. If Quarter 2 Commission errors are worse than Quarter 1 (especially in light of a normalized Quarter 1 score), then the subject displays an inability to maintain vigilance and sustained impulse control over time. These children typically show deterioration in classroom behaviors. If Quarter 2 is the only poor performance on the test, if the raw data show only one, two, or three errors, then it is likely that the result is by artifact.

19. Quarter 3 reflects the change in test conditions to a highly demanding target recognition task. Poor scores here are seen in children who cannot stop themselves in highly stimulating situations. ADHD children show no improvement from Quarter 3 to Quarter 4.

20. If Quarters 3 and 4 show a high number of raw Commission errors, review the patient's history for loss of consciousness, anoxia, seizure disorder, or other neuropsychological sequelae, especially for subcortical sequelae. If such a history does not support this hypothesis, then consider the possibility of malingering if the subject is an adult.

21. The Response Time (RT) score is the mean (average) of the response time for correct responses for each quarter, half, and total. If the raw score for any quarter, half, or the total is .000, the test is invalid. A raw average speed of .000 indicates that either the microswitch was not correctly installed, became unplugged, or is malfunctioning.

22. The RT is a response measure that is influenced by stimulant medications. Physicians (e.g., Corman & Greenberg, 1996) report that proper stimulant dosing leads to normalized RT scores. Neurofeedback therapists (e.g., Othmer & Othmer, 1992) also report an ability to improve RT through treatment and consider RT an important outcome measure.

23. RT is also slowed by those who need use cognitive strategies to complete the tasks of the test. These individuals use a "stop, think, act" model of functioning. This can be inferred by those whose prior quarter score was faster than the current one, but demonstrated task failure during that quarter. RT should be evaluated whenever any Omission or Commission score is abnormal. Many adolescents who have problems with attention processing but who have managed to develop a method for controlling impulses show this slow but accurate response pattern. Depressed patients show consistently slower response times across the entire test, coupled with near normal or normal RTV scores.

24. It is not uncommon to find a slightly higher score for Half 2 RT, given that there are more responses. However, a decline in RT for Half 2 coupled with normal Omission and Commission Half 2 scores is found in the individual who needs highly structured cognitive strategies to complete the highly demanding task. This is more often the case for the adolescent or adult who has a childhood history of ADHD but has managed to find a way to control his or her impulses. These subjects typically do not manifest abnormal scores on behavioral rating scales, except for those items that reflect behavior in early childhood. These subjects are reported to respond positively to stimulant medication trials (Corman & Greenberg, 1996).

25. Response Time Variability is a measure of response consistency. The RTV is the statistical variance of the mean of the response times for

correct responses. The wider the range of the RTV (in raw data) the greater the inconsistency of response. Scores below 85 reflect problems with consistency of response. Poor RTV scores, in the absence of other poor scores on the test, should always be treated seriously.

26. RTV for Quarters 1 and 2, when Quarters 3 and 4 are normal, reflect problems sustaining impulses in boring tasks. These children are often described as being fidgety in the classroom. Abnormal scores for RTV in the target infrequent condition is not seen as often as those for the target frequent condition.

27. When RTV is abnormal, always look at RTV Half 1 and RTV Half 2. Differences between halves can help you understand whether the patient has poor impulse control in boring (Half 1) or in demanding (Half 2) situations, or across the board. Response inconsistency is a hallmark of ADHD. RTV Total has been found to correlate to measures of hyperactivity and impulse control on behavioral rating scales (Forbes, 1998; Sporn, 1997).

28. RTV for the target frequent condition (Quarters 3 and 4) are impaired in subjects with head injury. In these cases, the RTV is extremely impaired. It is not uncommon to find raw data that show that the variance is greater than the response time mean in these cases. If RTV scores are extremely impaired in an adult subject, but there is no history of head injury, anoxia, or loss of consciousness, consider the possibility of malingering.

29. RTV is highly responsive to medication effects. It is also responsive to neurofeedback treatment. Stimulant medications in proper dosing normalize RTV scores.

30. If Quarter 2 is improved over Quarter 1, the subject does display an ability to contain impulses in boring situations over time. If Quarter 4 is improved over Quarter 3, then the subject demonstrates an ability to perform task learning in the demanding task condition.

31. A window from 200 microseconds prior to stimulus onset to 200 microseconds after stimulus onset is defined as an anticipatory response (AR). Response times faster than 200 microseconds are recorded as AR regardless of whether the subject correctly identified the target. This is an important note, as individuals who have acquired a rapid response time by training (such as athletes, video game players, etc.) often respond with quick, consistent responses.

32. The standardization sample display few, if any at all, AR. ADHD subjects do not necessarily show AR. Thus, when AR is greater than 4, caution is urged on test interpretation.

33. A MR is defined as pressing the microswitch more than once during a stimulus presentation. The response is automatically excluded from the

total possible for that quarter, half, or total. MR responses are also a measure of validity of an individual's protocol. MR were rarely found in the normative group and rarely occurred in the ADHD clinical sample group. More than 4 overall may be interpreted as invalidating the protocol.

34. Despite the importance of sustained attention in many day-to-day life tasks, the brief nature of many psychological tasks makes impairments in this area less of a factor in test performance. There are two classes of exceptions to this generalization, however. First, tests that take extended periods of focus (WCST, Category, Rey Figure) may be affected by abnormalities in sustained attention. Second, severe problems, especially when combined with impulsivity and hyperactivity, can interfere with the performance on nearly every test. When these problems are intermittent, this can cause uninterpretable and invalid patterns of scores across all tests.

References for Test of Variables of Attention (TOVA)

Corman, C. L., & Greenberg, L. M. (1996). *Medication guidelines for use with the Test of Variables of Attention.* Unpublished manuscript. Los Alamitos, CA: Universal Attention Disorders.

Downey, K. K., Stelson, F. W., Pomerleau, O. F., & Giordani, B. (1997). Adult attention deficit hyperactivity disorder: Psychological test profile in a clinical population. *Journal of Nervous and Mental Disease, 185*(1), 32–38.

Forbes, G. (1998). Clinical utility of the test of variables of attention in the diagnosis of attention deficit hyperactivity disorder. *Journal of Clinical Psychology, 54*(4), 461–476.

Greenberg, L. (1996). *Test of Variables of Attention: Clinical guide.* Los Alamitos, CA: Universal Attention Disorders.

Greenberg, L. M., & Waldman, I. (1993). Developmental normative data on the Test of Variables of Attention. *Journal of Child Psychology & Psychiatry, 34*(6), 1019–1030.

Leark, R. A. (1996). *Development of additional scales for the Test of Variables of Attention.* Poster presentation, Annual Meeting of the National Academy of Neuropsychologists: New Orleans.

Othmer, S. F., & Othmer, S. (1992). *Evaluation and remediation of attention deficits.* Unpublished manuscripts. Encino, CA: EEG Spectrum.

Sporn, M. (1997). *The use of the Test of Variables of Attention to Predict Attention Behavior Problems in Deaf Adults.* Unpublished dissertation. Washington, D. C.: Gallaudet University.

Weyandt, L. L., Rice, J. A., Linterman, I., Mitzlaff, L., & Emert, E. (1998). Neuropsychological performance of a sample of adults with ADHD, developmental reading disorder, and controls. *Developmental Neuropsychology, 14*(4), 643–656.

INTERMEDIATE VISUAL AND AUDITORY CONTINUOUS PERFORMANCE TEST (IVA)

The Intermediate Visual and Auditory (IVA) Continuous Performance Test (CPT) assesses difficulties in attention and impulsivity. This computerized test measures reaction times and error rates while different conditions are presented. It was developed to aid in the diagnosis of Attention Deficit Hyperactivity Disorder (ADHD). It requires one to sustain attention to a series of stimuli that tend to be boring, as well as inhibit one's response after a certain paradigm has been established. It assesses areas of performance including speed, stamina, vigilance, prudence, consistency, and off-task behaviors.

Interpretation

1. Test-taking behavior is one of the first things that should be evaluated. Double-clicking of the mouse signifies hyperactive behavior. Test comprehension and motivation to do well should be established at the beginning to ensure a valid test. It is essential to establish that the client understands what is to be done, is making adequate effort, and has the necessary sensory and motor skills to complete the test. These can be evaluated with the IVA session and through performance on other tests of motor (such as Finger Tapping or Purdue Pegboard), sensory (Sensory–Perceptual Examination), and comprehension (Receptive Speech, Comprehension).

2. Prudence measures the ability to stop and think about a situation before reacting to it. It is measured by the number of correct responses. The examinee is required to quickly inhibit a response to the foil after being presented a series of target responses. Those with low prudence scores are described as having problems with impulsivity and inhibition to a set response. They also can be described as being careless, neglectful, or overreactive in terms of response tendencies. Those with high Prudence scores are described as being cautious and careful.

3. Consistency measures one's ability to respond in the same fashion over time. In other words, it is a measure of reliability. This score is computed based on the general variability of reaction time to correct responses. Those with low Consistency scores are described as having difficulties sustaining attention which leads to incoherence, inconsistency, and undependable responses. When presented with repetitive, demanding, structured, or boring tasks, these individuals also tend to be very distractible and exert varied attention to tasks. However, those with high scores tend to exhibit purposeful, coherent, consistent, and dependable response sets and it may arise from the ability to inhibit distracting thoughts.

4. Stamina assesses fluctuations in one's speed of reaction time. This score can aid in determining if one will have difficulties maintaining effort throughout a task. It is known that the normal person's reaction time will slow by 6 percent during the test, and thus some decrease in

reaction time is normal. Limited attentional energy, problems maintaining speed of information processing, fatigue, weak response sets, and decreased attentional abilities are characteristic of those with low Stamina scores. In contrast, vigor, strength, and attentional endurance are characteristic of those with high Stamina scores.

5. Vigilance is measured by a missed response to a target during rare blocks. The person may be visually distracted and may miss the briefly displayed target. A person may daydream and avoid responding. Also, the person may get the target mixed up and not be able to discriminate it. Those with low Vigilance scores exhibit difficulties with remaining focused, discrimination, and attention. These scores may also reflect negligence or indifference. In contrast, those with high scores are described as being attentive and alert.

6. Focus is a measure of how alert and attentive the subject is. Low scores are characteristic of those who are capricious and unreliable in terms of attentional abilities, whereas those with high scores are described as being directed, having good concentration, and being conscientious. Individuals with high scores can also pay attention to only the most relevant stimuli required for the task, leading to less variability in reaction time.

7. Speed is defined as discriminatory speed of mental processing and is computed as the average reaction time for correct trials. Mental slowness is reflected by low Speed scores. Those with high Speed scores are described as being quick and rapid.

8. The Fine Motor Regulation Quotient (Hyperactivity) is a measure of fine motor agitation using the mouse. Those with low scores may be described as having poor self-control regarding motor abilities. These subjects will often double-click, click while instructions are being given, click randomly, and may click in anticipation. Their behaviors are often described as capricious, chaotic, and confusing. Those with higher scores exhibit control, and are orderly and peaceful.

9. Balance is calculated by determining if the client is relatively better in visual or auditory modalities. Balance scores of less than 85 indicate a visual dominance, while scores of 115 and higher indicate an auditory dominance. Those scores ranging from 85 to 114 reveal no dominance in any one area. Dominance in a certain area can be described as having a relative strength in that area of sensory modality in terms of mental processing.

10. The Readiness scale determines under which conditions individual subjects exhibit their fastest speed of mental processing. Faster readiness scores (>115) reflect a person who is able to respond faster when he or she has been given time to rest. Those with this type of response are described as being indolent or lazy, and are able to perform opti-

mally only when they have been allowed time to relax. Those with low Readiness scores (<85) are described as having faster reaction times when they have already been active for some time, and tend to be motivated by their own eagerness to be active. They tend to perform more poorly when they are not required to constantly sustain attention because their mind then begins to wander and they may "tune out."

11. Despite the importance of sustained attention in many day-to-day life tasks, the brief nature of many psychological tasks makes impairments in this area less of a factor in test performance. There are two classes of exceptions to this generalization, however. First, tests that take extended periods of focus (WCST, Category, Rey Figure) may be affected by abnormalities in sustained attention. Second, severe problems, especially when combined with impulsivity and hyperactivity, can interfere with the performance on nearly every test. When these problems are intermittent, this can cause uninterpretable and invalid patterns of scores across all tests.

References for the Intermediate Visual and Auditory
Continuous Performance Test (IVA)

Sandford, J. A., & Turner, A. (1996). *Intermediate visual and auditory continuous performance test: Administration manual.* Richmond, VA: Braintrain.

Snyder, P. J., & Nussbaum, P. D. (1998). *Clinical neuropsychology: A pocket handbook for assessment.* Washington, D. C.: American Psychological Association.

Taimela, S. (1991). Factors affecting reaction-time testing and the interpretation of results. (Special Issue: Part 2), *Perceptual and Motor Skills, 73*(3), 1195–1202

PACED AUDITORY SERIAL ADDITION TEST (PASAT)

The Paced Auditory Serial Addition Test (PASAT) is easily administered with the accompanying prepared audio tape. Total administration time is about 15–20 minutes. The PASAT is useful as a measure of information processing speed and sustained attention. However, the administration instructions and speed of presentation often overwhelm lower functioning patients. It is most useful in detecting subtle attention problems in patients who otherwise perform well on more traditional tests of sustained attention (i.e., visual/verbal span, continuous performance tests, cancellation tasks, etc.). This test is an excellent addition to a comprehensive attention battery.

Interpretation

1. Correct responses typically decline progressively across trials as speed of presentation increases. Thus the time per response will also pro-

gressively increase across trials. T-scores are useful in comparing the raw scores with population norms.

2. Scores that do not consistently decline indicate fluctuating attention or lack of sustained attention throughout the entire task. Patients with significant anxiety often display such inconsistent patterns of responding across trials.

3. Acute patients with mild head injury and/or post-concussion syndrome are likely to display reduced T-scores as the task demands increase. These scores typically return to normal within 1–3 months. A pattern such as this is indicative of reduced attentional capacity and processing speed consistent with a post-concussion syndrome.

4. The PASAT has minimal correlation with mathematical ability and general intelligence.

5. The PASAT is contraindicated in patients with severe psychiatric disturbance and those with motor speech deficits (dysarthria).

6. The PASAT has some benefit in detecting malingering, or lack of significant effort, by examining the number of errors or omissions that occur in the first third of each trial. In general, all patients display fewer of these errors in the first third of each trial and the number increases as the trial progresses. Therefore, response accuracy rarely remains consistent throughout the entire trial. Also, adjusted time per response does not usually remain consistent for all four trials.

7. Trials that differ by more than 0.6 seconds in adjusted time scores from all others are invalid and should be discarded.

8. If more than one trial differs by 0.6 seconds from all others the entire session should be considered invalid and/or unreliable.

9. The test should be considered invalid if the proportion of errors exceeds 10%.

10. The PASAT is generally a more cognitively difficult task than other measures of attention such as the TOVA, IVA, or Digit Span. Thus, impairment on the PASAT alone points to the active cognitive element as the cause of the problems rather than sustained attention and vigilance.

11. Deficits on PASAT, Digit Span, and Arithmetic when tests such as the TOVA and Spatial Span are intact may suggest problems with numbers rather than attentional problems.

12. The PASAT is more of an active concentration/attentional task while the TOVA and IVA combine periods of vigilance with simple motor responses. As such, an ability to do the PASAT but not the TOVA or IVA may relate to an inability to deal with periods of inactivity. Such clients often are able to do well as long as they are occupied, but when forced to wait or listen to others they may show impulsive or hyperactive-like behaviors.

13. Despite the importance of sustained attention in many day-to-day life tasks, the brief nature of many psychological tasks makes impairments in this area less of a factor in test performance. There are two classes of exceptions to this generalization, however. First, tests that take extended periods of focus (WCST, Category, Rey Figure) may be affected by abnormalities in sustained attention. Second, severe problems, especially when combined with impulsivity and hyperactivity, can interfere with the performance on nearly every test. When these problems are intermittent, this can cause uninterpretable and invalid patterns of scores across all tests.

References for Paced Auditory Serial Addition Test (PASAT)

Cicerone, K. D. (1997). Clinical sensitivity of four measures of attention to mild traumatic brain injury. *Clinical Neuropsychologist, 11*(3), 266–272.

D'Elia, L. F., Boone, K. B., & Mitrushina, A. M. (1995). *Handbook of normative data for neuropsychological assessment.* New York: Oxford University Press.

Gronwell, D., & Wrightson, P. (1981). Memory and information processing capacity after closed head injury. *Journal of Neurology, Neurosurgery, and Psychiatry, 44,* 889–895.

Sherman, E. M. S., Strauss, E., & Spellacy, F. (1997). Validity of the paced auditory serial addition test (PASAT) in adults referred for neuropsychological assessment after head injury. *Clinical Neuropsychologist, 11*(1), 34–45.

Spreen, O., & Strauss, E. (1991). *A compendium of neuropsychological tests: Administration, norms, and commentary.* New York: Oxford University Press.

Snyder, P. J., & Nussbaum, P. D. (1998). *Clinical neuropsychology: A pocket handbook for assessment.* Washington, D.C.: American Psychological Association.

SECTION X: TEST BATTERIES

THE LURIA–NEBRASKA NEUROPSYCHOLOGICAL BATTERY

The Luria–Nebraska Neuropsychological Battery (LNNB) is a method that integrates the qualitative information generated by the techniques of A. R. Luria with traditional American psychometric procedures. This hybrid approach takes elements from both significant traditions. The test has been found to have both a strong psychometric base as well as to provide the clinician with the opportunity to make numerous and valuable qualitative observations and discriminations of highly specific problems in clients that cannot be easily made with traditional psychometric instruments. The test battery itself provides a brief but comprehensive evaluation in less than 3 hours, which makes it practical to use in situations where time is limited and with impaired clients whose ability to be tested over long time periods is limited.

Interpretation

1. With the LNNB, there are many levels of client classification ranging from normal/abnormal to sophisticated analysis of the precise deficits and precise neurological causes of a given deficit.
2. The LNNB provides several independent methods to identify the possible presence of a brain injury. The first involves a comparison of the 12 basic skills along with the Pathognomonic Scale to the critical level (CL). More than three scales above the CL is indicative of brain injury.
3. Because the CL is dependent on age and education, the accuracy of this rule depends on the accuracy of the information. While age is rarely misstated in a significant fashion, education can be much more difficult to calculate. For example, the CL will overestimate the premorbid abilities of a client who has simply attended school for 12 years but was impaired as a result of retardation or brain injury. In such a case, the choice of a specific level of education for the formula often depends on the question being asked. If a clinician simply wishes to know how the person is performing in relation to other people with 12 years of educational opportunity, then using 12 is appropriate. If a clinician wishes to know if the person had a recent brain injury (since the end of school), then using the client's actual achievement level may be more appropriate. In addition, the test manual includes a formula for calculating the critical level from premorbid IQ levels.
4. A second method for identifying brain injury is to note the difference between the lowest and highest T-score. Normal individuals typically show less than a 20-point spread between the lowest and highest scores, with a few normals showing up to a 25-point difference. In such cases, the highest scores are often on Arithmetic or Writing (because of spelling). Brain-injured clients typically show greater variability. Using this information, score differences exceeding 30 points are considered clearly indicative of brain dysfunction. Ranges between the highest and lowest scores less than 30 but more than 20 are considered borderline, while ranges 20 and under are considered normal. The basic quantitative scales of the LNNB yield T-score profiles. Two-point codes (the highest two scales) and three-point codes (the highest three scales) can be determined to generate statistical descriptions of the client's most likely problems.
5. A high point pair of the Motor and Tactile scales is often seen in clients in whom there is lateralized impairment, often caused by a cerebral vascular accident of some kind. In general, these occurrences are cortical strokes, whose side can be reliably determined by the comparison of the left and right hemisphere scales. These strokes are generally

accompanied by severe cognitive deficits, the nature of which depends on lateralization of injury. In general, the scales representing those cognitive areas (e.g., Expressive Language) will show secondary elevations. Elevations on Motor and Visual are most often associated with anterior right hemisphere injuries. The client shows intact basic visual skills, but has trouble with more abstractive and visual reasoning tasks. Motor impairment is generally greatest on the left side of the body. Impairment elevations on the Rhythm scale may be seen as well, producing a Motor–Visual–Rhythm 3-point code. When the 2-point code is Motor/Rhythm, the lesion is generally more anterior than when the 2-point code is Motor/Visual. The Motor/Rhythm combination is generally associated with attentional problems, difficulties in emotional control or emotional recognition, poor insight, poor social skills (especially if the lesion is longstanding), and difficulties in following the relationships between sequences of events. This profile may also be seen in many subcortical injuries, including mild to moderate head injury.

6. Motor and Expressive Language high points are seen in anterior left hemisphere injuries, usually arising from a relatively serious problem such as a stroke or a fast growing tumor. Such clients have dysfluent speech. They may slur their words, speak haltingly, repeat sounds, and substitute sounds, which makes the client unintelligible. In extreme cases they may be mute or unable to communicate verbally at any level, although nonverbal communication, reading, and writing may be intact. Naming problems are frequently present and may be consistent with expressive aphasia, also called Broca's aphasia.

7. The Motor/Writing 2-point code is seen primarily in disorders where the dominant hand is dysfunctional. This result can be seen in lateralized subcortical disorders but can also be a peripheral disorder where the function of the arm is disrupted by spinal cord or nerve injuries, or fractures. When the disorder is in the brain, there are usually secondary attentional or arousal problems which will be noted in the testing process. When the injuries are peripheral, the deficits are generally limited to items that tap motor speed and coordination and tactile sensitivity. Thus, drawing is often disrupted as well as writing, along with the speeded items.

8. The Motor/Reading combination occurs most often in people who have a learning disorder (dyslexia) history. The occasional exception to this tendency is seen in individuals with multiple strokes, who may develop an acquired dyslexia from a small stroke along with more general motor problems.

9. The Motor/Arithmetic code type is seen in individuals with primarily

subcortical lesions who have motor and attentional problems. It is also seen in many individuals with preexisting arithmetic disorders, which occur in up to 30% of normal controls on the LNNB. In cases where an arithmetic difficulty is premorbid, it is best to ignore this scale and look for the 2-point code without Arithmetic included.

10. The Motor/Memory combination is nearly always seen in subcortical injuries. This deficit is common after mild to moderate head injuries. The clients have generally mild but pervasive motor problems as well as difficulty retaining information, especially with interference. They perform better with simple memorization tasks. They generally have little insight into their condition or the impact of their memory problems. Emotional lability and irritability is also common.

11. The Motor/Intermediate Memory 2-point code has a similar interpretation as for Motor/Memory, but the condition tends to be somewhat milder than when Motor/Memory is the 2-point code.

12. The Motor/Intelligence code type is rarely seen. It may represent preexisting problems or may reflect a multiinfarct or similar process (such as multiple tumors). It is very important with this and similar codes to discriminate what was preexisting, particularly if the testing is administered to assess the effects of an injury.

13. The Rhythm/Visual 2-point code is associated with defects in nonverbal processing. In mild elevations, this profile is associated with subcortical injuries which may affect the processing of items demanding attention or detail, while in more severe forms it is usually associated with lesions in the temporal/parietal areas of the right hemisphere where such processing is interrupted by the inability to analyze novel or less overlearned material.

14. The Rhythm/Receptive code is associated with problems in auditory processing. This code can be caused by poor hearing abilities therefore peripheral hearing loss must be ruled out as a possible cause. In the absence of a peripheral hearing loss, a bilateral central hearing loss must also be investigated. In the presence of adequate hearing, the deficit is most often associated with damage to the left temporal area but can also be seen in bilateral temporal injuries. In severe forms, this may represent a stroke or an open head trauma but can also be seen in a variety of degenerative processes.

15. The Tactile/Reading combination is often seen in left parietal injuries. These may be longstanding (as seen in learning disabilities), or more recent injuries that are generally along the lines of a stroke, open head injury, abscess, hemorrhage, or other condition that destroys brain tissue. These latter injuries are usually associated with other substantial

problems as well, although this may be seen as residual many years after an event.

16. The Visual/Receptive, Visual/Arithmetic, and Visual/Memory high point codes are often associated with right hemisphere problems, usually in the posterior areas. Such deficits can reflect an inability to do spatial processing and to visualize material, although the person may function well in terms of verbal skills (depending of course on the elevation of the entire profile). It is important that when any Arithmetic deficit is considered, one establish that the deficit is not a preexisting condition, but is the result of some type of more recent cerebral event.

17. A high point comprised of Receptive and Expressive may represent a breakdown of speech processes in general. This is most often seen in strokes and other disorders that destroy brain tissue, with lesser elevations reflecting residual deficits. These deficits are often associated with very high profiles, as these basic skills are necessary to understand the test instructions. Such a profile may also be seen in severe dementing processes as well.

18. The Receptive/Intelligence combination (with elevations on one or more of the achievement scales) reflects a more posterior injury than the Receptive/Expressive combination. This can be seen as the result of an adult-onset injury or may reflect longstanding learning disabilities or mental retardation. Such profiles are usually associated with substantial disabilities that affect day-to-day life.

19. Each scale can be divided into groups of items, which explore a specific aspect of the overall scale area. Item analysis involves focusing on these specific item groupings to evaluate contributions to the overall scale elevations. Consequently, more specific hypotheses of the underlying deficits are generated. This information can be used to modify the more statistically based interpretations generated from the high point codes, and provide more precise details of the specific problems.

References for the Luria–Nebraska Neuropsychological Battery

Chelune, G. J. (1982). A reexamination of the relationship between the Luria–Nebraska and Halstead-Reitan batteries: Overall with the WAIS. *Journal of Consulting and Clinical Psychology, 50,* 578–580.

Golden, C. J., Purisch, A. D., & Hammeke, T. A. (1985). *Luria–Nebraska Neuropsychological Battery: Forms I and II Manual.* Los Angeles: Western Psychological Services.

Makatura, T. J., Lam, C. S., Leahy, B. J., Castillo, M. T., & Kalpakjian, C. Z. (1999). Standardized memory tests and the appraisal of everyday memory. *Brain Injury, 13*(5), 355–367.

Mayes, A. R. (1995). The assessment of memory disorders. In A. D. Baddeley, B. A. Wilson, et al. (Eds.), *Handbook of memory disorders* (pp. 367–391). Chichester, England: John Wiley & Sons.

McKinzey, R. K., Roecker, C. E., Puente, A. E., & Rogers, E. B. (1998). Performance of normal adults on the Luria–Nebraska Neuropsychological Battery, Form I. *Archives of Clinical Neuropsychology, 13*(4), 397–413.

Moses, J. A., & Pritchard, D. A. (1999). Performance scales for the Luria–Nebraska Neuropsychological Battery-Form I. *Archives of Clinical Neuropsychology, 14*(5), 285–302.

Nagel, J. A., Harrell, E., & Gray, S. G. (1997). Prediction of achievement scores using the Luria–Nebraska Neuropsychological Battery Form II. *Psychological, 34*(1), 41–47.

HALSTEAD–REITAN NEUROPSYCHOLOGICAL BATTERY (HRNB)

The Halstead–Reitan is the oldest and best known of the major neuropsychological test batteries. There has been more extensive research on this battery than on any other neuropsychological instrument, with the possible exception of the Wechsler Intelligence Tests (which are traditionally included as part of the HRNB). The use of the battery is complicated by several different sets of unofficial norms and configurations. The most well accepted of these are those proposed by Reitan and Wolfson (1995) and by Heaton, Grant, and Matthews (1993).

Interpretation

1. The first level of interpretation provides global indicators of brain injury. The most effective single indicator is the Impairment Index. The first impairment index (HII) consisted of 10 measures, each classified as normal or abnormal. This was later reduced to seven scores (Tactual Performance Test-Total Time, TPT-Memory, TPT-Location, Category Test, Rhythm Test, Speech Sounds, and Finger Tapping). The Impairment Index is the percentage of these tests that fall into the "impaired" range. Impaired ranges for the HII tests include: TPT Total Time (>15.7 minutes), TPT Memory (<6 correct), TPT Location (<5 correct), Speech–Sounds (>6 errors), Rhythm (>5 errors), Category (>51 errors), and Finger Tapping (dominant hand <51 taps).

2. The Impairment Index will accurately classify some 90% of uncomplicated cases of verified brain injury when compared to normal controls. Accuracy rates are reduced when psychiatric controls are employed. The score is most likely to miss mild injuries, subcortical injuries, and cases of epilepsy. In addition to the Impairment Index, there are three other general indicators of organic damage: the Category Test, Trail Making Test-Part B, and TPT-Total Time. Cases where two or more of these indicators are abnormal have a high probability of brain injury. Russell, Neuringer, and Goldstein (1971) introduced a more complex and extended version of the HII known as the Average Impairment

Rating (AIR). This score correlates over .9 with the HII and they seem to have similar accuracy.

3. Pattern analysis within the tests of the battery are essential to the diagnosis of the HRNB. These are discussed within the sections on each of the HRNB tests.

4. Comparison of the left and right sides of the bodies on the TPT, Finger Tapping, Grip Strength, and the Sensory–Perceptual Examination are effective measures (about 80%) to identify the lateralization of specific lesions. The details of these comparisons are discussed within the sections on each test.

5. Right (nondominant) frontal injuries tend to be most difficult for the HRNB (as well as other tests) to diagnose. Signs of right frontal impairment on the HRNB include poor performance on the TPT-Nondominant Hand, TPT-Localization, Finger Tapping-Nondominant, Digits Backwards, Picture Arrangement, Seashore Rhythm Test, and the Category Test. It is not unusual for these performances to be impaired more by comparison to other performances rather than in absolute terms. The Impairment Index is often normal in these cases.

6. Left (Dominant) frontal injuries are more easily diagnosed, with signs including poor Finger Tapping-Dominant, TPT-Dominant, TPT-Total, Category Test, Trails B, Aphasia Examination (oral motor problems), Speech Sounds, and Similarities.

7. Posterior left (dominant) hemisphere injuries are usually easily recognized by problems on the Aphasia Examination (language, reading, and writing problems along with a lack of detail on the key, Category Test, dominant side on the Sensory Perceptual Examination, Speech Sounds, Finger Tapping-Dominant, Verbal IQ, Trails A and Trails B).

8. Posterior right (nondominant) hemisphere injuries are characterized by extensive deficits in the Tactual Performance Test-Total, Tactual Performance Test-Nondominant, Sensory Perceptual Examination-Nondominant, Aphasia Examination (spatial and drawing problems, especially distortions on the cross and the key), Performance IQ, Block Design, Object Assembly, Matrices, TPT-Memory, and TPT-Location.

9. Subcortical injuries are characterized by slowness and inconsistencies on TPT, Finger Tapping, and the Sensory–Perceptual Examination. Attentional problems may be seen on Digit Span and Digit Symbol. Other tests may be disrupted because of attentional rather than cognitive problems.

10. Patterns that include only motor and sensory deficits in the absence of any cognitive problems may indicate peripheral injuries or spinal injuries rather than injuries to the brain itself.

References for Halstead–Reitan Neuropsychological Battery (HRNB)

Arnold, B. R., Montgomery, G. T., Castaneda, I., & Longoria, R. (1994). Acculturation and performance of Hispanics on selected Halstead–Reitan neuropsychological tests. *Assessments, 1*(3), 239–248.

Bigler, E. D., & Tucker, D. M. (1981). Comparison of verbal IQ, tactual performance, seashore rhythm and finger oscillation tests in the blind and brain-damaged. *Journal of Clinical Psychology, 37*(4), 849–851.

Bornstein, R. A. (1983). Relationship of age and education to neuropsychological performance in patients with symptomatic carotid artery disease. *Journal of Clinical Psychology, 39*(4), 470–478.

Bornstein, R. A. (1985). Normative data on selected neuropsychological measures from a nonclinical sample. *Journal of Clinical Psychology, 41*(5), 651–659.

Bornstein, R. A. (1986). Classification rates obtained with "standard" cut-off scores on selected neuropsychological measures. *Journal of Clinical and Experimental Neuropsychology, 8*(4), 413–420.

Butters, M. A., Goldstein, G., Allen, D. N., & Shemansky, W. J. (1998). Neuropsychological similarities and differences among Huntington's disease, multiple sclerosis, and cortical dementia. *Archives of Clinical Neuropsychology, 13*(8), 721–735.

Choca, J. P., Laatsch, L., Wetzel, L., & Agresti, A. (1997). The Halstead category test: A fifty year perspective. *Neuropsychology Review, 7*(2), 61–75.

Charter, R. A., Dutra, R. L., & Lopez, M. N. (1997). Speech–Sounds Perception Test: Analysis of error types in normal and diffusely brain damaged patients. *Perceptual and Motor Skills, 84*, 1507–1510.

Dee, H. L., & Van Allen, M. W. (1972). Psychomotor testing as an aid in the recognition of cerebral lesions. *Neurology, 22*, 845–848.

Dikman, S. S., Heaton, R. K., Grant, I., & Temkin, N. R. (1999). Test–retest reliability and practice effects of Expanded Halstead–Reitan neuropsychological test battery. *Journal of the International Neuropsychological Society, 5*(4), 346–356.

Dunwoody, L., Tittmar, H. G., & McClean, W. S. (1996). Grip strength and intertrial rest. *Perceptual and Motor Skills, 83*, 275–278.

Ernst, J. (1987). Neuropsychological problem-solving skills in the elderly. *Psychology and Aging, 2*(4), 363–365.

Golden, C. J., & Anderson, S. M. (1977). Short form of the Speech Sounds Perception Test. *Perceptual and Motor Skills, 45*, 485–486.

Golden, C. J., Zillmer, E., & Spiers, M. (1992). *Neuropsychological assessment and intervention.* Springfield, IL: Charles C Thomas.

Haaland, K. Y., & Delaney, H. D. (1981). Motor deficits after left or right hemisphere damage due to stroke or tumor. *Neuropsychologia, 19*, 17–27.

Haaland, K. Y., Temkin, N., Randahl, G., & Dikmen, S. (1994). Recovery of simple motor skills after head injury. *Journal of Clinical and Experimental Neuropsychology, 16*(3), 448–456.

Halstead, W. C. (1947). *Brain and intelligence: A quantitative study of the frontal lobes.* Chicago: University of Chicago Press.

Hays, J. R. (1995). Trail making test norms for psychiatric patients. *Perceptual and Motor Skills, 80*, 187–194.

Heaton, R. K., Grant, I., & Matthews, C. G. (1991). *Comprehensive norms for an expanded Halstead–Reitan battery: Demographic corrections, research findings, and clinical applications.* Odessa, FL: Psychological Assessment Resources.

Heilbronner, R. L., Henry, G. K., Buck, P., & Adams, R. L. (1991). Lateralized brain damage and performance on Trail Making A and B, Digit Span Forward and Backward, and TPT Memory and Location. *Archives of Clinical Neuropsychology, 6*(4), 251–258.

Heilbronner, R. L., & Parsons, O. A. (1989). The clinical utility of the Tactual Performance Test (TPT): Issues of lateralization and cognitive style. *Clinical Neuropsychologist, 3*(3), 250–264.

Johnstone, B., Holland, D., & Hewett, J. E. (1997). The construct validity of the category test: Is it a measure of reasoning or intelligence? *Psychological Assessment, 9*(1), 28–33.

Keyser, D. J., & Sweetland, R. C. (1984). The Halstead–Reitan Neuropsychological Battery and Allied Procedures. In *Test Critiques*, Vol. I. Kansas City, MO: Test Corporation of America.

Leon, J., Pearlman, O., Doonan, R., & Simpson, G. M. (1996). A study of bedside screening procedures for cognitive deficits in chronic psychiatric inpatients. *Comprehensive Psychiatry, 37*(5), 328–335.

Lezak, M. (1995). Perception. In *Neuropsychological Assessment* (3rd ed.). New York: Oxford University Press.

Mercer, W. N., Harrell, E. H., Miller, D. C., Childs, H. W., & Rockers, D. M. (1997). Performance of brain-injured versus healthy adults on three versions of the category test. *The Clinical Neuropsychologist, 11*(2), 174–179.

Montazer, M. A., & Thomas, J. G. (1991). Grip strength as a function of repetitive trials. *Perceptual and Motor Skills, 73*, 804–806.

O'Donnell, J. P. (1983). Lateralized sensorimotor asymmetries in normal learning-disabled and brain-damaged youth adults. *Perceptual and Motor Skills, 57*, 227–232.

Prigatono, G. P., & Parsons, O. A. (1976). Relationship of age and education to Halstead test performance in different patient populations. *Journal of Consulting and Clinical Psychology, 44*(4), 527–533.

Reddon, J. R., Stefanyk, W. O., Gill, D. M., & Renney, C. (1985). Hand dynamometer: Effects of trials and sessions. *Perceptual and Motor Skills, 61*, 1195–1198.

Reitan, R. M., & Wolfson, D. (1989). The Seashore Rhythm Test and brain functions. *The Clinical Neuropsychologist, 3*, 70–78.

Reitan, R. M., & Wolfson, D. (1993). *The Halstead–Reitan neuropsychological test battery: Theory and clinical interpretation* (2nd ed.). S. Tucson, AZ: Neuropsychology Press.

Russell, E. W., Neuringer, C., & Goldstein, G. (1971). *Assessment of brain damage: A neuropsychological key approach*. New York: Wiley-Interscience.

Ryan, J. J., & Larsen, J. (1983). Comparison of three Speech Sounds Perception Test short forms. *Clinical Neuropsychology, 5*(4), 173–175.

Schear, J. M., & Sato, S. D. (1989). Effects of visual acuity and visual motor speed and dexterity on cognitive test performance. *Archives of Clinical Neuropsychology, 4*, 25–32.

Schwartz, F., Carr, A., Munich, R., Bartuch, E., Lesser, B., Rescigno, D., & Viegener, B. (1990). Voluntary motor performance in psychotic disorders: A replication study. *Psychological Reports, 66*, 1223–1234.

Searight, H. R., Dunn, E. J., Grisso, T., & Margolis, R. B. (1992). The relation of the Halstead–Reitan neuropsychological battery to ratings of everyday functioning in a geriatric sample: Clarification. *Neuropsychology, 6*(4), 394.

Snyder, P. J., & Nussbaum, P. D. (1998). *Clinical neuropsychology: A pocket handbook for assessment*. Washington, D. C.: American Psychological Association.

Stringer, A. Y., & Green, R. C. (1996). Stimulus imperception. In *A guide to adult neuropsychological diagnosis*. Philadelphia, PA: F. A. Davis.

Temkin, N. R., Heaton, R. K., Grant, I., & Dikmen, S. S. (1999). Detecting significant change in neuropsychological test performance: A comparison of four models. *Journal of the International Neuropsychological Society, 5*(4), 357–369.

Thompson, L. L., & Heaton, R. K. (1991). Pattern of performance on the tactual performance test. *Clinical Neuropsychologist, 5*(4), 322–328.

Welch, L. W., Cunningham, A. T., Eckardt, M. J., & Martin, P. R. (1997). Fine motor speed deficits in alcoholic Korsakoff's syndrome. *Alcoholism: Clinical & Experimental Research, 21*(1), 134–139.

Williams, J. M., & Shane, B. (1986). The Reitan–Indiana aphasia screening test: Scoring and factor analysis. *Journal of Clinical Psychology, 42*(1), 156–160.

Wood, D. G., & Bigler, E. D. (1995). Diencephalic changes in traumatic brain injury: Relationship to sensory perceptual function. *Brain Research Bulletin, 38*(6), 545– 549.

Young; K. L., & Delay, E. R. (1993). Seashore rhythm test: Comparison of signal detection theory and standard scoring procedures. *Archives of Clinical Neuropsychology, 8*, 111–121.

Appendix

Score Translations for Neuropsychological Data

Standard score	T-score	Percentile	Inverted T-score	Z-score	Scale score
150	83	99	17	3.33	20
145	80	99	20	3.00	19
140	77	99	23	2.67	18
135	73	99	27	2.33	17
130	70	98	30	2.00	16
125	67	95	33	1.67	15
120	63	91	37	1.33	14
115	60	84	40	1.00	13
110	57	75	43	0.67	12
105	53	63	47	0.33	11
100	50	50	50	0.00	10
95	47	37	53	−0.33	9
90	43	25	57	−0.67	8
85	40	16	60	−1.00	7
80	37	9	63	−1.33	6
75	33	5	67	−1.67	5
70	30	2	70	−2.00	4
65	27	1	73	−2.33	3
60	23	1	77	−2.67	2
55	20	1	80	−3.00	1
50	17	1	83	−3.33	0
45	13	1	87	−3.67	0
40	10	1	90	−4.00	0

Index

Aphasia Examination, 13, 99–103, 112, 116, 161, 168, 235
Arithmetic, 54, 105, 112, 125, 150, 153, 178, 182, 228
Arithmetic (LNNB-II), 34, 44–46, 101, 125, 150, 154, 158–160, 228, 230–233

Bender Visual Motor Gestalt Test, 19–20, 59, 61, 63–64, 65–70, 76, 80, 83–84, 87–88, 90–91, 93, 95, 96, 100, 120, 123, 124, 125, 188
Benton Visual Retention Test (BVRT), 23–25, 64, 68–69, 72–73, 83, 85–89, 90–91, 93, 94, 95, 96, 100, 110, 166, 168, 170, 181, 188, 190, 212, 214
Block Design, 9, 53, 59, 60–65, 67–72, 75–76, 80, 83–84, 87–89, 90, 93, 94, 95, 96, 97, 98, 113, 119, 120, 121, 122, 123, 124, 155, 164, 168, 169, 190, 214
Boston Naming Test (BNT), 30–31, 59, 98, 101, 102, 104, 106, 108–112, 116, 117, 122, 168, 181

California Verbal Learning Test (CVLT), 17, 192, 194, 195–199, 205
Category Test (CT), 3, 11–12, 60, 64, 73, 76, 80–81, 84, 93, 95, 96, 107, 112, 113, 117, 120, 122, 127, 129, 143, 161, 163, 164, 165, 166, 167–171, 173, 176, 177, 190, 212, 224, 227, 228
Clock Drawing Test (CDT), 22–23, 63–64, 68, 72, 81, 82–85, 87, 90–91, 93, 94, 95, 100
Comprehension, 54–55, 59, 101, 102, 103, 104, 105–108, 110, 122, 126, 164, 181, 225
Controlled Oral Word Association Test (COWAT), 31, 81, 102, 112, 113, 160–163, 165, 166, 169, 170, 173, 176, 177, 190, 212

Digit Span, 54, 94, 105, 121, 122, 123, 125, 129, 144, 164, 169, 178, 183–185, 186, 194, 198, 203, 207, 228
Digit Symbol, 53–54, 69, 88, 94, 123, 124–126

Expressive Speech Scale, 38–39, 101, 106, 109, 115–118, 161, 231, 233

Faces, 14–17, 166, 178, 179, 181, 190, 195, 199, 203, 207, 208–214
Family Pictures, 14, 178, 179, 190, 195, 199, 203, 207, 212, 213, 214–215
Finger Tapping Test (FTT), 11, 13, 63, 67–70, 72, 79–80, 88, 90–91, 93, 100, 123, 124, 130–133, 134, 135, 136, 138, 139, 140, 141, 142, 188, 225, 234–235

Grip Strength, 11, 13, 132, 134, 136, 137–141, 234–235

Halstead–Reitan Impairment Index, 234
Halstead–Reitan Neuropsychological Battery (HRB), 7, 11–13, 78–82, 99–103, 114–115, 128–133, 137–141, 144–146, 167–174, 234–238; see also specific tests: Aphasia Screening Test, Category Test, Finger Tapping Test, Grip Strength, Seashore Rhythm Test, Sensory-Perceptual Examination, Speech Sounds Perception Test, Tactual Performance Test, Trail Making Test
Hooper Visual Organization Test (HVOT), 32, 65, 69, 84, 88–89, 96, 97–99

Information, 59, 101, 102, 107, 108, 126
Intermediate Memory, 37–38, 215–217, 233

Intermediate Visual and Auditory Continuous Performance Test (IVA), 48–49, 81, 166, 170, 190, 202, 212, 224–227, 228

Logical Memory, 14–17, 179, 194, 195, 198, 199, 200–204, 205, 206, 207, 213, 214, 215
Luria–Nebraska Neuropsychological Battery II (LNNB-II), 32–47, 125, 141–143, 154–160, 215–219, 229–234; see also specific tests: Arithmetic Scale, Expressive Speech Scale, Intermediate Memory Scale, Memory Scale, Motor Functions Scale, Reading Scale, Receptive Speech Scale, Writing Scale

Matrices, 61, 64–65, 67–70, 76–77, 83, 87–88, 89–94, 95, 96, 109, 113, 119, 120, 121, 122, 123, 124, 126, 168, 190
Memory, 34, 39–40, 217–219, 232–233
Motor Functions, 34, 36–37, 141–143, 230–233

Paced Auditory Serial Addition Test (PASAT), 227–229
Peabody Individual Achievement Test-Revised (PIAT-R), 20–21, 60, 100, 104, 125, 146–151, 153, 158, 168
Peabody Picture Vocabulary Test-Revised (PPVT-R), 17–18, 58–60, 118, 119
Picture Arrangement, 60, 63–65, 68–69, 72, 88, 90, 108, 110, 121–124, 126, 129, 181
Picture Completion, 60, 65, 69, 88, 102, 109, 110, 121, 122, 123, 124, 125, 126–128, 164, 168, 181
Purdue Pegboard, 26, 68–69, 88, 123, 124, 131, 132, 133–137, 138, 139, 140, 141, 142, 188, 225

Raven's Matrices, 21, 63–64, 68–74, 76–77, 80, 83, 87–88, 89, 90–91, 94, 95, 96, 103, 109, 122, 150, 153, 168, 169, 188, 190
Reading, 102
Receptive Speech, 34, 46–47, 102, 110, 112, 115, 116, 118–121, 161, 164, 168, 181, 225, 232–233
Rey Auditory Verbal Learning Test (RAVLT), 21–22, 192–195, 198
Rey Complex Figure Test (CFT), 3, 27–29, 59, 61, 67, 81, 87, 90, 123, 129, 155, 166, 187–192, 212, 214, 224, 227, 228

Seashore Rhythm Test (SRT), 11–12, 114, 119, 123, 128–129, 234–235
Sensory-Perceptual Examination, 11, 13, 144–146, 225, 235
Similarities, 59, 102, 105, 110, 112–114
Spatial Span, 121, 122, 144, 182, 184, 214, 228
Speech Sounds Perception Test (SSPT), 11–12, 114–115, 116, 119, 129, 234–235
Standard Progressive Matrices (SPM), see Raven's Matrices
Stroop Color and Word Test, 29–30, 60, 73, 76, 81, 84, 93, 96, 112, 113, 163, 165, 166, 169, 170, 173, 174–177, 190, 212
Symbol Search, 72, 90, 93

Tactual Performance Test (TPT), 11–12, 63–64, 67, 69,70–72, 78–82, 84, 88, 90, 92, 93, 94, 95, 123, 124, 130, 131, 134, 146, 163, 165, 166, 170, 176, 177, 190, 212, 234–235
Test of Line Orientation, 18–19, 64, 66–67, 72–73, 74–78, 80, 83, 94, 96, 119, 120, 122, 123, 124
Test of Variables of Attention (TOVA), 47–48, 81, 94, 129, 144, 166,170, 191, 202, 212, 219–224, 228
Trail Making Test (TMT), 11, 64, 73, 76, 81, 84, 93, 95, 96, 112, 117, 122, 129, 155, 161, 163, 164, 165, 166, 169, 170, 171–174, 176, 177, 190, 212, 235

Verbal Paired Associates, 201, 202, 203, 204–208, 213, 214, 215
Visual Form Discrimination Test (VFDT), 31–32, 64, 68–69, 73, 76, 83–84, 88–89, 94–97, 103, 109, 110, 122, 125, 150, 153, 154, 181
Vocabulary, 58–59, 102, 103, 104, 107, 108, 110, 112, 126, 181

Wechsler Adult Intelligence Scale-Third Edition (WAIS-III), 14, 52–57, 58–59, 70, 80, 83, 102, 109, 116, 161, 168, 177, 178, 181, 182, 234; see also specific tests: Arithmetic, Block Design, Comprehension, Digit Span, Digit Symbol, Information, Matrices, Picture Arrangement, Picture Completion, Similarities, Vocabulary

Wechsler Memory Scale-Third Edition (WMS-III), 14–17, 54, 107, 177–183, 200–215; *see also* specific tests: Digit Span, Faces, Family Pictures, Logical Memory, Spatial Span, Verbal Paired Associates

Wide Range Achievement Test-Third Edition (WRAT-3), 60, 125, 149, 150, 151–154, 158

Wisconsin Card Sorting Test (WCST), 60, 64, 73, 76, 80–81, 84, 93, 95, 96, 107, 112, 113, 115, 117, 120, 122, 127, 129, 143, 161, 163–167, 170, 173, 176, 177, 190, 212, 224, 227, 228

Writing, 101, 156–157

CPSIA information can be obtained at www.ICGtesting.com
Printed in the USA
LVOW102138060213

319024LV00010B/145/A